Second Edition

Operating Room Nursing

Perioperative Practice

Linda K. Groah, RN, MS, CNOR
Assistant Director of Nursing
Kaiser Permanente Medical Center

Clinical Instructor
University of California School
of Nursing
San Francisco, California

with a chapter by
Lillian H. Nicolette, RN, MS, CNOR

Vice President of Perioperative Nursing
Surgical Staff
Philadelphia, Pennsylvania

APPLETON & LANGE
Norwalk, Connecticut/San Mateo, California

0-8385-7406-8

Notice: Our knowledge in clinical sciences is constantly changing. As new information becomes available, changes in treatment and in the use of drugs become necessary. The authors and the publisher of this volume have taken care to make certain that the doses of drugs and schedules of treatment are correct and compatible with the standards generally accepted at the time of publication. The reader is advised to consult carefully the instruction and information material included in the package insert of each drug or therapeutic agent before administration. This advice is especially important when using new or infrequently used drugs.

90 91 92 93 94 / 10 9 8 7 6 5 4 3 2 1

Prentice Hall International (UK) Limited, *London*
Prentice Hall of Australia Pty. Limited, *Sydney*
Prentice Hall Canada, Inc., *Toronto*
Prentice Hall Hispanoamericana, S.A., *Mexico*
Prentice Hall of India Private Limited, *New Delhi*
Prentice Hall of Japan, Inc., *Tokyo*
Simon & Schuster Asia Pte. Ltd., *Singapore*
Editora Prentice Hall do Brasil, Ltda., *Rio de Janeiro*
Prentice Hall, *Englewood Cliffs, New Jersey*

Library of Congress Cataloging-in-Publication Data

Groah, Linda K.
   Operating room nursing : perioperative practice / Linda K. Groah.
  --2nd ed.
     p. cm.
   Includes bibliographical references.
   ISBN 0-8385-7406-8
   1. Operating room nursing. 2. Therapeutics, Surgical. I. Title.
   [DNLM: 1. Intraoperative Care--nurses' instruction. 2. Operating
Room Nursing. 3. Surgical Nursing. WY 162 G873o]
   RD32.3.G76 1990
   610.73'677--dc20
   DNLM/DLC   90-209
   for Library of Congress   CIP

Acquisitions Editor: Marion K. Welch
Production Editor: Elizabeth Ryan
Designer: Janice Barsevich
Cover: Michael J. Kelly
PRINTED IN THE UNITED STATES OF AMERICA

*Dedicated to my mother,
whose love and encouragement
has been instrumental throughout
my life.*

Contents

Preface

This book was written to define the role of the professional registered nurse in the operating room and to assist in identifying and articulating that role to colleagues, legislators, and consumers.

A historical perspective is used to assist the neophyte and experienced nurse in understanding how the perioperative role has evolved. The past is significant in identifying the future.

One primary emphasis of the first edition was the use of the nursing process. In the second edition Chapter 5 has been expanded to include the cross cultural/ethnic patient, and the ambulatory surgery patient.

The components of nursing diagnosis, expected outcomes, and nursing orders must be an integral part of the perioperative nurse's role. Routine use of these components will stimulate nurses to assume more professional roles and assist in identifying how medicine and nursing can complement each other's role in caring for the surgical patient.

NEW FEATURES

Included in the second edition are new topics that have relevance for perioperative nursing practice. Chapters 1 and 4 review the role of perioperative nursing in the ambulatory surgery setting and discuss the expanded role of the nurse serving as the first assistant. The discussion of nursing research in Chapter 1 is expanded to include how perioperative nurses are validating current recommended practices and the outcomes of patient care. Research conducted by perioperative nurses is cited, whenever relevant, throughout the text as this is key in validating perioperative nursing practice.

Chapter 2 identifies the latest design and construction options for inpatient and ambulatory surgery settings. The outline of the policy and procedure manual in Chapter 3 has been expanded to include current requirements of licensing bodies and the philosophy has been expanded to include a contemporary "service philosophy."

Chapters 4 and 16 discuss the relevant changes in Joint Commission on Accreditation of Healthcare Organization standards for operating rooms, the "agenda for change," and identifies how a quality assurance program can be implemented in an operating room. A method of credentialing perioperative nurses is identified in Chapter 16.

Chapters 6 and 7 have been expanded to include information on AIDS and universal precautions. In addition, Chapter 7 identifies problems resulting from construction of new facilities or remodeling of existing facilities and discusses the changes in recommended practices such as the use of shoe covers and cover gowns.

Chapter 8 discusses the use of sterilization containers and the regulations regarding ethylene oxide exposure. New antiseptics and the use of prosthetic fingernails are discussed in Chapter 9.

Chapter 13 has been expanded to include a discussion about tourniquets, and the use of autologous blood transfusions. Sutures have been updated to reflect new products. The discussion in Chapter 14 on dressings includes the new techniques of occlusive and biologic coverings.

Chapter 15 provides an expanded discussion of caring for the postoperative patient using new technology such as pulse oximetry. Documentation during this critical phase of the patient's recovery has been enhanced to include an example of a form.

The health care environment is undergoing tremendous changes and pressures. One area of prime concern is finance. The operating room manager and staff nurses must place an emphasis on cost containment through discriminate analysis of all policies and procedures. This analysis is essential to make certain that the dollars available for nursing care are spent appropriately.

Throughout the text, professional aspects of perioperative nursing are interwoven with the technical skills necessary for providing sophisticated care for patients undergoing surgical intervention.

The author wishes to express grateful appreciation and thanks to all the practitioners who have used this book and provided valuable suggestions for this second edition; to Lillian Nicolette, who revised the chapter on Postoperative Care; to the nursing staff at Kaiser Permanente whose daily practice serves as a role model for perioperative nurses; and to Elizabeth Ryan and other editors whose editorial assistance was invaluable in producing this second edition.

It is the author's hope that this text will assist perioperative nurses in their functions as clinicians, administrators, teachers, and investigators.

Linda K. Groah, RN, MS, CNOR

PART ONE

The Perioperative Nurse and the Environment

Chapter 1

Historical Perspective of the Perioperative Role

Surgery is as old as the human being. Archaeologists have found skulls that date back to 350,000 BC with evidence that surgical procedures were performed then. The earliest scientific document ever brought to light on the subject is a treatise on surgery. This work, the *Edwin Smith Papyrus*, conceived in ancient Egypt in about 3000 BC, is one of the most remarkable books in the history of surgery. Besides describing clinical methods then in use, it contains accurate observations on anatomy, physiology, and pathology.[1]

Hippocrates, "The Father of Medicine," born about 460 BC, wrote more than 70 books on medicine and surgery. In one of these books entitled *On the Surgery*, he discusses the operating room in detail.

The items he relates to surgery are the patient; the operator; the assistants; the instruments; the lights, where and how; the time; the manner; and the place. Hippocrates refers to using an assistant when he discusses instrumentation[2]:

> The instruments, and when and how they should be prepared, will be treated of afterwards; so that they may not impede the work, and that there may be no difficulty in taking hold of them, with the part of the body which operates. But if another gives them, he must be ready a little beforehand, and do as you direct.

We do not know who this other person was, only that Hippocrates potentially recognized the value of using an assistant during surgery. There is little mention of the surgical assistant in the literature until the late 1800s.

HISTORY OF OPERATING ROOM NURSING

1873–1900

In 1873, there were three nursing training schools opened in the United States, patterned after Florence Nightingale's school at St. Thomas Hospital in London. They were Bellevue in New York City, the Connecticut Training School in New Haven, and the Boston Training School (later called the Massachusetts General Hospital Training School) (Figs. 1–1, 1–2). The Bellevue Report of 1875 listed lectures on "Surgical Instruments and Preparation for Operation," "Bandaging," and "Haemostasis."[3]

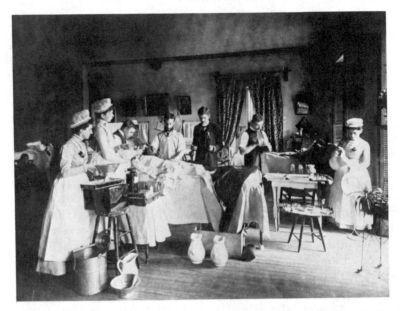

Figure 1-1. Operating room, Bellevue Hospital, 1870. *(The Bettmann Archive.)*

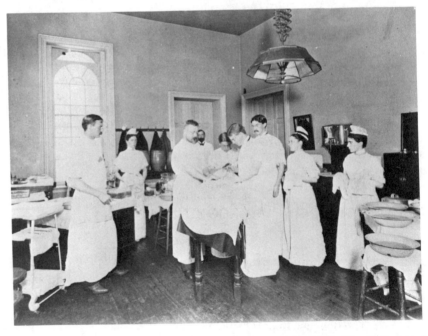

Figure 1-2. Operating room, St. Luke's Hospital, New York, 1880. *(The Bettmann Archive.)*

In *History of Nursing*, James J. Walsh wrote the following regarding the period around 1880[4]:

> The demand for nurses, properly trained, was not felt in the hospitals generally throughout the country until Lister's revolutionary discovery of the value of antisepsis in surgery . . . made it absolutely necessary that nurses should be of such an intellectual calibre and development as would permit them to be trained in the prevention of infection through absolute cleanliness.

In 1889, William H. Welch, pathologist; William S. Halsted, surgeon; and Sir William Osler, internal medicine set up Johns Hopkins University in Baltimore to train doctors and nurses. Operating room nursing was identified as an area of specialization and thus became nursing's first specialty.[5]

During that same year, at the Boston Training School, a lecture on bacteriology was added to the curriculum. In 1891, students were given the responsibility for cleaning and sterilizing instruments for Saturday operations. By 1896, student nurses were sent to assist with Saturday operations.[6]

1900–1920

Soon after the turn of the century, several factors radically changed the role and the identity of the surgical nurse. Advances in anesthesia made it possible to extend operating time and to reduce the surgical mortality rate. Therefore, more surgical procedures were performed (Figs. 1–3, 1–4, 1–5). Due to the increase in surgical procedures, a graduate nurse was placed in charge of the surgical amphitheaters and student nurses began to assist regularly with operations and etherizing.[6]

In 1901, Martha Luce of Boston described duties of an operating room nurse as numerous. They require a knowledge of the principles of asepsis, careful attention to details, and much forethought in the preparation of supplies.[7]

> The care of the operating room includes dusting with clean, damp cloths; polishing of glass, tables and utensils, regulation of the temperature and ventilation of the room. In addition to the daily cleaning, it is desirable to use a solution of corrosive sublimate (1 to 3000) before an operation, especially before a Laparotomy, and all the basins to be used for sterile water or any of the antiseptic solutions should be thoroughly cleansed with the same strength of corrosive solution.
>
> The surgeon's retiring room must be kept in perfect order. Gowns, sheets, towels and sponges have to be folded in the regulation way and pinned securely. Gauze sponges of two or three sizes can be made by carefully folding cut gauze in such a way that all the edges are securely turned in and no sewing is necessary. The sponges are counted before being put in packages.
>
> The instruments for all operations are selected by the surgeon or his assistant, and, with the exception of the knives, are wrapped in cotton cloth for sterilization. The knives are cleaned with soap and water, ether and alcohol (95%). They are wrapped in separate sterile towels and boiled three minutes, but the rest of the instruments are boiled one-half hour in water in which a small amount of bicarbonate of soda has been added.

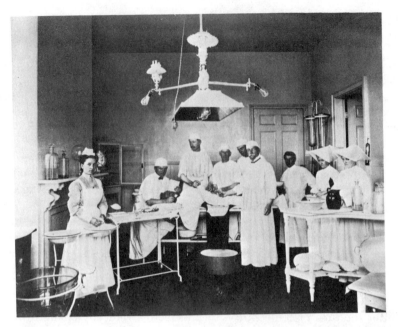

Figure 1-3. Operating room in Mobile, Alabama, 1900. *(The Bettmann Archive.)*

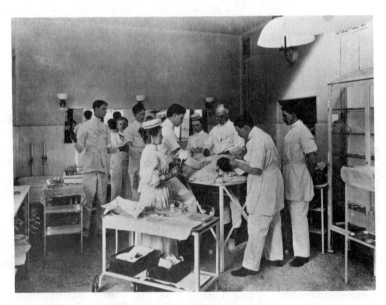

Figure 1-4. Professor Charles McBurney (1845–1913) operating in Roosevelt Hospital, New York, 1901. *(The Bettmann Archive.)*

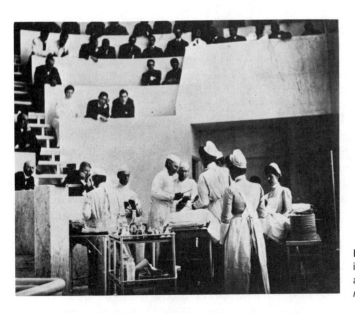

Figure 1–5. Dr. Halsted operating in Johns Hopkins' new amphitheater, 1905. *(The Bettmann Archive.)*

Most surgeons have individual preferences in the choice of needles, ligatures, etc. and it is the duty of the operating room nurse to acquaint herself with these preferences and to carefully prepare what each requires for his use.

Rubber gloves are tied together in pairs with pieces of cotton bandage on which is marked the wearer's name. A few cots should be included, to be used in case a glove finger becomes punctured.

The operating room nurse is responsible for every detail of the preparation, including the careful instruction of her assistant nurse. If all has been well done, it will prevent awkwardness and delay during the process of the operation.

Leila Clark Woodbury wrote in 1903 that[8]:

Surgical nursing is a subject of such almost unlimited extent that volumes might be written on it. I shall endeavor to give the requirements of a surgical nurse; a brief outline of bacteriology and the relationship this science bears to surgery; the care of the surgical case, and some additional notes of things learned by experience.

One of the areas Woodbury cited was in regard to the patient's mental state[8].

As a rule, the preparations and, perhaps, the unfamiliar surroundings of a hospital tend to make the patient apprehensive and really in a pitiable frame of mind. A good nurse with tact can, by a few cheerful or encouraging words, divert the thought of the patient, or, at least relieve her fears of the ordeal in store for her.

Another area Woodbury identified was economy[8].

> In all parts of her work a surgical nurse who practices economy is doubly valuable. There is no department of nursing where this may be practised to greater advantage than in the care of a surgical case. Many of the materials used in this work are expensive, and a nurse by thought and good judgement may be able to lessen enormously the expense necessary at such a time.

By 1900, the surgeons were wearing sterile scrub suits, and surgical scrubs were being performed by all members of the surgical team. Following the scrub, sterile gloves were worn to protect the hands until surgery was started, and then they were removed. In 1905, it was determined that skin could not be sterilized so rubber gloves were worn throughout the procedure. In this same year it was recommended that the instrument nurse wear a sterile gown.

Around 1907, the use of head coverings was advocated; and by 1914, the use of surgical masks for surgeons, assistants, and the sterile nurse was gaining acceptance.

It was during these two decades that the roles of the "circulator" and the "scrub" nurse began to emerge. The nurse who remained sterile is referred to in the literature as the scrubbed nurse, suture nurse, washed-up nurse, sterile glove nurse, tray nurse, instrument nurse, sponge nurse, and setting-up nurse. The surgeon insisted that this individual be the senior member of the nursing team. However, by 1910, nursing authorities agreed that the nurse who remains unsterile, or circulates, runs the operating room and must be the senior, more experienced nurse. They also suggested that only a trained nurse and not a student could fill this role; however, the role of the scrub nurse could be performed by a student if necessary.[9]

1920–1940

During this period it was common for student nurses, under the direction of a graduate nurse or a senior student, to provide most of the patient care. Students spent part of their training in the operating room and were expected to function effectively. In many instances it was considered acceptable for students to function in the role of the circulator after minimal experience. One author in the *American Journal of Nursing* advised that, "The student nurse whose three months' training is completed then continues the work of the non-sterile (circulating) nurse for one month."[10]

Early in this period, there were no standards or curriculum guide available to identify how a nurse should be trained. Frequently, the nurse in charge of the area would be the only registered nurse present and would be expected to perform the training of students in addition to her other duties.

In 1927, the *American Journal of Nursing* published an article entitled "The Operating Supervisor and Her Qualifications." The operating supervisor was to show "a high sense of responsibility to the patient, the peculiarities of the surgeon, and to instruct young nurses."[11]

In 1919, the National League of Nursing Education included in their standard curriculum a section on "Operating Room Technic." It was intended to be a guide and was not considered mandatory for schools to implement. In that first standard were included

10 hours of instruction in operating room technique and bacteriology and 20 hours in surgical diseases. Aided by this and specific pointers published in nursing journals, the head nurses were able to fulfill their teaching assignments.[6]

In 1933, the Subcommittee on Surgical Nursing of the Education Committee of the National League for Nursing Education outlined a master curriculum plan for an advanced course in operating room technique and maintenance of standards. It was the first attempt to standardize the level of nursing care in the operating room by a national organization. The curriculum listed the following objectives[12]:

1. To instruct the student in the relation of the operative procedure to the patient's safety and progress
2. To improve thoughtfulness and skill in the nursing care of patients in the operating room
3. To improve understanding of operating room technique, routines and develop an appreciation of the scientific basis for them
4. To acquaint the student with the special supervisory problems of the operating room
5. To aid the student in organizing a teaching program in the operating room

This curriculum was to serve as a model for training operating room nurses during the next decade.

The Depression resulted in a decrease of the patient census in most hospitals; therefore, hospitals had to reduce the number of nurses they employed. In addition, many schools of nursing were forced to close due to a lack of necessary financial resources. Consequently, the number of graduate and student nurses was declining by 1940.

1941–1945

When America entered World War II, many nurses left hospital positions to join the Armed Forces. This situation resulted in an acute nursing shortage in the United States. Hospitals found it necessary to train ancillary personnel to take the place of the graduate and student nurses who had once been the traditional work force. For example, in the operating room, orderlies were being used as circulators.[13]

During World War II, mobile field hospitals were developed to care for the wounded in direct combat areas. To augment the necessary staff needed for these hospitals, the Armed Forces developed programs to train corpsmen and nurses to function in field hospitals.

Army nurses assigned to surgery needed additional training to meet the demands of the field and evacuation hospitals. To fulfill this demand, a 12-week postgraduate course in operating room technique was established at Cushing General Hospital in Framingham, Massachusetts. The course included basic principles such as gowning and gloving. In addition, it was expanded to cover fluid therapy, including plasma and whole blood transfusions; care of patients in shock or respiratory or cardiac failure; and methods of administering general, spinal, intravenous (IV), or rectal anesthesia.[14]

The term "operating room technician" was created to apply to those personnel trained to assist in surgery. The theory usually taught by Army and Navy nurses included not only how to function in the scrub and circulating roles but also how to serve as an anesthetist and first assistant. In field hospitals, the operating room technician worked under the direction of the surgeon until the nurses arrived. However, on board combat ships where nurses did not serve, the corpsmen, under the medical officers' supervision, not only set up and ran the operating room, but also trained other corpsmen. The work of the corpsmen during World War II was well-known, and word of their excellent service is reported in the nursing literature.[15]

World War II resulted in reorganization in hospitals, such as the development of centralized sterile and reprocessing departments and the increased use of nonprofessionals to perform tasks formerly identified as nursing responsibilities.

1946–1960
The changes in the roles and the identity of operating room personnel brought about by World War II provided the major focus on staffing during the immediate postwar years. With an increasing shortage of nurses, many hospitals hired operating room technicians who had been trained while in the Armed Forces to fill vacancies in the operating rooms. Hospital administrators began to question, "In view of the still acute shortage of both professional and practical nurses is it right to utilize, in a definitely technical field, persons who are trained in the bedside care of the sick?"[16]

The nursing literature indicated that operating room technicians were to perform "certain routine duties" under the direct supervision of a graduate nurse and that this would then allow the graduate nurse to carry out more complex nursing activities.[17]

Hospitals and adult education programs established training programs to meet the increased demand for operating room technicians.

It was during these postwar years that nursing educators began to question whether the operating room rotation was essential to the learning experience of the student nurse. Despite attempts by some educators such as Alexander[18] and Shaltis[19] to prove that this rotation was essential, the general atmosphere of uncertainty had the effect of limiting the development of sound curricula and would eventually result in eliminating the operating room rotation.

In January 1949 in the midst of these transitions, 17 operating room supervisors from New York City identified the need for an organization to meet routinely to pool knowledge and exchange ideas on their area of specialization. The result of this unprecedented independent nursing meeting was the Association of Operating Room Nurses (AORN).

The primary aims of this association were[20]:

1. To stimulate operating room nurses in other parts of the country to form similar groups
2. To be a specific group to pool and share nursing knowledge and technology
3. To provide the surgical patient with optimum care through a broad educational program
4. To make a body of knowledge available to operating room nurses

5. To motivate experienced operating room nurses to share their expertise with others

6. To be an association for the benefit of all professional operating room nurses

The first national conference of AORN was held in February 1954, with the major topic "Where Do We Belong?" Through this peer support, operating room nurses began to identify themselves as leaders, supervisors, and teachers.

In 1957 following repeatedly denied attempts to affiliate with the National League For Nursing Education and the American Nurses Association, AORN became an independent national organization.[20]

The future development of operating room nursing as a specialty would be synonymous with the growth of AORN.

1960–1970

In 1960, AORN published the first issue of its official journal, *OR Nursing*. Published bimonthly, this journal was dedicated to[21]:

Promote the goals of the Association; present scientific, clinical, technical and organizational information of interest to O.R. nurses; provide means for the exchange of ideas among members; and, when indicated, will be the spokesman for the Association on professional problems that confront the membership.

With the January–February issue of 1963, the name of the publication was changed to the *AORN Journal*. Being alert and sensitive to a variety of needs and demands that operating room nurses were experiencing, AORN began to publish this journal monthly in 1967.

During the 1960s, one of AORN's major concerns centered on the shortage of operating room nurses and on the best use of trained paramedical personnel in the operating room.

In 1965, AORN, ANA, and the National League for Nursing met to recommend standards and guidelines for the selection, instruction, and training of operating room technicians. As a result of this group's decisions, AORN produced a manual, *Teaching the Operating Room Technician* in 1967.[22]

In 1968, the AORN House of Delegates directed the Board of Directors to structure an allied association, the Association of Operating Room Technicians (AORT). During its infancy, this organization was guided by the AORN–AORT Advisory Board. The Advisory Board was dissolved in 1973, and AORT continued as an independent organization.[23] In that same year, they changed their name to Association of Surgical Technologists (AST). Later, the title of operating room technician was changed to surgical technologist.

In 1969, the following definition of professional operating room nursing was adopted[24]:

Professional nursing in the operating room is the identification of the physiological, psychological and sociological needs of the patient and the development and implementation of an individualized program of nursing care that coordinates the nursing actions, based on the knowledge of the natural and behavioral sciences, to restore or maintain the health and welfare of the patient before, during and after surgical intervention.

The objective of clinical practice of professional operating room nursing was identified: "to provide a standard of excellence in the care of the patient before, during and after surgical intervention."[24]

Together, the definition of operating room nursing and the objectives for clinical practice provided direction for the practitioners of professional operating room nursing.

1970–1980

Since the inception of the organization, AORN's primary focus had been education for operating room nurses. However, the scope of the organization was expanded during this decade in response to the need for national standards, official policies, and position statements.

One of the first resolutions adopted in 1973 pertained to the necessity for a registered nurse in the operating room. With the adoption of this resolution, AORN accepted the role of consumer advocate and determined how the functions of registered nurses justify their presence in this critical nursing area. Included in the rationale were the following statements[25]:

The registered nurse has knowledge, experience, and responsibility that prepare her to:

1. Independently assess patient needs, therefore implementing nursing intervention.
2. Make collaborative decisions relative to total intraoperative care.
3. Make decisions and take action in emergency situations.
4. Establish and maintain inter- and intradepartmental functioning for continuity of care.
5. Provide for and contribute to patient safety through control of his internal and external environment, biological testing, and product evaluation.
6. Assist the patient with the management of anxiety through the application of the principles of biological, physical, and social sciences.
7. Provide efficient patient care in the operating room through organizational skills, preoperative and postoperative visits, and sound principles of management.
8. Conduct and participate in research projects directed toward improvement of patient care through the application of scientific principles.
9. Control hospital costs through budget preparation and implementation.
10. Participate in architectural design of operating suites effecting efficiency and quality in patient care.
11. Participate in supervision and instruction of ancillary and allied health personnel in the operating room.
12. Evaluate and modify the quality of patient care within the operating room.

In an effort to further assure excellence in patient care and to validate the outcome of nursing care in the operating room, an ad hoc committee of AORN developed a nursing audit tool. Published in 1974, this tool outlined one method of evaluation in which actual patient care rendered is compared with the standards of care as defined by departmental policies and procedures. By development of this program, operating room nurses identified their continued concern to provide the patient with optimum nursing care (see Chapter 16).

In 1975, AORN formulated a statement of policy indicating that the circulator must at all times be the professional registered nurse. The rationale for this policy statement was based on the following[26]:

Patients undergoing surgery experience physical and psychosocial trauma. Not only are most patients unconscious during this time, but they are also completely powerless and unable to make decisions concerning their welfare. The patient is entering what is probably the most alien environment he has ever known and is removed from personal contact of family and friends as well as that of other hospital care personnel. His physical and psychological needs have reached ultimate proportions. At this critical time, patients need much more than technical caretakers; they need professional nurses.

In response to the need for standards by which the quality of patient care could be measured, AORN and ANA collaborated on the development of the "Standards of Nursing Practice: Operating Room." These standards, published in 1975, focus on the process of nursing practice and are directed toward providing continuity of nursing care through preoperative assessment and planning, intraoperative intervention, and postoperative evaluation (see Chapter 5).

Concurrently the Technical Standards Committee of AORN formulated and published the "Standards of Technical and Aseptic Practice: Operating Room."[27] Although optimal, these standards are realistic and achievable and serve as a guide for developing institutional policies and procedures.

"The Standards of Administrative Nursing Practice: Operating Room" were published in 1976.[28] These structural standards together with the previously published standards provided a method by which the quality of nursing administration in the operating room could be evaluated.

In 1976, the AORN Board of Directors appointed a task force to define the role of nurses in the operating room. This task force was to identify a universal definition of operating room nursing practice that was to include the integration of both the technical and professional functions.

In 1978 at the 25th AORN Congress, the House of Delegates adopted the following definition of operating room nursing in its Statement of the Perioperative Role[29]:

The perioperative role of the operating room nurse consists of nursing activities performed by the professional operating room nurse during the preoperative, intraoperative and postoperative phases of the patient's surgical experience. Operating room nurses assume the perioperative role at a beginning level dependent on their expertise and competency to practice. As they gain knowledge and skills they progress on a continuum to an advanced level of practice.

As a result of accepting this definition, operating room nurses became the first nursing specialty to define its role (see Chapter 5).

The task force included with its report recommendations for implementing the perioperative role and implications of this role for the future. Among those recommendations were[29]:

1. Develop continuing education programs to implement the perioperative role.
2. Discuss with nurse educators curricula changes as related to the perioperative role.
3. Explore matters pertaining to socioeconomic and political issues as they relate to implementation of the perioperative role of the operating room nurse.
4. Operating room nurses must accept the challenge of professional achievement and attain certification.

In 1979, AORN contracted with the Professional Examination Service of New York to offer the first voluntary certification examination for operating room nurses. The purposes of the certification program are[30]:

1. Demonstrate concerns for accountability to the general public for nursing practice.
2. Enhance quality patient care.
3. Identify professional nurses who have demonstrated professional achievement in providing care for patients during surgical intervention.
4. Provide employing agencies with means of identifying professional achievement of an individual practitioner.
5. Provide personal satisfaction for practitioner.

1980-1990

During this decade, the health care industry was in the midst of the greatest challenge it had ever faced. The challenge focused on increased health care costs, advancements in medical technology, the public's increased knowledge of health care, and the abundant supply of providers and facilities in the health care field. A combination of an oversupply of hospital beds, competition from hospital and nonhospital providers, and the increasing pressures applied by third-party payers stimulated many hospitals to adopt new delivery systems. In pursuing these strategies, hospital administrators discovered that ambulatory surgery provided care of equal quality at much lower cost. Perioperative nurses continuing to assume a leadership role in the care of all surgical patients moved into these centers as administrators and clinicians.

The concept of ambulatory surgery was not new. At a meeting of the British Medical Association in 1909, J. H. Nichol, MD reported that he had performed 7320 operations on an ambulatory basis at the Royal Glasgow Hospital for Children in England. He reported that his surgical results were as good as those for inpatients.[31]

The 1960s saw advancements in anesthetic and surgical techniques that increased the safety of ambulatory surgery. In addition, ambulatory surgery was found to be more convenient for both the patient and physician and cost savings were noted.

In 1962, the University of California at Los Angeles developed a hospital-based ambulatory surgery program. In 1970, Wallace Reed, MD and John Ford, MD of Phoenix, Arizona established the Surgi-Center, a free-standing ambulatory surgery center. These two centers paved the way for further developments in ambulatory surgery. In 1983, there were 239 ambulatory surgery centers and by 1988, that number had grown to 983 with 1.8 million surgeries being performed in these facilities.[32]

It has been suggested that 20% to 40% of all surgeries performed in the United States could be safely performed in an ambulatory setting. Estimates vary, but market analysts predict that, during the 1990s, 60% of all surgical care will be provided on an ambulatory basis.[33]

Perioperative nursing care in the ambulatory surgery environment proved to be both stimulating and challenging. Due to the relatively brief encounter with the patient, the operating room nurse's knowledge of the nursing process, technical proficiencies, and teaching skills involving both the patient and family members must be highly refined and sophisticated. In addition, an ability to adapt the Recommended Practices and Standards of Care to this environment is important, as are good organizational skills. The ambulatory surgery nurse must also be flexible as he may be responsible for providing nursing care in all three phases of the perioperative role: preoperatively, intraoperatively, and postoperatively.

The role of the professional operating room nurse expanded into yet another arena, as the functions of the first assistant began to be practiced by operating room nurses. In 1980, the house of delegates adopted a Statement on the Role of the First Assistant. This statement included that in the "absence of a qualified physician, the registered nurse who possesses appropriate knowledge and technical skills is the best qualified nonphysician to serve as the first assistant."[34]

In 1984, the statement was refined and the following definition of the RN First Assistant was adopted[35]:

> The RN first assistant to the surgeon during a surgical procedure carries out functions that will assist the surgeon in performing a safe operation with optimal results for the patient. The RN first assistant practices perioperative nursing and has acquired the knowledge, skills, and judgment, necessary, to assist the surgeon, through organized instruction and supervised practice. The RN first assistant practices under the direct supervision of the surgeon during the first assisting phase of the perioperative role. The first assistant does not concurrently function as a scrub nurse.

The inclusion of the role as part of perioperative nursing practice provided the professional component previously absent in this role and served as the momentum for AORN in collaboration with ANA to seek indirect reimbursement from Medicare for these services. Their attempts were unsuccessful in 1986 and 1988.

During the 1980s, operating room nurses continued to expand their role and take on new responsibilities. As this occurred, the AORN Board of Directors charged the Nursing Practices Committee to review the Statement of Perioperative Nursing Practice. The 1978 definition of nursing in the operating room was too restrictive because it addressed the individual practitioner rather than the scope of nursing practice in the operating room. The term *perioperative nursing practice* was determined to be more descriptive than the term *perioperative role*. This revised statement was adopted[36]:

> The registered nurse in the operating room is responsible for providing nursing care to surgical patients. Perioperative is used as an encompassing term to incorporate the three phases of the surgical patient's experience. This includes the preoperative, intraoperative and postoperative periods. Practice refers to expected behavior patterns and technical activities performed during the preoperative, intraoperative, and postoperative phases.
>
> Perioperative nursing practice is flexible and diverse and includes a variety of nursing roles that incorporate both behavioral and technical components of professional nursing. The scope of practice for each individual perioperative nurse may include, but is not limited to, roles such as scrub person, circulator, manager, educator, and first assistant. The perioperative nurse delivers care through the use of the nursing process as reflected in the "Standards of Perioperative Nursing Practice" in a manner that is cost effective without compromising quality of care.

Nursing research gained momentum during the 1980s and perioperative nurses conducted clinical research to test the body of knowledge used in implementing patient care and to validate the recommended practices. A resolution on operating room nursing research adopted in 1983 committed AORN to support research through educational activities and earmarking funds for projects related to perioperative nursing. This was reinforced in 1988 when the AORN Board of Directors adopted a Policy, Plan, and Priority Statement on Nursing Research.

This statement placed a priority on validating through research the current recommended practices for perioperative nursing. The focus of research the organization committed to support was the generation of scientific knowledge that would enable perioperative nurses to develop recommended practices and desired patient outcome. The priorities identified were[37]:

1. Identify and classify nursing practice phenomena specifically related to perioperative care
2. Develop instruments to measure perioperative nursing outcomes
3. Identify perioperative nursing practices that will ensure quality care for the surgical patient while maintaining cost-effectiveness
4. Identify perioperative nursing practices that will ensure quality care for the surgical patient experiencing complex multisystem health care problems
5. Provide effective care in alternative health care delivery systems
6. Design educational programs to prepare perioperative nurses for practice in evolving delivery systems
7. Identify perioperative ethical issues and develop models for resolution

The numerous milestones achieved during this period and this policy statement on research would provide direction for the organization and for perioperative nursing during the next decade.

THE FUTURE OF PERIOPERATIVE NURSING

The role of the professional operating room nurse has expanded beyond the confines of the surgical suite; however, a new role may emerge in the future. This new role might appropriately be titled "Perioperative Nurse Practitioner." In this role, the professional registered nurse will provide the preoperative care performing patient assessments, obtaining baseline laboratory data, and referring abnormal data (not consistent with the patient's current health state) to the physician for diagnosis and treatment. Intraoperatively the perioperative nurse practitioner will have the clinical responsibility of the first assistant, or will function as the scrub or circulating nurse.

Postoperatively, this nurse practitioner will provide routine postoperative care, evaluate patient outcomes, and prior to discharge, will provide the necessary education to the patient and the significant others. In this role, the perioperative nurse will be in private practice and will be reimbursed directly for services. Through the development of this role, surgeons will have time to devote to complex surgical procedures.

Surgical intervention will continue to expand its technical base by the application of the laser beam and computers. Perioperative nursing will continue to be a vital link between technical advances and effective humanistic care in a variety of nontraditional settings.

Through this historical review of perioperative nursing, it is noted that the progress this nursing specialty has made is due to the momentum of the national association. There are approximately 83,000 professional operating room nurses in the United States; of that number, 37,450 are members of AORN.[38] Perioperative nurses, questing for excellence and serving as the surgical patient's advocate, will continue to be a vital force in the changing health care scene.

REFERENCES

1. Zimmerman LM, Veith I. *Great Ideas in the History of Surgery.* New York: Dover Publications; 1967
2. *The Genuine Works of Hippocrates;* Adams F, trans ed. New York: William Wood & Co; 1929:7–10
3. Stewart IM. *Education of Nurses.* New York: Macmillan; 1944
4. Walsh JJ. *History of Nursing.* New York: P.J. Kennedy; 1929
5. Clemons B. Lister's Day in America. *AORN J.* 1976; 24:47
6. Metzger RS. The beginnings of OR nursing education. *AORN J.* 1976; 24:80
7. Luce M. The duties of an operating-room nurse. *Am J Nurs.* 1901; 1:404–406
8. Woodbury LC. Surgical nursing. *Am J Nurs.* 1903; 13:688

9. Van Syckel J. The operating room technique of St. Luke's Hospital, New York. *Am J Nurs.* 1910; 10:636

10. Sister Bertilla M. Operating room routine: The training of students. *Am J Nurs.* 1924; 24:380

11. Lockwood C. The operating supervisor and her qualifications. *Am J Nurs.* 1927; 27:97

12. Advanced course in surgical nursing. *Am J Nurs.* 1933; 33:1186

13. King C. Planning the day's work in the operating room. *Am J Nurs.* 1942; 42:396

14. Poole R. Army course in operating room technic. *Am J Nurs.* 1945; 45:270

15. Danys A. The navy trains operating room technicians. *Am J Nurs.* 1945; 45:727

16. Bell HS. Practical nurses in the operating room. *Am J Nurs.* 1952; 52:582

17. Ferris S. Training operating room technicians pays. *Am J Nurs.* 1955; 55:691

18. Alexander EA. There's a lot to learn in the OR. *Am J Nurs.* 1949; 49:584–586

19. Sholtis LA. Operative aseptic technic in the basic curriculum. *Am J Nurs.* 1949; 49:116–118

20. Driscoll J. 1949–1957: AORN in retrospect. *AORN J.* 1976; 24:142

21. West EJ. Our official journal. *OR Nurs.* 1960; 1:23

22. *The AORN Story.* Denver: The Association of Operating Room Nurses; 1973

23. National AORT advisory board is dissolved. *AORN J.* 1973; 18:42

24. Definition and objective for clinical practice of professional operating room nursing. *AORN J.* 1969; 10:44

25. Delegates approve statements on RN and nursing student in OR, institutional licensure, abortion. *AORN J.* 1973; 17:188–189

26. Delegates approve statements, resolutions at the twenty-second congress. *AORN J.* 1975; 21:1068

27. AORN standards: OR wearing apparel, draping and gowning materials. *AORN J.* 1975; 21:594

28. Standards of administrative nursing practice: Operating room. *AORN J.* 1976; 23:1202

29. Operating room nursing: Perioperative role. *AORN J.* 1978; 27:1165

30. Hercules PR, Kneedler JA. *Certification Series Unit 1: Certification Process.* Denver: Association of Operating Room Nurses; 1979

31. O'Donovan T. Hospital ambulatory surgery in 1980s. *Hosp Health Serv Admin.* 2. 1981; 26:21

32. Prospective Payment Assessment Commission. Medicare Prospective Payment and the American Health Care System Report To The Congress. Washington, DC: Prospective Payment Assessment Commission; June, 1989: 48

33. Curtin L. Ambulatory surgery: Organization, finance, and regulation. *Nurs Manage.* 1984; 15:22–24

34. Association of operating room nurses house of delegates statement on first assisting. *AORN J.* 1980; 31:451

35. Association of operating room nurses taskforce defines first assisting. *AORN J.* 1984; 39:403

36. Association of operating room nurses a model for perioperative nursing practice. *AORN J.* 1985; 41:193

37. AORN policy, plan and priority statement on nursing research. *AORN J.* 1988; 48:437–438

38. Novak D, Schmaus D. The OR nurse universe study. *AORN J.* 1988; 48:26

Chapter 2

Introduction to the Surgical Suite

DESIGN OF THE SURGICAL SUITE

It is important that the perioperative nurse understand the design and the construction of the surgical suite, as this will aid in the effective and efficient use of the facilities.

DETERMINATION OF THE NUMBER OF OPERATING ROOMS

A number of complicated formulas have been developed as aids for determining the appropriate number of rooms in a surgical suite. The simple 5% formula is a good starting point for planning. This formula states that the number of rooms should equal 5% of the total number of surgical beds. Thus, for a 200-bed hospital with 100 surgical beds, there should be 5 or 6 operating rooms. Cystoscopy and endoscopy rooms are not included in this count.[1]

Variations on this formula are determined by the following factors:

1. Review of historical data for the preceding 5 years to examine:
   a. Number of surgical procedures performed
   b. Type of surgery performed
   c. Average length of surgical procedures
   d. Distribution of inpatient versus outpatient procedures
   e. Number of emergency surgeries performed
2. The hours and the days of the week the operating rooms will be available for scheduled surgical procedures
3. The number of critical-care beds available for surgical cases
4. The flow of patients, supplies, equipment, and personnel into and out of the area
5. The current and future surgical needs of the community
6. The utilization rate of the existing operating rooms
7. The future trends in surgical technology

The utilization rate is derived by determining the relationship between the actual hours of surgery and the potential hours of surgery that would be performed if all rooms were used 100% of the time during the normal scheduled hours of surgery. A 75% to 80% room use is considered optimal and usually constitutes justification for adding additional operating rooms.[2]

DESIGN AND PLANNING OF SURGICAL SUITE COMPONENTS

The construction of a new surgical suite may occur in any of the following:

1. Renovation of existing facilities
2. Expansion of existing facilities
3. Construction of a new facility

Construction of the surgical suite will be discussed in the following three components:

1. Traffic patterns
2. Surgical support systems (the environment)
3. Communication system

Traffic Patterns

The surgical suite should be isolated from the mainstream of corridor traffic in the hospital. The suite should be adjacent to the recovery rooms and in an area easily accessible to central supply, pathology, radiology, blood bank, and critical-care areas. The flow of traffic should be such that contamination from outside the suite is excluded, and within the suite a separation of clean and contaminated areas should exist. Traffic control design is aided by designing the three-zone concept. The three zones are the unrestricted, the semirestricted, and the restricted areas. The unrestricted area includes the patient reception area, locker rooms, lounges, and offices. The semirestricted areas include the storage areas for clean and sterile supplies, work areas for storage and processing of instruments, and corridors to restricted areas of the suite. The restricted area includes all areas where personnel are required to wear surgical masks (see Chapter 7).

Early in the planning stages, a decision must be made in regard to handling all materials. If the central supply department is located in an area with convenient access to the operating rooms, consideration may be given to removing support functions (i.e., processing of instruments and supplies) to that department. If the department is not located on the same floor, access may be accomplished via a conveyor, monorail, elevator, or dumbwaiter, or any combination of these methods. When this method of processing is used, there must be two separate methods of transportation, one to remove contaminated supplies from the operating rooms and one to transport clean and sterile items from the central supply department to the surgical suite. Supplies prepared outside the surgical suite should be transported to the operating room in closed or covered carts. Soiled items and trash should be contained in a closed impervious system for transportation to the processing or disposal site. If trash and linen are to be picked up at intervals from the surgical suite, a separate room should be constructed for this activity.

The advantage of this system is the reduction in the total cost of capital expenditures and maintenance because there is no duplication of equipment (such as ultrasonic cleaners, washer–sterilizers, and cart washers). The disadvantage is that the control of instruments and supplies is removed from the operating rooms, and, therefore, an increase in the inventory of instruments and equipment is often necessary. In addition to the initial cost of installing the transport system, routine maintenance costs must be considered as well as an alternative method of transporting supplies and equipment in the event of a malfunction. This system reportedly works well and is cost effective in a surgical suite of less than eight operating rooms.

Surgical Support Systems (The Environment)

There are four basic designs for surgical suites:

1. Central corridor or hotel plan
2. Double corridor or clean core plan
3. Peripheral corridor or race track
4. Grouping, cluster, or pod plan

The central corridor plan is effective when only two to four operating rooms are required. In this plan, all the operating rooms and support areas are accessible from a single corridor.

The double corridor plan results in a U-shape or T-shape architectural arrangement and is used in designing 5 to 15 operating rooms.

The peripheral corridor plan (Fig. 2–1) provides a corridor around the surgical suite and a clean central core where instrument packs are prepared and from which distribution of materials to the rooms occurs. The patient and the surgical team enter the operating room via the clean corridor and leave by way of the peripheral corridor. This plan requires that an elaborate traffic pattern be developed in an attempt to enforce this concept; however, in practice, these patterns are not followed. Valuable storage space is frequently sacrificed for the peripheral corridor and, as a result, this area is frequently used to store equipment and supplies.

The cluster plan of four operating rooms (Fig. 2–2) with a peripheral corridor and a central support area with access to each operating room is widely accepted in designing large surgical sites. It is more efficient than the central or double corridor because all operating rooms are close to the supply source. It is the most adaptable to expansion because additional clusters can be added with little disruption to the existing facilities.

With all four designs a holding area for surgical patients may be constructed. Prior to entering this area the patient may be transferred onto an operating room stretcher or surgical table in a vestibular exchange area. This is done on the premise that hospital bacteria may be tracked into the operating room on the wheels of the cart. There is, however, no hard evidence to impute this practice for being a cause of surgical infection.[3]

The preoperative area (holding area) is designed to support the patient awaiting surgery. Ideally, it should be a separate room in the surgical suite or immediately adjacent to it. The area should be quiet and restful, away from direct traffic flow, and provide privacy and seclusion. Talk and noise should be kept to minimum. The area should be equipped with an emergency cart, drugs, defibrillator, oxygen, and suction devices. Access to the emergency alarm system is essential.

The preoperative area has gained importance as increasing numbers of patients are not admitted to the hospital the evening prior to surgery. The nurse in the preoperative area conducts a preoperative assessment, collecting baseline data that will be important to the nurses caring for the patient postoperatively. The assessment should include re-

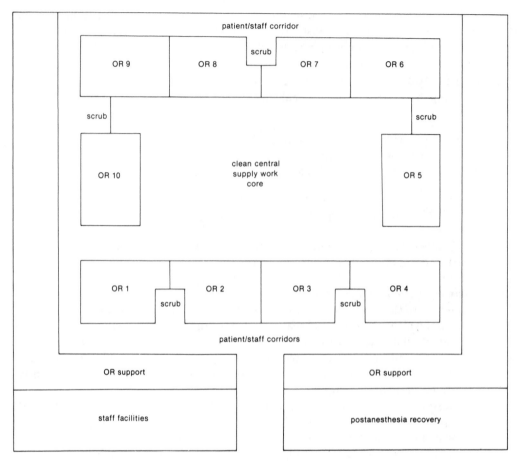

Figure 2-1. Peripheral corridor design. (*Adapted from Chvala C. O.R. supervisor's role in planning the surgical suite. AORN J. 1976; 23(7):1242, with permission.*)

cording of vital signs, notation of the conditions or symptoms presented that necessitate surgical intervention, and any psychological stresses the patient may be experiencing. Postoperative teaching may be included in the preoperative area for ambulatory surgery patients or their significant others. The medical record is checked for accuracy, laboratory data reviewed, and the preoperative checklist completed. In addition, the patient receives premedication, and the surgical shave preparation is performed. Other procedures such as inserting catheters and starting IV lines may also be performed in this area.

If effectively managed, a preoperative area can improve the efficiency of the operating room by reducing the preparation time required once the patient is taken into the operating room. During periods of inactivity, the preoperative area nurse can telephone or visit the previous day's patients to discuss any concerns or impressions they may have regarding their surgical experience.

Significant bacterial contamination may occur as a result of the surgical team (at-

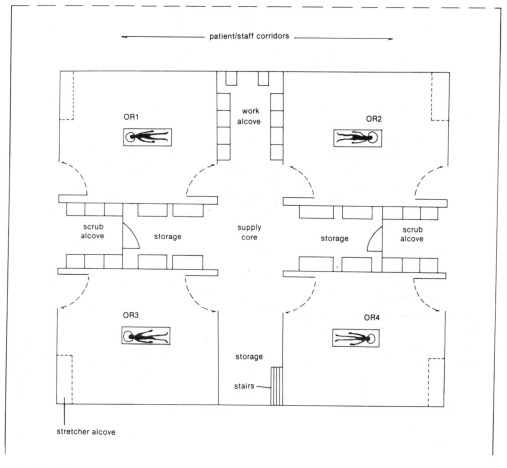

Figure 2-2. Basic modular design. (*Adapted from Chvala C. O.R. supervisor's role in planning the surgical suite. AORN J. 1976;23(7):1243, with permission.*)

tired in clean scrub clothing) mixing with individuals in street clothing. Therefore, it is preferable that entry into the locker/change area precede entry into the surgical lounge or office area. Only those individuals in surgical attire should be permitted in the lounge and office area. This may require that office space be maintained in the unrestricted area as well as in the restricted area.

Another common mix of traffic can be observed in the handling of supplies. Outside cartons unloaded directly from delivery trucks must be removed before the contents are delivered to the surgical suite for storage. Therefore, a "staging area" is required. In this area, inner cartons or packages should be removed from the outer cartons before materials are distributed to the surgical suite. Corrugated cardboard cartons have been found to harbor gas gangrene bacilli, silverfish, and cockroaches. Therefore, these cartons should not be permitted to enter the surgical suite under any circumstances.

The overall traffic patterns in and out of the suite should be controlled by the central desk personnel. A pass-through window located in this area will reduce the need for traffic to enter the interior corridors of the surgical suite. If the suite is large and has more than one entrance or exit area, the use of closed-circuit television located in the remote areas will assist the central desk personnel in monitoring all traffic.

Interior Design of the Surgical Suite. The design of the surgical suite should allow two, three, or four rooms to share a substerile area and scrub facilities. The standard operating room is rectangular or square in shape and should be 20 × 20 × 10 or similar dimensions that provide a floor space of 400 square feet (approximately 37 square meters). Operating rooms designed for surgical services requiring additional equipment such as cardiac or neurosurgery will require rooms 20 × 30 × 10, or a floor space of 600 square feet (approximately 60 m^2). Rooms designed for endoscopy and outpatient surgery require only 18 × 18 × 10, or a floor space of 324 square feet (approximately 29 m^2).

Fire-resistant, hard, smooth, nonporous surfaces are used for floors, walls, and ceilings as these surfaces are easy to clean and do not readily permit adherence of bacterial particles. The material must be able to withstand repeated washings with germicidal cleaners. The surface should be as free as possible of seams, joints, and crevices. For many years ceramic tile was used for the walls. However, because the grouting between the tile was rough, it was shown to harbor bacteria and therefore is no longer used. Materials currently used include laminated polyester with an epoxy finish, hard vinyl covering that can be heat-sealed leaving no seams, and panels of ceramic glass sealed to eliminate seams. Stainless steel or Formica guards at corners help avoid damage, as do guard rails on corridor halls. The only requirement for color is that it should be free from glare. Although traditionally cool pastels have been used, recently, a wide variety of warmer tones has been introduced.

The ceilings are sound absorbent and are either a polyester film or metal-faced ceiling tile.

Floor coverings should be conductive unless a variance from the appropriate local or state agencies is obtained. Many institutions have made the commitment not to use flammable anesthetic agents and, therefore, have obtained this variance. If a variance is not obtained, the floor must meet the requirements of the National Fire Protection Association Standard 56A (NFPA 56A). A wide variety of conductive and nonconductive floor coverings are available including stone terrazzo, plastic terrazzo, linoleum, asphalt, and a variety of hard plastic materials. The material used should be seamless, and have the ability to withstand flooding and wet vacuuming. The color should be such that if a needle is dropped it will be easily visible. The wall-to-floor junction should be curved or concaved to facilitate adequate cleaning.

Each operating room has recessed cabinets for supply storage. These cabinets contain standard supplies in the same location in all operating rooms with a designated area reserved for special instruments and supplies used for the operations usually performed in that room. The cabinets are usually stainless steel with sliding glass doors. All shelves in the surgical suite and its support areas should be of the wire type. Solid shelving readily accumulates dust whereas wire shelving permits air circulation, and, therefore, dust accumulation is negligible.[4] One cabinet in the operating room may have a pegboard to hang items on, such as parts for the surgical table.

A pass-through cabinet stocked from the outside of the room and used from the inside is also being used. A truck on wheels serves as a bank of shelves and is moved to a central area for restocking and cleaning. A latch system prevents the inside and outside doors from being open at the same time unless the latch is released. Carts restricted to a procedure or a surgical specialty may be stocked appropriately and moved into the operating room for a specific operation. This eliminates the need to perform these procedures only in designated rooms.

If central supply personnel process all the instruments, the operating rooms may use a case cart system. With this system an enclosed cart containing all the necessary supplies for a specific surgical case is sent to the operating room. At the end of the procedure, the cart is sent back to the central supply department for reprocessing. If this system is used, fewer cabinets need to be constructed within the operating rooms.

Ideally, doors in the operating room should be of the sliding variety. This eliminates air turbulences created by swinging doors and reduces the potential for microorganisms to become airborne. The doors should be surface mounted to allow for adequate cleaning, and the frame should be at least 5 feet wide.

Airborne microbial contamination can occur in the operating room. An effective ventilation system is necessary to minimize contamination from this source. Currently, it is required that there be 20 air exchanges per hour; 4 of these changes must be fresh air. The air is cleaned by either bag-filtered or high-efficiency particulate air filtered (HEPA) systems. HEPA filters are capable of filtering 99% of all particles larger than 0.3 micron. The air may need to be modified with an air conditioning system to maintain a temperature of 20° to 24°C (68° to 75°F) and a humidity level of 50% to 55%. Maintaining humidity at this level aids in reducing static electricity, prevents the possibility of an explosion, and reduces bacterial growth.

The inlet vent is located at the ceiling, and air leaves the room through outlets located in the walls at floor level. The air pressure within each operating room is greater than that in the substerile rooms, the scrub area, and the corridors. This 10% positive pressure forces air out of the rooms and prevents air from the support areas from entering the operating rooms. To maintain this positive pressure, the doors of the operating rooms must be kept closed.

In the past few years, there has been increased emphasis on the hazard that may exist from chronic exposure of anesthetists and other operating room personnel to low concentrations of vapors of commonly used volatile liquid inhalation anesthetic agents.

Certain anesthetic gases such as the halothanes are not biodegradable beyond the molecular stage, and therefore are not filtered out of recirculated air. As a result, it is necessary to employ a scavenging system to rid the air of escaped gases. This may be done by one of the following methods: (1) direct passage to the outside from the anesthetic area, (2) aspiration by the air exhaust system of the room, (3) aspiration by a dedicated or shared vacuum system, and (4) by vacuum pump to the outside.[5]

Laminar air flow or unidirectional flow systems where there are as many as 600 air changes per hour have demonstrated substantial reductions in the number of airborne bacteria in the operating rooms. However, no substantial evidence has been found showing that these results can be translated into a reduced operative-wound infection rate, and the question of the value of the various types of laminar flow remains controversial.[6]

It has been demonstrated that the use of ultraviolet radiation of the operative field during surgery can reduce the postoperative wound infection in refined clean cases.[7] If ultraviolet radiation is used, protective cream, goggles, and headgear must be used to prevent irritation and potential damage to the eyes and the skin of all members on the surgical team. The ultraviolet lights require special care and maintenance to ensure their effectiveness. The intensity must be measured daily with a calibrated meter. The ultraviolet output depends on the temperature, the cleanliness of the lamps, and the humidity level in the room. The lamps must be protected from chilling by the ventilation system, and the humidity must not exceed 55% or the effect of ultraviolet radiation declines markedly. The film of grime that collects on the lamps must be removed twice a week.

General room illumination is provided by incandescent or deluxe cool white fluorescent lamps. Fluorescent lamps give much less radiant heat than incandescent lamps, and they have a relatively longer life. When fluorescent lamps are used, the fixtures are designed to reduce radio frequency interference to a level that will not interfere with electronic equipment used during surgery. The support lighting should be a uniformly distributed level of 200 footcandles, with provisions for reducing the level.[8]

The surgical light should be a single-post ceiling-mounted unit (Fig. 2–3). Track lights are not as acceptable because the tracks are inaccessible for cleaning and therefore may harbor microorganisms that will fall out each time the light is moved. The light should not produce any dense shadows that would prevent the surgeon from visualizing the surgical field.

The radiant heat produced must be minimized for the protection of surgically exposed tissue and for the comfort of the surgeons and assistants. The approved amount of light should raise the tissue temperature no more than 2°C. The acceptable radiant energy level can be tested by painting a 1-cm round spot in india ink on the back of the wrist and focusing the light on the spot. If the spot is uncomfortable after 1 minute, the radiant energy level may be harmful to delicate tissues, such as the brain.[8] Halogen lights generate less heat than do other types of lights.

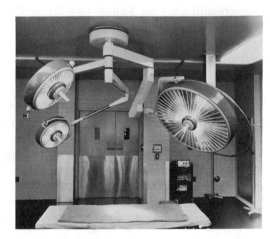

Figure 2-3. Single-post ceiling mounted surgical light. (*Courtesy Chick Surgical Systems, Greenwood, S.C.*)

In addition, the light should be near daylight in color to reduce visual fatigue. The surgical light should be capable of providing a minimum of 2500 footcandles (27 kilolux) directed to the center of a 78-square-inch pattern (800 square centimeters), 8 inches in diameter on a surgical table with the top 39 inches (97 cm) from the floor. There should be 500 footcandles at the edge of the circle.[8]

Variable pattern sizes are provided by a focusing control or by moving the light closer to or farther from the surgical incision. Variable voltage transformer or intensity control provides additional lighting when it is necessary for difficult procedures. These transformers allow selection of any voltage up to 140 volts. Consistently operating surgical lights above the normal voltage and turning the light on in the high voltage area will reduce the lamp's life.

Recent recommendations indicate that protection should be given against a total lamp failure, for example, by the use of multiple lamps in a single lighthead, or by multiple lightheads. If a single lamp is used, it should be changed routinely to avoid failure during a surgical procedure.

Additional lighting for two-team surgeries may be obtained by adding additional lightheads or satellites that extend from the primary mounting.

Freestanding portable light and fiber-optic light sources used for a headlight or as part of a sterile instrument must be in accordance with NFPA 56A. A fiber-optic unit used in a sterile field must be capable of sterilization or encasement in a sterile sleeve. If the light source is actually intended for insertion in the wound, the irradiance should be no more than 25,000 μW/cm.[8]

Headlights are frequently used by surgeons to supplement overhead surgical lights or provide light from angles that overhead lights cannot achieve. They are particularly useful for seeing in small, narrow, or deep cavities where the beam of light must be parallel to the surgeon's line of sight. Typically, it consists of a headlight mounted on a headband, a cable, and a power or light source. There are two common styles of headlights: a coaxial type and a direct type. The coaxial type projects a beam forward or down from a location directly between the surgeon's eyes, and the direct type projects a beam generally downward from a location on the forehead. Cable size, durability, and ease of maintenance are important factors to be considered in evaluating headlights.

X-ray view boxes should be recessed into the wall and located in the line of vision of the surgeon standing at the operating table.

Electrical Requirements. When flammable gases are used by the anesthesiologist, all electrical outlets and fixtures located less than 5 feet above the floor must meet explosion-proof code requirements, as identified in NFPA 56A. Grounded outlets installed above the 5-foot level may result in electrical cords running down the wall and across the floor to the equipment. There is a potential hazard for surgical team members of falling or tripping on the cords. Rigid or retractable ceiling service columns, located conveniently in the operating rooms, have assisted in controlling this hazard. The columns are equipped with vacuum, compressed air, oxygen, nitrous oxide, nitrogen, and electrical outlets. The location of two columns per operating room increases the flexibility in regard to positioning the operating room table.

Due to the decrease in the use of flammable anesthetic agents, fires and explosions in operating rooms have been reduced to a minimum. The hazard that now exists is electrical (i.e., macroshock and power failure).

Equal-potential grounding and isolated power systems were installed in operating rooms to protect patients and personnel from electrical hazards. The equal-potential grounding system insured that the patient or the personnel and the equipment were grounded to only one ground. This eliminated potential voltage differences between the patient or the personnel and the equipment, thus eliminating shocks. The isolated power system has an alarm that is activated at the 2-milliampere level. This warning system indicates when inadvertent grounding of the isolated circuits has occurred and alerts personnel to potential equipment failure or to defective equipment. These panels limit the shock personnel may receive to 2 milliamperes. Controversy regarding the cost versus the benefits of these panels has resulted in their deletion from NFPA 76B.

Multiple electrical outlets should be available from separate circuits. This minimizes the possibility of blown fuses or faulty circuits shutting off all electricity at a critical moment.

In the event of an interruption in the normal electrical supply source, an electrical generator must provide emergency power within 10 seconds to identified areas in the operating room. This usually includes designated outlets in each operating room, the surgical lights, the corridors, and the communication system.

Additional Fixed Equipment. Careful consideration should be exercised before purchasing additional fixed equipment. In the past few years, it has been in vogue to mount in the ceiling microscopes, x-ray tubes, image intensifers, cryosurgery units, and various other pieces of equipment (Fig. 2–4). Such fixed equipment requires that the operating rooms be unavailable for surgery during all necessary repairs and replacements or that these activities be performed on overtime pay status.

Equipment requiring tracks, similar to surgical lights, is a potential source of contamination as tracks are difficult to clean and therefore harbor dust and microorganisms that may fall out each time the equipment is moved. Recessing the tracks into the ceiling will minimize this as a potential source of contamination.

Television cameras mounted in one corner of the operating room can project a full view of the operation to a monitor at the control desk. Thus, the progress of all surgical procedures can be determined without an on-site visit by the charge nurse.

For teaching purposes, television cameras may be mounted on the surgical lights. The surgical procedure is then viewed from a remote area. This practice provides an excellent view of the surgical field and eliminates visitors from the operating room.

A closed-circuit television system may also relay images between the operating rooms and the pathology and radiology areas. Wall screens enable the surgeon to view the results of microscopic sections or x-ray films and to discuss the pathology with these consultants.

Furniture and Accessory Equipment. Furniture and equipment should be made of a conductive material and have conductive castors or conductive tips. Stainless steel is

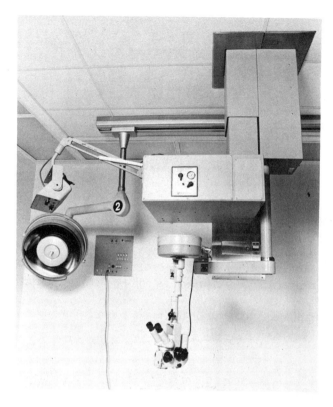

Figure 2-4. Microscope support column. (*Courtesy American Sterilizer Company, Erie, Pennsylvania.*)

frequently used in manufacturing furniture for the operating room as it is durable and easily cleaned. Standard equipment in the operating room may include:

1. *Operating Room Table.* Operating room tables are available as movable or with a fixed base. The fixed-base table is available with interchangeable table tops to meet the needs of specific surgical specialties (Fig. 2–5). The standard operating room table has three or more hinged sections that can be flexed at the articulating sections of the body. The table can be turned from side to side or placed in Trendelenburg's or reverse Trendelenburg's position, and the height is adjustable.

   Accessory equipment (such as shoulder braces, knee crutches, stirrups, or leg holders and armboards) is designed to stabilize or brace the patient in the desired position and to provide flexibility in positioning patients. Armboards are rigid in construction, fit flush with the table pad, and lock within a 90° radius. The basic head section is removable, and special head rests can be substituted. A foot extension may be added for additional length to accommodate the tall patient. An x-ray penetrable tunnel top may be placed on the operating room table to allow the insertion of x-ray cassette holders at any position along the table. The mattress and the armboards are covered with conductive rubber.

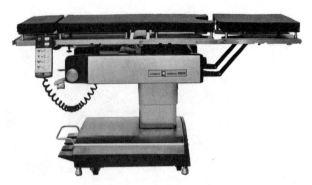

Figure 2-5. Surgical operating table with x-ray penetrable top. Tables are operated by remote control, electro-hydraulic control or manual control. (*Courtesy American Sterilizer Co., Erie, Pennsylvania.*)

Special operating tables (Fig. 2–6) are available for genitourinary, ortho-pedic, and ophthalmologic surgery. All the tables are operated manually or electrically and have a brake for stabilization.

2. *Mayo Stand.* The base of this stand slides under the operating room table; the rectangular top is used for instruments and sutures in constant use during the surgical procedure.

3. *Back Table.* This table supplements the use of the mayo stand by providing extra space for instruments, drapes, and sutures that may be required during surgery.

4. *Overhead Table (Gerhardt Table).* Various sizes and designs of overhead tables are available. The overhead table combines the mayo stand and the back table. It slides over the operating room table and provides a large surface area for the scrub assistant. One of the advantages of this table is that the scrub nurse never has to turn away from the sterile field.

5. *Ring Stand.* The ring stand is covered with a sterile drape, and a sterile basin is placed inside the ring. This basin may be used for rinsing the powder from gloves or for rinsing instruments soaked in glutaraldehyde. (The basin must be

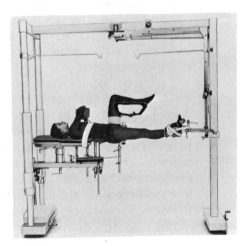

Figure 2-6. Orthopedic surgical table. (*Courtesy Chick Orthopedic, Greenwood, S.C.*)

removed immediately after use and must not be used as a "splash basin" during surgery.)

6. *Kick buckets in wheeled bases.* These buckets are lined with plastic bags and are used by the scrub team to discard soiled sponges.
7. *Linen and waste hamper frames.*
8. *Sitting stools, standing platforms, or steps.*
9. *Additional small tables* may be available to perform additional patient preparation.
10. *Poles or hangers for IV solutions.*
11. *Suction.* Each operating room must have at least two sources of suction, one for the anesthesiologist and the other for the operative site. Current construction provides for two or more suction sources to the operative site to accommodate two-team surgeries.
12. *Anesthesia machine* with a table or cart for additional drugs and supplies (Fig. 2–7).
13. *Desk Area.* This may be built into the recessed cabinets or wall mounted. Current construction is also providing a surface area for a computer terminal in each operating room. These computers are being used to generate patient changes and to maintain current inventory information.

Substerile Area and Scrub Room. Two or more operating rooms may be located around a substerile and scrub room area. Contamination of sterile supplies may occur from aerosol contaminants when members of the surgical team are scrubbing; therefore, the scrub room must be separated from the substerile area. The substerile area may

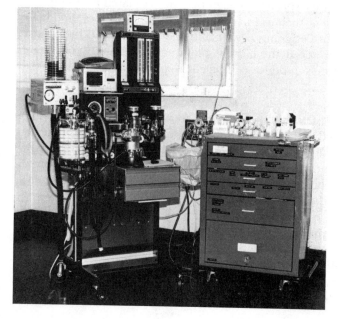

Figure 2-7. Anesthesia machine and cart for additional supplies.

contain cupboards for storing sterile supplies, a sink with a work area, an autoclave or a washer–sterilizer, blanket-solution–warmer, and a small refrigerator for drugs and solutions. The decentralization of these activities increases the efficiency of the operating rooms by decreasing the amount of time required to travel to a central location.

Central Processing Area or Workroom. If the processing of instruments remains in the operating room suite, the functions of decontaminating, preparing, packaging, and sterilizing are located in a central area. In this situation, the room is divided into a contaminated or "cleanup" area where all instruments and supplies are received following surgical procedures and a clean area or "instrument room" where the instruments are processed through the ultrasonic cleaner and then stored or wrapped for sterilization.

The use of pass-through washer–sterilizers and gravity conveyor belts in this area reduces the need to physically move the instruments from one area to another.

The clean area may also contain sterilizers that open into the next room—the sterile storage area.

The sterile storage area maintains a stock supply of sterile items such as gloves, instruments, sponges, catheters, and dressings. The shelves are preferably of the free-standing style. This allows supplies to be placed on the shelf from one side and removed from the other; therefore, rotating of supplies occurs automatically. The lowest shelf is 8 inches from the floor and the highest at least 18 inches from the ceiling. All shelves are at least 2 inches from the outside walls.[9]

The size of the sterile storage area will vary with the number of disposable products being used. Generally, disposable products require more storage area than do reusable products.

Storage Areas. The need for storage space is frequently underestimated by architects. Therefore, large pieces of equipment such as image intensifiers, microscopes, and laser machines occupy the corridors. In designing new facilities, storage should be located throughout the suite and should exceed the current requirements. Rapidly changing needs and technology will ultimately produce equipment requiring additional storage space.

Housekeeping Facilities. An area within the operating room is identified for the storage of supplies and equipment used in terminal cleaning. Providing adequate storage for this support service ensures that the equipment is used only within the operating rooms. Rooms containing hopper sinks for disposing of suction material and equipment required for cleaning between cases should be located at various points in the suite. For efficiency, they should serve not more than three to four rooms.

Surgical Waiting Room and Signage. Provision should be made to incorporate facilities for relatives and significant others waiting during surgery. Consistent with the philosophy of keeping only essential traffic in the area of the surgical suite, this space is best located one floor above or below the surgical suite.

If the waiting room is located on the same floor as the operating rooms, it should not have a view of the main entrance into the surgical suite or the recovery room because anxious relatives tend to move into and cause congestion of these areas.

The area should have an information desk where families can obtain information regarding the progress of surgery or the recovery of the patient. Direct telephone lines with these two locations will assist in the communication process.

Carefully designed and coordinated signage and directional graphics throughout the operating room suite will greatly enhance the flow of staff, patients, and visitors.

Communication System

A reliable communication system is an important link between the operating rooms and the control desk. The system chosen should be capable of differentiating between a routine call and a call requiring emergency assistance. For emergency activation, the system should have a foot or knee switch as well as a hand switch. To supplement the audible call into the operating room, each unit should have the ability of being switched off and of having a call light activated. This variation can then be used when patients are awake or when the surgeon requests that the intercom be turned off (i.e., during microsurgical procedures). In addition to the control desk, each operating room should have direct communication with the surgical pathology and radiology areas. This provides for direct consultation between the physicians in these areas.

The substerile area should have an auxiliary intercom system that provides communication directly to the recovery room, the central processing area, and the control desk.

The control desk should have connections with the blood bank, pathology area, radiology area, recovery room, anesthesia workroom, central processing area, holding area, all corridors, operating room administrative offices, and locker and lounge areas.

Telephone jacks installed in each substerile area provide for the telephone to be answered in multiple locations. This is especially useful when secretarial assistance is unavailable. Depending on the institution, direct telephone lines ("hot lines") may be a valuable connection with the emergency room and the intensive care unit.

As technology and surgical procedures become more complex, many institutions are installing telephones in each operating room. This allows the surgical team to communicate directly with ancillary areas without going through the control desk.

Music has long been recognized as a form of therapy in managing physical and emotional illness; however, the use of music in the operating room remains a controversial subject. The disadvantage identified most frequently is the distraction associated with music in the work setting; for this reason it is important that each speaker have an on/off switch and a volume control. The use of earphones for each patient would eliminate the music as a potential source of distraction for team members. Music should be played while patients are under anesthesia as musical vibrations have an effect on the subconscious mind.[10]

The benefits of music for patients and personnel are the following[11]:

1. Music creates a warmer, more pleasant environment for the patient and the staff.
2. Music provides a diversion distracting the patient from strange sights and treatments.

3. The patient undergoing regional anesthetic becomes less restless because discomfort from positioning muscle strains is lessened and time passes more quickly.
4. The use of headsets muffles extraneous noises and may also keep the patient from overhearing inappropriate conversation.
5. Members of the surgical team work in closer harmony because of decreased levels of tension and fatigue.
6. Appropriate rhythms may stimulate rapid, coordinated movements.
7. The monotony of preparation and cleanup procedures is reduced, contributing to staff morale and efficiency.
8. The use of music in the recovery period may result in a shortened and more pleasant postanesthetic recovery.

Research indicates a significant decrease from preoperative to postoperative anxiety for patients who listen to music intraoperatively.[12]

The philosophies of the operating room committee and the hospital administration on the use of music should be discussed prior to a decision being reached in regard to music in the surgical suite. If music is incorporated into the suite, the most appropriate system is Muzak. Muzak is a centralized system of recorded music that can be purchased commercially and connected to the communication system. Guidelines for the use of the system must be established and communicated to all members of the surgical team. Specific procedures related to decontamination of the earphones after each use must be outlined.

If managed appropriately, music can be a valuable adjunct during the perioperative period by providing additional emotional support to the patient.

AMBULATORY SURGERY FACILITIES

Operating rooms and recovery areas in an ambulatory surgery facility will require the same mechanical and electrical support systems as previously discussed. In addition to the areas defined in an inpatient operating room, there will be a need for a business office, examination rooms, toilet facilities, laboratory, x-ray, and admission area.

Patients electing to use an ambulatory surgical facility are more demanding of amenities—such as adequate waiting areas, toilet rooms, and privacy in treatment and consultation rooms. Easy access to the facility is essential, as is adequate parking and clearly marked entry points. Sensitive use of building materials, room finishes, color, lighting, furniture, artwork, and plants can contribute greatly to an atmosphere that promotes patient confidence and well-being.[13]

REFERENCES

1. Laufman H. Planning the surgical environment. *Contemp Surg.* 1974; 5:15
2. Operating Room Resource Utilization: Chicago Area Findings and Recommendations. Chicago: Chicago Hospital Council; 1976

3. Altemeier WA et al. *Manual on Control of Infection in Surgical Patients*. Philadelphia: JB Lippincott Co; 1976:203

4. Laufman H. Surgical hazard control: Effect of architecture and engineering. *Arch Surg.* 1973; 107:562

5. Laufman H. Operating room air. *J Surg Prac.* 1979; 8:16

6. Altemeier WA et al. *Manual on Control of Infection in Surgical Patients*, 2nd Ed. Philadelphia: JB Lippincott Co; 1984:273

7. Hart D, Nicks J. Ultraviolet radiation in the operating room: Intensities used and bactericidal effects. *Arch Surg.* 1961; 82:449

8. Beck WC et al. *Lighting for Health Care Facilities*. New York: Illuminating Engineering Society of North American; 1985:17–22

9. Garner J. *Guidelines for prevention of surgical wound infections 1985;* Guidelines for the Prevention and Control of Nosocomial Infections. Atlanta, Ga; Communicable Disease Center. 1985:6

10. Halpern S. *Tuning the human instrument*. Belmont, Ca; Spectrum Resident Institute; 1978:1

11. MacClelland D. Music in the operating room. *AORN J.* 1979; 29(2):258

12. Moss V. Music and the surgical patient. *AORN J.* 1988; 48(1):67

13. Burns L. *Ambulatory Surgery: Developing and Managing Successful Programs*. Rockville, MD: Aspen; 1984:124

Chapter 3

Administration of the Surgical Suite

The administration of perioperative nursing practice is the coordination of all functions relating to the nursing care of surgical patients.[1] The title of the individual responsible for the administration and supervision of the nursing service varies with the organization's complexity. The person to whom that individual reports also varies. In large, complex environments the title may be nursing director of the operating rooms, director of surgical services, or assistant director of nursing services. Here the daily supervision of personnel is delegated to a supervisor or an assistant supervisor.

In smaller or less complex organizations where the volume of administrative responsibility is less time consuming, the individual may have the title of operating room supervisor or head nurse.

Throughout this text the term *nurse manager* will be used to identify the individual ultimately responsible and accountable for managing the surgical suite.

In large, complex organizations it has become increasingly popular for the nurse manager of the operating room to report to the hospital administration rather than to the director of nursing services. When this occurs, the nurse manager of the operating room must establish communications with other nursing leaders within the institution and maintain an awareness of current events and trends in nursing practice.

Regardless of the title given to the nurse manager, this person is expected to coordinate all the nursing functions related to the nursing care of surgical patients.

In 1976, AORN originally published "The Standards of Administrative Nursing Practice: Operating Room" in the *AORN Journal*. The format was revised in 1982. These practices are intended to serve as guidelines for the development of a reliable means of producing good administrative care.

PERFORMANCE DESCRIPTIONS

Regardless of the size or nature of the setting, every nurse administrator has three major areas of responsibility. They are the management of:

1. Patient care
2. Human resources
3. Operational management

Components of each of these responsibilities are included in performance descriptions for the nurse manager and the supervisor. The nurse manager has ultimate responsibility for the overall functioning of the unit including fiscal management and long-range planning, whereas the operating room supervisor has responsibility for the daily clinical functions of the unit. In large, complex units the assistant supervisor is responsible for specific functions of the unit such as supervision of the ancillary personnel and acts as the administrative head in the absence of the supervisor.

It is essential that nursing administrators collaborate and cooperate for the effective and efficient functioning of the department. Concise performance descriptions will assist in this process by identifying lines of authority and responsibility. Examples of job descriptions follow.

Nursing Director, Operating Rooms and Post Anesthesia Care Unit

Minimum Qualifications

1. Current licensure as a registered nurse
2. Current certification in basic cardiopulmonary resuscitation
3. Master's degree in nursing administration or business management with 3 years of experience in operating/postanesthesia care units (PACU), 2 years of which have had an administrative component, or

    Baccalaureate degree in nursing with 5 years of experience in operating/PACU rooms, 3 years having had an administrative component, or

    Equivalent combination of education and experience with skills, knowledge, and abilities essential to the successful performance of the duties assigned to the position

General Description. Within the guidelines of the institutional philosophy, the Nursing Director of the Operating Rooms and PACU carries ultimate administrative authority and responsibility for the nursing services provided surgical patients. The Nursing Director is accountable for creating a social system that fosters the participation of the nursing staff in the assessment, planning, implementation, and evaluation of professional practice to ensure safe, efficient, and therapeutically effective nursing care. This includes organizational programming, goal setting, and policy development.

Responsibility and Accountability. The Nursing Director is accountable to the Associate Director of the Hospital and is expected to develop and maintain a constructive working relationship with the operating room committee.

Responsibilities

I. *Administration:* The Nursing Director, Operating Room and PACU is responsible for the organization, administration, and control of the operating and recovery rooms.
   A. *Planning*
      1. Assumes final responsibility for the formulation and the implementation of a nursing philosophy and objectives congruent with the stated goals of the institution

2. Is responsible for the development of policy, procedures, and staffing patterns essential to the achievement of the philosophy and the objectives. Reviews and revises these annually to meet trends in nursing practice and patient services
3. Is responsible for planning future needs of departments, including the following areas:
   a. Personnel
   b. Program development
   c. Facilities
   d. Equipment
   e. Relationships with other clinical units
   f. Relationships with hospital support services
4. Involves appropriate medical staff and administrative staff in the planning process
5. Is responsible for developing and implementing the operating and capital budgets; this includes providing for personnel, supplies, equipment, and evaluating their current level of effectiveness
6. Is responsible for evaluation of programs and patient care activities
7. Assumes primary planning responsibility in designing new facilities or in remodeling existing facilities
8. Is responsible for unit compliance with regulating standards such as JCAHO* and State licensure requirements

B. *Management*
   1. Is responsible for developing an organizational structure, assigning responsibilities and delegating authority that will facilitate safe, effective, and efficient care for the surgical patient
   2. Provides leadership and support to administrative nurses in developing and maintaining effective relationships with the medical staff
   3. Establishes and maintains standards of nursing care within the departments
   4. Analyzes and evaluates nursing care in relation to the established standards
   5. Is responsible for the scope of nursing practice and its mode of delivery within the departments
   6. Functions as a facilitator to ensure the provision of adequate resources so that nursing objectives can be met in the most cost-effective manner (scheduling of surgical procedures and staff)
   7. Is responsible for collaborating on standards of performance for the following support services:
      a. Environmental Services
      b. Material Services
      c. Laundry
      d. Building Management

---

*JCAHO is the Joint Commission on Accreditation of Health Care Organizations.

8. Is responsible for monitoring monthly fiscal reports, using this information to change departmental practices when appropriate
9. Is responsible for controlling costs and maximizing patient revenues by supervising the processing of appropriate charge documents
10. Acts as a resource to administrative nurses for problem identification and resolution
11. Develops and supports multidirectional communication systems both intradepartmentally and interdepartmentally
12. Is responsible for the recruitment of nursing personnel; this includes defining qualifications, interviewing, hiring, and maintaining staff at appropriate levels consistent with a departmental affirmative action program
13. Is responsible for departmental personnel policies that provide for job satisfaction, professional growth, development, and retention of employees
14. Is responsible for the maintenance of positive relationships with all departments of the hospital
15. Interprets and disseminates information on hospital-wide policies and new programs and other pertinent information to administrative nurses
16. Contributes to the development of institutional programs and policies through participation in nursing director meetings
17. Initiates contact with and responds to community agencies to translate the philosophy and the objectives of perioperative nursing
18. Campus committees: participates as an active member of campus committees as assigned by the hospital administration
19. Serves as a resource and a consultant for all visiting nursing personnel, other departments, community hospitals, and community agencies on operating room practices and procedures
20. Maintains awareness of professional issues at the local, state, and national levels that affect the delivery of nursing services

C. *Supervision*
1. Is responsible for developing the roles and the responsibilities of the positions that report directly to the Nursing Director
2. Is responsible for guiding, counseling, and supporting the administrative nurses in the effective use, supervision, and development of the staff, including the following:
   a. The design of job roles and job responsibilities
   b. Performance evaluation for all staff
   c. Assurance that all staff personnel actions are consistent with personnel policies
3. Provides direction and supervises orientation programs and weekly staff development sessions
4. Contributes to the development of programs appropriate to meet the changing needs of the surgical population, assuring the provision of adequate services that are relevant and accessible

5. Promotes professional growth by actively contributing to the development of employees through delegation, supervision, and education
6. Is responsible for evaluating the performance of the administrative staff
7. Oversees the supervision of professional activities of nursing staff and supportive nursing personnel
8. Consults and supervises the departmental quality assurance program and disaster plan
9. Is available to all personnel for guidance, counseling, and advice as needed
10. Supervises the collection of all required records and reports: OR records, monthly statistics, patient charges, unusual occurrence reports, personnel records, and payroll records

II. *Clinical Practice*
1. The Nursing Director is expected to have knowledge of all surgical specialties
2. When appropriate, provides direct patient care

III. *Education*
1. Assumes an active role in the educational process that prepares nurses for professional perioperative nursing by serving as consultant to the postpreparatory course in perioperative nursing (Fig. 3–1)
2. Obtains a nonsalaried clinical appointment at a school of nursing and collaborates with the faculty in the development of an area of concentration in the operating room; assumes responsibility for direct teaching in this program
3. Serves as a faculty member for students choosing the operating room as an independent study
4. Serves as preceptor on operating room management for students
5. Serves on committees as appointed by the Dean of the School of Nursing
6. Participates in professional nursing organizations and in educational programs, including workshops, seminars, and institutes

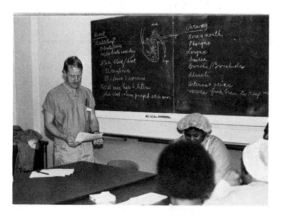

Figure 3–1. Education of the ancillary staff is the responsibility of professional staff members.

IV. *Research*
   1. Actively promotes and participates in appropriate research activities related to professional nursing practice and nursing administration
   2. Critically examines and facilitates use of valid nursing research in nursing service and administration
   3. Cooperates in research projects conducted by other health care disciplines

Operating Room Supervisor

Minimum Qualifications

1. Current licensure as a registered nurse, current certification in basic cardiopulmonary resuscitation
2. Master's degree in nursing or business management, with at least 3 years of recent clinical experience, including at least 1 year in a position with a management component, or

   Baccalaureate degree in nursing with 5 years of recent clinical experience, including at least 2 years in a position with a management component, or

   Diploma or associate degree with 5 years of recent clinical experience, including 3 years in a position with a management component, or

   Equivalent combination of education and experience with skills, knowledge, and abilities essential to the successful performance of the duties assigned to the position
3. Ability to assume departmental responsibility in the absence of the Nursing Director, Operating Rooms and PACU

General Description. The Operating Room Supervisor has 24-hour line responsibility for the operating rooms. This responsibility includes the supervision of administrative and clinical nurses, hospital assistants, surgical technicians, and clerical personnel.

Responsibility and Accountability. The Operating Room Supervisor is accountable to the Nursing Director of the Operating Rooms and PACU and is expected to develop and maintain a constructive working relationship with the physicians and the support service personnel of the hospital.

Responsibilities

I. *Administration:* The Operating Room Supervisor is responsible for the management, the supervision, and the support of the operating rooms.
   A. *Planning*
      1. Assists other administrative and clinical nurses in planning for the future needs of the unit including the following areas:
         a. Personnel
         b. Program development

    c. Equipment

    d. Relationships with other clinical units

    e. Relationships with hospital support services

2. Understands and uses knowledge of departmental philosophy and objectives in directing activities of the department

3. Participates in the annual budget planning process

4. Participates in the evaluation of departmental programs and patient care activities

5. Collaborates with the Nursing Director on special projects and other assignments as needed

B. *Management*

1. Is responsible for the maintenance of effective and efficient patient care in the operating rooms

2. With the assistance of the Nursing Director of the Operating Rooms and PACU, provides leadership and support to other administrative and clinical nurses in the following areas:

    a. Developing and maintaining effective relationships with medical staff

    b. Developing and maintaining effective and efficient staffing patterns for the delivery of patient care

3. Is responsible for the maintenance of positive relationships with other units of the hospital

    a. Develops and supports effective working relationships with:

        1) Inpatient nursing

        2) Ambulatory care nursing

        3) Building management

        4) Environmental services

        5) Material services

        6) Laundry

    b. Assists the Supply Coordinator in implementing administrative decisions that involve support services

    c. Assists the Biomedical Equipment Coordinator in implementing physical plant projects

4. Initiates and supports activities to control costs

5. Acts as a resource to administrative and clinical nurses for problem identification and problem resolution within the unit

6. Determines the need for and makes recommendations concerning new or revised policies and procedures for the department

7. Ensures that existing policies and procedures are understood and implemented

8. Follows up on unusual occurrences or employee—patient incident reports

9. Participates in the reclassification process and in salary administration as delegated by Nursing Director

10. Through professional publications, library facilities, lectures, workshops, and seminars, is aware of current trends in nursing and health care management

C. *Supervision*
1. Collaborates with the Nursing Director in developing the roles and the responsibilities of the positions reporting directly to the Operating Room Supervisor
2. Is responsible for guiding, counseling, and supporting the administrative and clinical nurses in the effective use, supervision, and development of the staff, including the following:
   a. Job responsibilities
   b. Proper conduct of performance evaluations for all staff
   c. Assurance that all staff personnel actions are consistent with the personnel policies of the hospital
3. Is available to all personnel for guidance, counseling, and advice as needed
4. Communicates effectively with the staff and ensures that all necessary information is disseminated
5. Holds individual staff members accountable for assigned responsibilities through annual performance evaluations, conferences, and contractual agreements for staff reporting directly to the Operating Room Supervisor

D. *Policies and Projects*
1. Interprets and disseminates information on hospital-wide policies and new programs and other pertinent information to all operating room personnel
2. Provides communication to the Nursing Director on problems encountered by personnel with hospital or departmental policies and systems
3. Contributes to the development of programs and policies through participation in regular administrative meetings
4. Committees: Participates as an active member or chairman on departmental or hospital committees

II. *Clinical:* The Operating Room Supervisor is expected to be clinically competent in at least five surgical specialties.
   A. *Practice*
   1. Assessment
      a. Performs a preliminary assessment of patients upon arrival in the OR, as required
      b. Collaborates with the clinical nurses in assessing the number and levels of personnel required to care for a specific patient population
      c. Collaborates with the Assistant Operating Room Supervisor in assessing the number of ancillary* employees required for the department
      d. Assesses the surgical schedule and ensures adequate staffing for planned procedures
      e. Assesses the need for changes in the number and levels of personnel and makes recommendations to the Nursing Director
      f. Assesses the clinical and administrative skills of the personnel directly responsible to the Operating Room Supervisor

---

*Ancillary employees are identified in this text as hospital assistants, orderlies, and clerical employees.

2. Planning
   a. Collaborates with the Administrative Nurses in developing department goals and objectives and makes recommendations to the Nursing Director
   b. Approves changes in the staff time schedule and communicates these to payroll clerk
   c. Collaborates with the medical faculty in planning daily surgical schedule
3. Implementation
   a. Provides support for administrative staff and/or clinical nurses in the effective use, supervision, and development of the staff
   b. Coordinates relevant patient care and clerical activities as indicated by the surgical schedule
   c. Ensures compliance with professional nursing standards and recommended practices
   d. Monitors compliance with relevant regulatory standards and licensure and makes recommendations to the Nursing Director
   e. Assists in the evaluation of new equipment and supplies
   f. Monitors the quality of environmental and support services, supplies, and equipment; and makes recommendations to the Supply Coordinator or Biomedical Equipment Coordinator
   g. Collaborates with the Assistant Operating Room Supervisor in using the skills of ancillary employees
   h. Assists in intraoperative nursing care as determined by the workload and the availability of alternate resources
4. Evaluation
   a. Collaborates with the Assistant Operating Room Supervisor and the staff in determining the outcome of patient care activities via the quality assurance program
   b. Evaluates the effectiveness of paraprofessional support activities and makes appropriate changes
   c. Evaluates the environment where patient care activities take place and makes appropriate changes
B. *Education*
   1. Uses principles of adult learning in educating staff and students
   2. Students
      a. Collaborates with the Clinical Nurses in meeting the objectives of the students assigned to the operating room
      b. Upon request assumes responsibility for direct teaching
   3. Staff
      a. Collaborates with the administrative staff and Clinical Nurses in identifying specific staff development needs of employees
      b. Arranges for the reasonable implementation of employee-identified plans for present or future job needs that are consistent with departmental policy

      c. Encourages participation in and contributes to weekly staff develop-
ment sessions

      d. Collaborates with the staff development instructor and the Nursing Di-
rector in conducting regular staff meetings to discuss patient care and
departmental issues

      e. Acts as a resource person in providing incidental teaching to all person-
nel as indicated

  C. *Research*

    1. Is familiar with research methods and actively participates in nursing re-
search projects

    2. Identifies and supports opportunities for research in the patient care area

    3. Cooperates in research projects conducted by other health care disciplines

    4. Uses research findings to recommend or initiate change

Assistant Operating Room Supervisor

Minimum Qualifications

1. Current licensure as a registered nurse, current certification in basic cardiopulmonary resuscitation

2. Master's degree in nursing with 2 years of recent clinical experience, including
at least 6 months in a surgical specialty, or

   Baccalaureate degree in nursing with 3 years of recent clinical experience, including at least 1 year in a surgical specialty, or

   Diploma or associate degree with 5 years of recent clinical experience, or

   Equivalent combination of education and experience with skills, knowledge, and
abilities essential to the successful performance of the duties assigned to the position

3. Ability to assume 24-hour line responsibility for the operating rooms in the absence of the Operating Room Supervisor

General Description. The Assistant Operating Room Supervisor has responsibility for
the ancillary staff in the operating rooms and for the quality assurance program. In
addition, the Assistant Operating Room Supervisor assumes 24-hour line responsibility
for the operating rooms in the supervisor's absence.

Responsibility and Accountability. The Assistant Operating Room Supervisor is accountable to the Operating Room Supervisor for all responsibilities except the quality
assurance program. Accountability for the quality assurance program is to the Nursing
Director of the Operating Rooms and PACU.

Responsibilities

I. *Administration:* The Assistant Operating Room Supervisor is responsible for the
management, the supervision, and the support of the ancillary staff and the quality assurance program.

A. *Planning*
  1. Participates with administrative and clinical nurses in planning for the future needs of the unit, including the following areas:
     a. Personnel
     b. Program development
     c. Equipment
     d. Interdepartmental relationships
     e. Intradepartmental relationships
  2. Understands and uses knowledge of the departmental philosophy and objectives in directing activities of the ancillary staff
  3. Participates in the annual budget planning process
  4. Participates in the evaluation of departmental programs and activities of the ancillary staff
  5. Collaborates with the Operating Room Supervisor on special projects and other assignments as requested

B. *Management*
  1. Is responsible for the effective and efficient functioning of the ancillary staff
  2. Acts as a resource to administrative and clinical nurses for problem identification and resolution in regard to ancillary job functions
  3. Determines the need for and makes recommendations concerning new or revised policies and procedures in relation to ancillary job functions
  4. Ensures that existing policies and procedures are understood and implemented by the ancillary staff
  5. Participates in the reclassification process and salary administration as delegated by the Nursing Director
  6. Is aware of current trends in nursing and health care management through professional publications, library facilities, lectures, workshops, and seminars

C. *Supervision*
  1. Is responsible for developing the roles and the responsibilities of the ancillary staff
  2. Is available to the ancillary staff for guidance, counseling, and advice as needed
  3. Communicates effectively with the ancillary staff to ensure that all necessary information is disseminated
  4. Holds the ancillary staff accountable for assigned responsibilities through annual performance evaluations and conferences
  5. Contributes to the development of programs and policies through participation in regular administrative meetings

D. *Quality Assurance Program*
  1. Serves as chairman of the quality assurance committee for the operating rooms
  2. Modifies and adapts audit tools to meet the needs of changing standards, policies, or procedures within perioperative nursing
  3. Submits to the Nursing Director the outcome of nursing audits with suggested action

4. Annually evaluates the quality assurance program and establishes future goals
5. When appropriate, collaborates to develop and implement intradepartmental quality assurance programs
6. Maintains an awareness of current trends and developments of quality assurance requirements

II. *Clinical:* The Assistant Operating Room Supervisor is expected to be clinically competent in at least five surgical specialties.

A. *Practice*

1. Assessment
   a. Uses previous clinical experience and knowledge to assess the needs of the surgical patient as required
   b. Collaborates with administrative and clinical nurses to assess the number of ancillary employees required for the department, and makes recommendations to the Nursing Director

2. Planning
   a. Collaborates with the Operating Room Supervisor in developing departmental goals and objectives and makes recommendations to the Nursing Director
   b. Collaborates with the In-service Instructor in planning for quality assurance activities

3. Implementation
   a. Provides direct nursing care to specific patients to:
      1) Explore areas of patient problems
      2) Provide experience necessary for increasing clinical competency
      3) Enhance interdisciplinary relationships by demonstrating clinical competence
   b. Collaborates with clinical nurses to develop, implement, and evaluate models of patient care
   c. Implements clinical programs designed to use ancillary services that will facilitate the efficient and effective delivery of patient care
   d. Assists in evaluating new equipment and supplies
   e. Collaborates with the Operating Room Supervisor in using the skills of ancillary personnel

4. Evaluation
   a. Evaluates the outcomes of patient care activities via the quality assurance program
   b. Evaluates the effectiveness of ancillary support activities and collaborates with the Operating Room Supervisor on appropriate changes
   c. Evaluates the effectiveness of departmental policies and procedures. Collaborates with supervisor in recommending changes to nursing direction

B. *Education*

1. Uses adult learning principles in developing educational programs
2. For staff education:

      a. Develops and implements orientation program for ancillary personnel
      b. Collaborates with administrative and clinical nurses to plan appropriate learning experiences for ancillary personnel
      c. Is responsible for conducting semimonthly educational programs for the ancillary staff
      d. Develops resource material to facilitate the teaching–learning process of ancillary personnel
      e. Collaborates with the Operating Room Supervisor for reasonable implementation of employee-identified plans for present or future job needs that are consistent with departmental policy
      f. Acts as a resource person in orienting personnel to the quality assurance program and the duties of ancillary personnel
      g. Participates in staff meetings to discuss patient care and departmental issues
   3. Students
      a. Upon request assumes responsibility for direct teaching
      b. Participates in the evaluation of student clinical experiences and communicates with clinical faculty
C. *Research*
   1. Is familiar with research methods and actively participates in nursing research projects
   2. Identifies and supports opportunities for research in the patient care area
   3. Cooperates in research projects conducted by other health care disciplines
   4. Uses research findings to recommend or initiate change

SUPPORT POSITIONS

Many institutions have identified two additional positions to assist the nursing administration staff to manage the nonnursing and indirect care activities. These positions are

   1. Supply Coordinator
   2. Biomedical Equipment Technician

The primary responsibilities of the Supply Coordinator include 24-hour responsibility for the ordering, receiving, storage, and distribution of all supplies used in the operating rooms. Additional responsibilities include coordination of services from the following departments: environmental services, material services, laundry, building management, and purchasing.

The Biomedical Equipment Technician is responsible for installing, inspecting, performing preventive maintenance of, and repairing equipment used in the operating room. Additional responsibilities include developing and implementing equipment control and safety maintenance programs, conducting educational programs for staff members, and advising the nurse manager on equipment purchases.

Previous operating room experience is a valuable asset in both these positions; however, this requirement may be waived. The Supply Coordinator must be accountable to the nurse manager, as collaboration in regard to the purchasing of supplies is essential. The Biomedical Equipment Technician may be employed by the clinical engineering department; however, the operating room must take priority over all other responsibilities.

In less complex institutions, these two positions may be combined in a Supply and Equipment Coordinator. When this occurs, the clinical engineer employed by the hospital must be relied upon for maintaining and inspecting all complex medical equipment and instrumentation.

To illustrate the potential scope of these two positions, examples of the job descriptions are included.

Supply Coordinator—Operating Rooms

Minimum Qualifications

1. Current licensure as a registered nurse and current certification in basic cardio-pulmonary resuscitation
2. Master's degree in nursing with 2 years of recent clinical experience, including at least 6 months in a surgical specialty, or

   Baccalaureate degree in nursing with 3 years of recent clinical experience, including at least 1 year in a surgical specialty, or

   Diploma or associate degree with 5 years of recent clinical experience
3. Master's degree in business administration with extensive knowledge of surgical supplies, instruments, equipment, and inventory control, or equivalent combination of education and experience with skills, knowledge, and abilities essential to the successful performance of the duties assigned to the position

General Description. The primary responsibilities of the Supply Coordinator include 24-hour responsibility for the ordering, receiving, storage, and distribution of all supplies used in the operating and recovery rooms. Additional responsibilities include coordination of services with the support departments of environmental services, material services, laundry, building management, and purchasing.

Responsibility and Accountability. The Supply Coordinator is accountable to the Nursing Director of Operating Rooms and PACU, and is expected to develop and maintain a constructive working relationship with the administrative and clinical nurses, physicians, support services, and vendors.

Responsibilities

A. *Planning*
   1. Collaborates with administrative nurses in planning for the future needs of the unit in the following areas:
      a. Environmental services
      b. Material services
      c. Laundry

      d. Building management

      e. Purchasing

  2. Collaborates with the administrative and clinical nurses to plan for:

      a. Quantity and quality of supplies required for direct and indirect patient care activities in the OR and the PACU

      b. Cost-effective use of all supplies

      c. Systematic methods of evaluation for new and/or improved products

      d. Annual supply and expense budget

  3. Initiates and supports activities to control costs (i.e., staff development sessions, communication book)

  4. Acts as a resource to administrative and clinical nurses regarding procurement of new supplies

  5. Ensures that existing procedures in regard to ordering, receiving, storage, and distribution of supplies are understood and implemented

  6. Through professional publications, meetings, and discussions with sales representatives, maintains an awareness of current trends in product development and their impact on direct and indirect nursing care activities

  7. Collaborates with the Nursing Director on special projects and other assignments as requested

B. *Management*

  1. Is responsible for collaborating with administrative nurses to evaluate and revise, where appropriate, the standards established in the following areas:

      a. Environmental services

      b. Material services

      c. Laundry

      d. Building management

      e. Purchasing

  2. Is responsible for collaborating with the administrative nurses to identify changing unit requirements that will affect the delivery of services by the following areas:

      a. Environmental services

      b. Material services

      c. Laundry

      d. Building management

  3. Is responsible for the ordering, receiving, storage, and distribution of all supplies

  4. Monitors usage of all supplies and adjusts stock levels quarterly according to the changing needs of departments

  5. Evaluates the effectiveness of all vendors and communicates to purchasing areas of concern

  6. Collaborates with the Nursing Director of Operating Rooms and PACU in developing an annual supply and expense budget

  7. Maintains expenditures within the limits of the established budget, communicating areas of excess expenditures to the Nursing Director for discussion and action

      8. Based on the evaluation of new and improved products, recommends to the administrative and clinical nurses items for purchase

      9. Responsible for the maintenance of positive relationships with other units of the hospitals and clinics

  C. *Supervision*

      1. Is responsible for developing the roles and the responsibilities of the employees reporting directly to the Supply Coordinator

      2. Holds staff members accountable for assigned responsibilities through annual performance evaluations and conferences

  D. *Communications*

      1. Disseminates information regarding the availability of supplies and other pertinent information to all operating room personnel

      2. Communicates routinely with administrative and clinical nurses regarding the status of all orders

      3. Contributes to the development of programs and policies through participation in weekly in-service sessions

      4. Provides communication to the Nursing Director on problems encountered in all areas of responsibility

      5. Committees

        a. Participates on the hospital and clinics product evaluation committee

        b. Serves as chairman of the departmental cost effectiveness committee

      6. Acts as administrative liaison with other departments to facilitate problem solving and the delivery of support services

Biomedical Equipment Technician (BMET)

Minimum Qualifications

      1. Bachelor's degree in electronics or a related field with emphasis in equipment maintenance and safety, with 2 to 5 years of experience with a biomedical equipment technology program, or

      Registered nurse with a bachelor's degree in a physical science, natural science, or nursing area with 2 to 5 years of related work experience (hospital experience is desirable), or

      Equivalent combination of education and experience with skills, knowledge, and abilities essential to the successful performance of the duties assigned to the position

General Description. The primary responsibilities of the BMET include installation, inspection, preventive maintenance, and major repair of equipment used by the operating and recovery room facilities. Other primary responsibilities consist of developing and implementing equipment control and safety maintenance programs and conducting educational programs for both students and staff.

Responsibility and Accountability. The BMET is accountable to the Nursing Director of Operating Rooms and PACU and is expected to develop and maintain a constructive working relationship with the administrative and clinical nurses, physicians, support service personnel, and vendors.

Knowledge, Skills, and Abilities

1. Considerable knowledge of electricity, electronics, mechanics, hydraulics, optics, and fiberoptics
2. Considerable knowledge of hazards and applicable safety standards and performance requirements related to biomedical instrumentation
3. Working knowledge of the operation, the underlying physiological principles, and the practical and safe clinical applications of patient care equipment
4. Considerable knowledge of anatomy, physiology, medical terminology, physics, and chemistry as related to biomedical instrumentation
5. Knowledge of state and federal codes as they relate to equipment used in operating and recovery rooms
6. Considerable skill in interpreting schematics, wiring diagrams, operational specifications, and illustrative drawings
7. Ability to recognize, analyze, and correct difficulties in biomedical instrumentation
8. Ability to work in a highly demanding technical, academic, and mental environment; the work performed is of a precise nature requiring long periods of concentration; may work under extreme stress caused by the nature of the position, which involves life-support equipment and the necessity of meeting deadlines set by surgeons and staff
9. Considerable skill in working with and supervising outside repair personnel, plant engineering personnel, nursing personnel, medical staff, and salespersons

Responsibilities

1. Installs, inspects, troubleshoots, repairs, or calibrates diagnostic and therapeutic medical equipment
2. Designs and implements modifications to improve the efficiency and the safety of biomedical instrumentation
3. Tests and repairs biomedical equipment, being certain that all new and repaired instruments are properly inspected before they are put into service
4. Provides effective periodic routine inspection of equipment and preventive maintenance and calibration of all biomedical equipment
5. Evaluates effectiveness of planned maintenance programs
6. Modifies equipment and makes system changes in accordance with manufacturer's guidelines
7. Makes scheduled inspections and tests necessary to maintain conformance to code requirements and documents this activity
8. Provides emergency service for biomedical equipment

9. Is responsible for surveillance of warranty and service agreements
10. Assists the Staff Development Instructor in the training of personnel in safe operation of equipment and in planning accident prevention programs for the staff
11. Provides written information for the policy and procedure manual regarding equipment operation and safety
12. Participates in accident and incident investigation to define causes, takes corrective action, and evaluates effectiveness of accident prevention programs
13. Maintains a reasonable perpetual inventory of replacement parts and standby equipment to minimize delay in service
14. Works closely with the Environmental Health and Safety Electronics/Safety Consultant regarding the development and the implementation of the biomedical equipment program in the operating and recovery rooms
15. Maintains and updates the inventory of equipment and space
16. Conducts the annual facilities and equipment inventory
17. Assists the Nursing Director in preparing and reviewing expense budgets for repairs, repair parts, and physical plant expenses
18. Collaborates with Clinical Nurses in developing the annual equipment and facilities budget for recommendation to Nursing Director
19. Advises the Nursing Director of long-term needs for acquisition of major items of equipment
20. Submits specifications for major equipment purchases to the Nursing Director
21. Evaluates the quality and the effectiveness of major equipment purchased for the units
22. Collaborates with Administrative Nurses to plan schedules for maintenance and renovation projects with minimum interruption to patients and staff
23. Acts as liaison with other departments to facilitate problem solving and the delivery of support services
24. Develops prototype equipment when suitable equipment is not commercially available
25. Collaborates with the Nursing Director to ensure that proper requirements are met in new construction and in renovation projects, and monitors this activity
26. Maintains knowledge of current developments applicable to biomedical specialization
27. Performs related work as assigned

PHILOSOPHY, PURPOSES, AND OBJECTIVES FOR PERIOPERATIVE NURSING

The philosophy of the operating room is consistent with the institution's philosophy and is developed with participation by all levels of departmental personnel. Once developed, the philosophy should be published and interpreted to all members of the operating room staff. In addition, it should be included in orienting all new employees.

The philosophy is reviewed annually and is revised to reflect changes in the hospital's goals and developments in perioperative nursing practice. One example of an operating room philosophy, that of the University of California Hospital and Clinics, is as follows[2]:

> The Operating Room's primary mission is to assess surgical patients in order to develop, implement, and evaluate comprehensive, cost-effective nursing care for them. To effectively serve our patients, we will develop individualized plans of care that reflect the patients' ethnic, cultural, and social diversity. We will work together with mutual respect and courtesy to blend technical knowledge and professional skills in implementing these plans for effective perioperative patient care, as well as in providing a climate for effective teaching, implementation of innovative new programs, and the conduct and application of research. We believe:
>
> 1. We have as our primary responsibility the assessment of surgical patients in order to develop, implement, and evaluate comprehensive nursing care guided by professional recommended practices.
> 2. Cost benefit analysis should precede implementation of recommended practices.
> 3. We have a responsibility to serve as patient advocates and to ensure observation of the Patient's Bill of Rights.
> 4. Perioperative nursing practice is essential to facilitate effective care for the surgical patient.
> 5. Patients should have individualized plans of care that reflect their ethnic, cultural, and social diversity.
> 6. Surgical intervention not only alters physiological functions, but may also generate stress, anxiety, and/or discomfort that can disturb individuals, families, and significant others.
> 7. We are responsible for contributing to the continuity of patient care by collaborating with other health care disciplines.
> 8. We are responsible for supporting programs that will enable health care practitioners to provide excellence in patient care.
> 9. We are responsible for developing an inservice program that will enhance the skills, knowledge, and abilities of our staff.
> 10. We are responsible for supporting the pursuit of nursing research to improve nursing practice and patient care.
> 11. We are responsible for developing courteous colleagial relationships characterized by mutual respect and understanding.

Purposes

After the philosophy of nursing care has been formulated, it is essential to develop a set of purposes. These purposes state the activities or actions that will be implemented in accordance with the philosophy and are defined in much greater detail than the articles of the philosophy:

- To define and implement a comprehensive nursing care program in the operating room
- To provide the medical staff with facilities, personnel, and a suitable climate for surgical intervention in disease treatment

If these are the purposes, the way they are performed, the frequency, and the methods used, will be determined by the objectives for nursing care.

Objectives

Objectives should be positive statements that are reasonable, attainable, and measurable.

The importance of identifying objectives is that they will become criteria for the evaluation of nursing care. Through constant emphasis on these objectives and their daily use by the administrative and clinical nursing staff members, the nursing care of patients will approximate the kind of care envisioned in the philosophy (Fig. 3–2).

- The objective of perioperative nursing is to provide patient-centered nursing care. Nurses shall view implementing the perioperative role as their primary responsibility.
- The patient's pertinent signs and symptoms will be observed, evaluated, and documented with appropriate nursing action initiated.
- The care the patient receives will be provided by the collaborative efforts of the nursing personnel and the medical staff.
- Equipment and supplies will continually be evaluated to ensure that cost-effective items are available for all surgical procedures.
- Employees will be encouraged to develop to a high level of proficiency. Educational programs will be planned to encourage individual motivation and to enhance knowledge.
- An environment conducive to nursing research will be fostered. Results of nursing research will be used to initiate change.

Policies and Procedures

The operating room has written policies and procedures that serve as guidelines for action and decision making. Policies and procedures are written to protect patients and personnel from injury; to meet local, state, and federal regulations with regard to licensure; to coincide with community standards; and to meet the standards of the JCAHO.

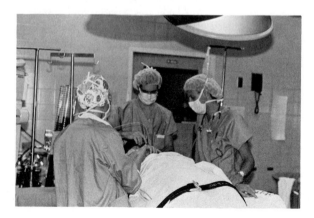

Figure 3-2. Collaborative efforts by nursing personnel and medical staff are essential to effective patient care.

The policies and the procedures are written by appropriate members of the department and approved and dated by the nurse manager. They are reviewed, revised, and updated at least annually to reflect changes in technology and perioperative nursing practice.

The operating room policy and procedure manual should include but not be limited to the following:

1. Ambulatory surgery
2. Admission of patient to operating room
3. Alarm systems
4. Anesthesia
   a. Equipment
   b. General
   c. Local, care of the patient
5. Aseptic technique
6. Attire, surgical
7. Banks
   a. Blood
   b. Cartilage
   c. Eye
   d. Skin
8. Bowel Technique
9. Bullet handling
10. Call, guidelines for
11. Cardiac arrest
12. Catheterization, bladder
13. Charges, OR
14. Circulating nurse responsibilities
15. Cleaning and maintenance of equipment
16. Consent for surgical intervention
17. Counts
   a. Sponge
   b. Needle
      1) Micro
      2) Regular
   c. Instruments
18. Disaster plan
   a. Internal (fire, nuclear material)
   b. External
19. Discharge planning
20. Disinfecting and processing of instruments and supplies

21. Documentation of perioperative nursing care
22. Donor organs, retrieval
23. Draping for surgical procedures
24. Drugs
   a. IV solutions
   b. Controlled substances
      1) Dispensing
      2) Counting
   c. Pharmacy
      1) Requisitions
      2) Stock supply
   d. Multiple-dose vials
25. Electrosurgical machines
   a. Grounding
   b. Maintenance
   c. Hazards
26. Emergency power source
27. Estimation and recording of blood loss
28. Gowning and gloving
29. Housekeeping
   a. End-of-case cleaning
   b. Terminal cleaning
30. Hypothermia machine
   a. Guidelines for temperature setting
   b. Maintenance
   c. Hazards
31. Implants, sterilization
32. Incident reports
33. Instruments, care and handling
34. Lasers
   a. Safety
   b. Documentation
35. Loaning of instruments and supplies
36. Local anesthesia, care of the patient

37. Operating room rules and regulations
38. Organizational chart
39. Orientation of new personnel
40. Patient charges
41. Personnel policies
    a. Attendance
    b. Continuing education
    c. Evaluation
    d. Overtime
    e. Sick leave
    f. Parental leave
    g. Leave of absence
    h. Vacation
42. Philosophy and objectives of perioperative nursing
43. Positioning for surgical procedures
44. Postmortem care
45. Preventive maintenance
46. Quality assurance program
47. Radiation exposure
48. Records
    a. Anesthesia
    b. Operating room
    c. Charges
    d. Requisitions for other services
49. Scheduling of surgical procedures
    a. Elective
    b. Urgent
    c. Emergency
50. Scrub assistant responsibilities
51. Surgical shave preparations
52. Surgical skin preparations
    a. Patients
    b. Staff
53. Specimens (collection and disposition)
    a. Amputation
    b. Bone
    c. Cadaver organs
    d. Calculi
    e. Cartilage
    f. Criminal evidence
    g. Cultures
    h. Frozen sections
    i. Prosthetic devices
    j. Tissue
    k. Urine
    l. Washings
54. Sterilization
    a. Ethylene oxide
    b. Steam
    c. Packaging
    d. Shelf life
55. Sterilizers
    a. High speed
    b. Washer
56. Tourniquets
57. Traffic control
58. Transportation of the patient to the surgical suite
59. Ultrasonic cleaner
60. Ultraviolet light in the OR
61. Valuables of patients
62. Visitors
    a. Operating room
    b. PACU
    c. Preoperative area
63. X-ray in the OR

REFERENCES

1. Standards of administrative nursing practice: Operating room. *AORN J.* 1982; 23(7):1202
2. *Philosophy for Perioperative Nursing Care.* San Francisco: University of California Hospital and Clinics: 1987

Chapter 4
Developing a Clinical Series

Traditionally, the system of rewarding clinical competency was to move the nurse away from clinical practice and into the administrative role of head nurse. This position's responsibilities required that the nurse learn and implement a new set of skills, those of management. This prevented or interfered with the nurse's retention of clinical skills.

A nontraditional approach to staffing that rewards clinical competence is a clinical series. This concept provides vertical promotion for the competent practitioner and does not require a move away from the clinical setting.

The objectives of a clinical series are the following:

1. Establishes career patterns that provide for quality nursing care
2. Provides for recognition and placement of the highly skilled nurse practitioner in direct care activities[1]
3. Identifies levels of nursing competence
4. Provides realistic and measurable expectations for practice that serve as guides for the evaluation of practice and advancement within the series
5. Acknowledges nurses' educational preparation for varying levels of practice both in the formal and informal setting
6. Provides a method that allows the nurse practitioner to set his or her own goals
7. Increases the expertise of the nursing staff
8. Assists in recruiting and retaining highly qualified nurse practitioners

Essential to the success of a clinical series is the identification of all the nonnursing tasks performed by nurses and the subsequent training of ancillary personnel to assume these duties. This includes restocking the operating rooms, outdating sterile supplies, preparing routine and special instruments or supplies for sterilization, and inventory of supplies. Delegating these tasks is cost effective and allows nurses to practice nursing.

In developing a clinical series, the depth of knowledge upon which nursing decisions are based, the scope of practice, and the degree of responsibility and accountability for patient care must be identified for each level. The definition of the perioperative role and the continuum (see Chapter 5) on which perioperative nurses function—from basic competency to excellence—provides the framework for the job descriptions.

Therefore, in a five-level clinical series, level one is the student role, and level two includes the operational staff nurses with basic perioperative skills. The variation in the roles is in the minimum qualifications, and in the degree of responsibility and accountability for implementation of the behaviors as identified in the job description. Level three includes the intermediate practitioner whose professional intraoperative skills have advanced and who assumes additional responsibilities for patient care activities within one surgical specialty. Level four functions as an advance-level clinician and assumes a leadership role for one or more surgical specialties. Level five is identified as a clinical specialist and is responsible for the continuing education program for the staff and the orientation of new employees and is a resource individual for the other levels.

CLINICAL NURSE I

Minimum Qualifications

1. Current license as a registered nurse
2. Current certification in basic cardiopulmonary resuscitation

General Description
A registered nurse who, under the close supervision of a preceptor, works in controlled patient care situations and performs established nursing procedures for individual patients within an assigned surgical specialty.

Responsibility and Accountability
The Clinical Nurse I is responsible to the Clinical Nurses II through V and the Administrative Nurses. This is the entry-level classification for the nurse without experience. This level is used only for the duration of the probationary period.

CLINICAL NURSE II

Minimum Qualifications

1. Current license as a registered nurse
2. Six months of clinical experience or completion of a postgraduate course in perioperative nursing
3. Current certification in basic cardiopulmonary resuscitation

General Description
Under supervision, the Clinical Nurse II implements established nursing interventions using current clinical knowledge, and may provide care for patients with special problems. Provides leadership for other nursing service personnel. This is the operational level for nurses with more than 6 months of experience.

Responsibility and Accountability
The Clinical Nurse II is responsible for all nursing care behavior as described and is accountable to Clinical Nurses III through V and Administrative Nurses.

Behaviors

I. *Nursing Process*
  A. Assessment
    1. Obtains nursing history from available resources in the surgical suite (i.e., patient, patient record, anesthetist, and surgeon). The nursing assessment identifies and documents common variables and unusual problems affecting care and serves as a guide for the development of an individual nursing care plan. The assessment data will:
      a. Include identity of patient, baseline data pertaining to preoperative status
      b. Include the physiological condition of the patient (i.e., laboratory values, allergies, level of consciousness)
      c. Include the patient's perception with regard to impending surgical intervention
      d. Include the psychological status of the patient
      e. Verify side and site of surgical procedure
    2. Identify abnormal diagnostic data
    3. Identify potential intraoperative patient problems, symptoms, and behavioral changes in relation to:
      a. Models of nursing care pertaining to the surgical procedure and the anesthesia technique
      b. Individual patient needs
  B. Planning
    1. Develops and documents a nursing care plan (using the assessment data) that:
      a. Integrates the plans for surgical intervention and anesthetic management
      b. Establishes achievable and measurable goals
      c. Applies knowledge of basic nursing sciences in nursing intervention
    2. Involves the patient and significant others in developing a nursing care plan that reflects the Patient's Bill of Rights
    3. Plans patient care with other members of the health team
    4. Identifies immediate and long-term implications of nursing activities including, but not limited to, positioning; placement of the electrosurgical grounding device; sponge, needle, and instrument counts; aseptic technique
    5. Adjusts the nursing care plan to the changing needs of the patient
    6. Uses models of patient care and physician preference cards in preparing for specific operative procedures
  C. Implementation
    1. Identifies priorities and implements nursing care based on the nursing care plan
    2. Collaborates in implementing the surgeon's plan of care during the intraoperative period

    3. Collaborates in the implementation of the anesthesia management during the intraoperative period
    4. Assigns appropriate aspects of care to selected members of the nursing team (i.e., surgical technologist, hospital assistants)
    5. Guides care given by selected members of the nursing team
    6. Coordinates the activities of other disciplines to implement the individual patient care plan
    7. Functions as a scrub nurse or circulating nurse during the intraoperative phase
    8. Documents intraoperative care
    9. Uses safe methods of handling equipment and uses supplies judiciously

D. Evaluation
    1. Evaluates the patient's immediate response to the care plan and surgical intervention in the PACU discharge area
    2. Revises the nursing care plan to meet the changing needs of the patient
    3. Evaluates and documents the outcomes of the patient care plan through observation and interview
    4. Collaborates with other disciplines to revise the patient care plan according to the changing needs of the patient

II. *Teaching*

A. Patient
    1. Communicates the rationale for nursing interventions to the patient
    2. Collaborates with the patient to identify individual informational needs and to assess learning readiness
    3. Uses principles of learning and teaching to meet individual informational needs that involve the patient or other supporting people
    4. Refers specific learning needs of the patient to other members of the health team (i.e., PACU nurse, unit nurse, surgeon)
    5. Validates the learning needs of the patient by consulting with Clinical Nurses III
    6. Documents the patient's learning needs
    7. Implements and assists others to implement the planned teaching strategies
    8. Evaluates and revises the teaching strategies in relation to the appropriateness of the patient's response

B. Staff and Students
    1. Functions as a positive role model for professional nursing students
    2. Contributes to the learning experiences of professional nursing students in cooperation with other members of the team and the instructor
    3. Assists paraprofessional personnel on the nursing team to identify their need for learning basic tasks
    4. Participates in teaching, guiding, and evaluating the performance of paraprofessional personnel
    5. Communicates the rationale for nursing interventions to staff and students

III. *Communication*
    A. Patient
        1. Applies effective interviewing skills to obtain information from the patient that is necessary to plan, implement, and evaluate nursing care
        2. Communicates accurate information about the nursing care plan to the patient
        3. Applies basic verbal and nonverbal communication skills to identify and reduce anxiety in the patient. Documents the patient's needs and responses
        4. Maintains confidentiality in communications and documentations
    B. Staff
        1. Interacts effectively with other team members to keep them informed of changes in the patient's condition
        2. Documents pertinent information clearly and accurately and reports to the appropriate individual
        3. Participates in the development of models of patient care and departmental conferences and serves on committees
IV. *Evaluation*
    A. Staff
        1. Participates in performance appraisal by providing data in the assessment of clinical performance
        2. Participates in the evaluation of models of patient care and procedure cards
        3. Participates in the identification of unsafe patient care practices and assumes responsibility for intervention
    B. Other
        1. Participates in formal self-evaluation by identifying areas of strengths, limitations, and future goals
        2. Seeks supervision of performance when appropriate
        3. Participates in educational programs and workshops to increase professional competence and to meet personal needs and goals
        4. Understands the legal implications of nursing actions

CLINICAL NURSE III

Minimum Qualifications

1. Current licensure as a registered nurse
2. Diploma or associate degree with 2 years of recent clinical experience, or

   Baccalaureate degree in nursing with 1 year of recent clinical experience, or

   Master's degree in nursing with 6 months of recent clinical experience, or

   Equivalent combination of education and experience
3. Recent clinical experience includes demonstrated efficiency scrubbing and circulating in at least five surgical specialties

4. Current certification in basic cardiopulmonary resuscitation
5. Maintains 10 clinical ladder hours every 6 months

General Description

Under general supervision, the Clinical Nurse III provides care to patients within a surgical specialty. This position assumes clinical responsibility for a surgical specialty by providing teaching, clinical supervision, and evaluation of other nursing service personnel assigned to the specialty.

Responsibility and Accountability

The Clinical Nurse III is responsible for all behaviors described in the level III job description and is accountable to the Clinical Nurse IV and the Administrative Nurses.

Behaviors

  I. *Nursing Process*
   A. Assessment
      1. Assesses the needs of the surgical patient by obtaining a nursing history from available resources on the surgical unit (i.e., patient, chart, primary nurse, other team members, patient's significant others) or during the preoperative work up
      2. Performs physical assessment of the patient that includes, but is not limited to:
         a. General physical condition
         b. Disabilities or physical handicaps (i.e., prosthesis, special physical needs with regard to transportation, positioning, instrumentation)
         c. Relevant laboratory values
         d. Allergies
         e. Present medications
      3. Performs psychosocial assessment of the patient that includes but is not limited to:
         a. Determining the patient's knowledge and understanding of the proposed surgical procedure and expected outcomes
         b. Determining the presence of any psychosocial problems that might affect surgical nursing care
      4. Identifies the relationship in data collected to the identified problem of the patient
      5. Analyzes the initial assessment and revises the assessment based on the patient's behavior
      6. Evaluates nursing care using the current patient assessment tool
      7. Identifies patient's problems and establishes priorities for the nursing care plan
      8. Uses previous clinical experience and knowledge to anticipate potential patient care problems.

B. Planning
  1. Develops individual patient care plans by:
     a. Using the opportunity to involve the patient's significant others in the preoperative assessment
     b. Participating in educational conferences with the patient and their significant others
     c. Translating assessment findings into a nursing diagnosis amenable to nursing intervention
     d. Identifying and documenting expected outcomes for planned nursing actions
     e. Planning and prescribing nursing actions for a surgical specialty
     f. Planning strategies for solving patient and nursing care problems with other members of the health team during the preoperative assessment
  2. Makes recommendations for staffing pattern of a surgical specialty to provide for patient care during an 8-hour period
  3. Uses past clinical experience and knowledge to solve immediate patient care problems and to make appropriate referrals.
C. Implementation
  1. Implements nursing action by either giving direct care or by delegating and supervising responsibility
  2. Assists in implementing new policies or procedures and provides support for those already established
D. Evaluation
  1. Evaluates the outcome of nursing interventions by performing a postoperative evaluation on the surgical unit
  2. Uses evaluation data in collaborating with members of the surgical team to influence the revision of patient care planning for a surgical specialty
  3. Uses data obtained from patient and significant others during the postoperative assessment to reevaluate patient care
  4. Monitors the judicious use of supplies and the safe handling of equipment
II. *Teaching*
A. Patient and Significant Others
  1. Plans preoperative teaching in cooperation with unit nurses to meet the learning needs of the patient and significant others
  2. Implements and assists others to implement the planned strategies
  3. Evaluates and revises the preoperative teaching in relation to the response of the patient and significant others
  4. Plans referrals in cooperation with unit nurses to other members of the health team to meet specific learning needs of the patient and significant others
B. Staff
  1. Works directly with new employees to see that planned orientation to a surgical specialty is carried out
  2. Assists with identification of learning needs for the new employee

3. Implements the planned orientation to a surgical specialty by working directly with new employees
4. Evaluates the orientation plan and recommends changes to Clinical Nurse IV

C. Students
1. Serves as a preceptor in the orientation of students to a surgical specialty
2. Plans and delivers a lecture within a surgical specialty
3. Participates in assigning students to individual patients
4. Evaluates learning experiences in a surgical specialty and informs students and faculty of opportunities
5. Supervises students' performance of specific nursing skills and helps them to develop nursing care plans
6. Contributes to the evaluation of the students' clinical experience by providing data to the faculty

III. *Communication*
1. Observes changes in behaviors of the patient and the staff and makes self available for problem solving
2. Helps patients and staff identify existing problems and explores with them the outcomes of alternative choices
3. Identifies potential problems of patients and staff and plans appropriate action
4. Communicates changes in models of patient care and physician preference cards to all staff members
5. Recognizes own limitations and uses appropriate resources for referral of patients and staff
6. Communicates information about staff's learning needs to Clinical Nurses IV and V
7. Demonstrates involvement and participates in work-related group activities

IV. *Evaluation*
1. Assesses the competencies of personnel assigned to area of responsibility
2. Collaborates with Clinical Nurse IV in the evaluation of all levels of nursing personnel
3. Participates in the evaluation of nursing care through participation in quality assurance programs or other appropriate review processes

V. *Leadership*
1. Collaborates with Clinical Nurse IV to:
   a. Identify budget needs of a surgical specialty required to support the established nursing care standards and to implement new procedures
   b. Evaluate the quality of and proper use of:
      1) Preoperative assessments
      2) Nursing care plans
      3) Models of patient care
      4) Physician preference cards
      5) Policies and procedures
      6) Supplies, equipment, and instrumentation

2. Collaborates with the Supply Coordinator to:
    a. Procure supplies
    b. Identify cost of requests for the annual supply budget
3. Collaborates with the Biomedical Technician to:
    a. Develop the annual equipment budget
    b. Evaluate the quality and the effectiveness of equipment used by a surgical specialty
4. Serves as a member of the departmental cost containment committee and assists in evaluating new supplies, equipment, and instruments
5. Functions as a Charge Nurse on an identified shift
VI. *Research*
    1. Identifies recurrent nursing problems and questions their adaptability to research methodology
    2. Cooperates in the data collection for research projects conducted by nurses and other health care disciplines
    3. Uses research findings for planning and implementing nursing care

CLINICAL NURSE IV

Minimum Qualifications

1. Current licensure as a registered nurse
2. Diploma or associate degree with 3 years of recent clinical experience, including at least 1 year in a surgical specialty, or

   Baccalaureate degree in nursing with 2 years of recent clinical experience, including at least 1 year in a surgical specialty, or

   Master's degree in nursing with 1 year of recent clinical experience, including at least 6 months in a surgical specialty, or

   Equivalent combination of education and experience
3. Recent clinical experience includes demonstrated efficiency in implementing the perioperative role in the majority of surgical specialties
4. Current certification in basic cardiopulmonary resuscitation
5. Maintains 15 clinical ladder hours every 6 months

General Description

Under general direction, the Clinical Nurse IV develops patient care standards; assesses the health needs of patients; and plans, implements, and evaluates care for patients in one or more surgical specialty. This level uses specialized knowledge and skills for direct patient care, for teaching patients or staff, and for evaluating the clinical performance of nursing service personnel. Assumes limited administrative responsibility for clinical activity. Acts as a resource person within the organization. May perform duties of lower-level Clinical Nurses.

Responsibility and Accountability

The Clinical Nurse IV is responsible for nursing care behaviors described in the level IV job description and is accountable to the Administrative Nurses.

Behaviors

I. *Nursing Process*
  A. Assessment
   1. May consult in the development of individual patient and nursing care plans during the preoperative assessment in the home, clinic, physician's office, or preoperative work up to:
     a. Identify complex patient problems, including physiological and psychosocial changes that may affect behaviors and responses to surgical intervention
     b. Identify the physiological, psychological, and environmental factors affecting the patient
     c. Identify the interrelationships of these factors
     d. Identify current coping mechanisms and their effectiveness
     e. Identify patient support systems and their effectiveness
   2. Assesses the level of practice required to provide nursing care for specific patients
  B. Planning
   1. Plans for direct patient care based upon:
     a. Identification of required level of clinical practice
     b. Identification of patients with unusual physiological and psychological problems
     c. Identification of complex family and social interaction problems
     d. Identification of a need to study a group of patients in order to identify common problems of patients
   2. Identifies potential problems of patients based on the nursing diagnosis
   3. Collaborates with the Clinical Nurse V to identify the level of practice needed to care for specific patients
  C. Implementation
   1. Demonstrates a high level of clinical expertise in one or more surgical specialties
   2. Provides nursing care for patients having complicated surgical procedures
   3. Assesses interaction and coordination with other members of the health care team
   4. Serves as a positive role model for staff, students, and other members of the health care team
  D. Evaluation
   1. Evaluates and revises staff assignments based on the needs of a specific patient population
   2. Performs postoperative evaluation in the home, the clinic, or the physi-

cian's office, and uses data obtained from the patient and significant others to reassess patient care

II. *Teaching*
A. Patient and significant others
    1. Collaborates with the Clinical Nurse V to formulate written objectives based on the teaching and learning needs of specific groups of patients
    2. Collaborates with the Clinical Nurse V to evaluate and revise teaching based on the responses of the patient and family
    3. Assists the staff to:
        a. Use and adapt teaching standards to set goals for individual patient teaching plans, developed in collaboration by the nurse, the patient, and the family
        b. Cooperate with teaching plans designed to promote the efforts of the patient toward health-sustaining behavior
        c. Use teaching strategies suitable for the learning abilities of the individual patient
        d. Evaluate the outcomes of the teaching plan and the strategies developed for the individual patient
B. Staff
    1. Collaborates with the Clinical Nurse V to develop written objectives for a planned orientation to a surgical specialty
    2. Collaborates with the Clinical Nurse V to adapt the planned orientation program to the identified learning needs of the new employee
    3. Collaborates with the Clinical Nurse V to evaluate and revise the orientation program based on the needs of a changing patient and employee population
    4. Collaborates with the Clinical Nurse V to plan appropriate learning experiences for all levels of staff by:
        a. Assessing the ongoing learning needs of the staff
        b. Setting mutual goals with the staff
        c. Identifying learning experiences to meet patient care needs and work-related interests of staff
    5. When teaching, uses a variety of strategies appropriate to the setting
    6. Evaluates the outcomes of learning experiences based on communication from the staff and the Clinical Nurse V
    7. Acts as a resource person for clinical care problems in a variety of settings within the institution
    8. Participates in formal teaching programs
C. Students
    1. Cooperates with student nursing programs by:
        a. Serving as a preceptor for students at a variety of learning levels
        b. Limiting expectations of students to include only those behaviors appropriate for the level of the students' experience and the objectives for clinical performance

  c. Participating in formal teaching sessions

  d. Participating with the faculty in evaluation of student clinical experience

 2. Cooperates with the teaching programs for all health care disciplines and serves as a positive role model

III. *Communication*

 1. Provides counseling and guidance for patients, significant others and staff

 2. Mediates staff conflict

 3. Arbitrates differences between staff after encouraging direct encounter concerning the conflict

 4. Advises the staff to set standards for behavior

 5. Participates in unit meetings where the staff can openly discuss work-related problems and participates in offering suggestions for change

 6. Schedules individual conferences with Clinical Nurse III to focus on professional counseling and establishment of career goals

 7. Participates in interdisciplinary patient care planning conferences

 8. Informs other departments of special patient problems to ensure continuity of care

IV. *Evaluation*

 1. Participates in evaluation of all levels of personnel and makes recommendations for retention and salary increases

 2. Completes written performance appraisals at specified intervals for nursing personnel as assigned

 3. Participates in the evaluation of Clinical Nurse V

 4. Uses the evaluation methodology as a learning experience for staff by providing:

  a. Positive reinforcement of described behaviors as specified in the job description

  b. Mutually contracted goals for change in staff behaviors

  c. Resources for achievement of goals

V. *Leadership*

 1. Identifies budget needs required to support the established nursing care standards and to implement new programs in area of responsibility

 2. Monitors the implementation, the quality, and the proper use of:

  a. Preoperative assessments

  b. Nursing care plans

  c. Models of patient care

  d. Policies and procedures

  e. Teaching protocols

  f. Supplies, equipment, and instrumentation

 3. Develops, evaluates, and revises models of patient care based on:

  a. The needs of a changing patient population

  b. Expanding body of nursing knowledge

  c. Increasingly complex technology

 4. Negotiates with the Supply Coordinator and the Biomedical Technician to

provide the necessary support that facilitates the delivery of safe and effective patient care
5. Contributes to the development of policies and procedures through participation in Clinical Nurse IV meetings
6. Participates in the clinical series reclassification process
7. Collaborates with the Assistant Operating Room Supervisor in using the skills of the ancillary employees
8. Participates in intradepartmental and interdepartmental committees
9. Functions as an Administrative Nurse on weekends and holidays

IV. *Research*
1. Identifies and communicates areas of potential research (i.e., patient or nursing care problems) to Clinical Nurse V or other appropriate disciplines
2. Observes recurrent nursing problems and assesses their adaptability to research methodology
3. Negotiates with the nursing faculty to cooperate or collaborate in research projects

CLINICAL NURSE V

Minimum Qualifications

1. Current licensure as a registered nurse
2. Master's degree in nursing with 2 years of clinical experience in the operating room, or

   Doctorate of nursing or a relevant discipline, or

   An equivalent combination of education and experience
3. Current certification as a basic cardiopulmonary resuscitation instructor
4. Maintains 20 clinical ladder hours every 6 months

General Description

Under general direction, the Clinical Nurse V designs and conducts educational programs and clinical research. She or he (1) assists the Clinical Nurse IV in evaluating current nursing practice, in developing the necessary methodologies, and in implementing the standards of nursing care; (2) provides 24-hour clinical consultation regarding difficult patient management problems; (3) assesses the clinical educational needs of the staff and implements appropriate educational programs.

Responsibility and Accountability

The Clinical Nurse V is responsible for the behaviors describes in the level V job description and is accountable to the Nursing Director, Operating Rooms and PACU.

Behaviors

   I. *Nursing Process*
     A. Assessment
        1. Uses specialized clinical knowledge to assess the needs of the patient undergoing surgical intervention
        2. Assists in developing, modifying, and adapting the assessment tool to meet the needs of the surgical patient
        3. In collaboration with the Clinical Nurse IV, assesses the social system of the work setting to identify directions for change in the delivery of nursing care services for the surgical patient
     B. Planning
        1. Identifies the basic nursing needs of patients and the abilities of the nursing personnel to fulfill those needs
        2. With the Clinical Nurse IV, identifies the level of practice required to provide quality nursing care for a surgical specialty
     C. Implementation
        1. Gives direct care to patients to:
           a. Orient new employees to perioperative role
           b. Explore areas of the patient's problems
           c. Identify learning needs of staff
           d. Provide content necessary for increasing clinical competency
           e. Enhance interdisciplinary relationships by demonstrating clinical competence
        2. Collaborates with the Administrative Nurse IV to submit the request to the Nursing Director for the number of personnel required to care for surgical patients
     D. Evaluation
        1. Uses systematic methods of scientific inquiry to investigate the long-term consequences of nursing interventions
           a. Observes practice
           b. Reviews guidelines for practice and helps develop new and revised tools
        2. Evaluates the milieu in which care is given and makes recommendations for change
  II. *Teaching*
     A. Patients and significant others
        1. Collaborates with the Clinical Nurse IV to formulate written objectives based on the teaching and learning needs of specific groups of patients
        2. Evaluates and revises teaching guidelines based on the needs of a changing patient population or surgeon's preference
     B. Staff
        1. Develops written objectives for the orientation program of the professional staff
        2. Collaborates with the Clinical Nurse IV to formulate written objectives

based on the learning needs of new employees rotating through a surgical specialty

3. Collaborates with the Clinical Nurse IV to adapt the structured orientation to meet the identified learning needs of the new employee
4. Evaluates and revises the departmental orientation program based on the needs of a changing patient and employee population
5. Collaborates with the Clinical Nurse IV to plan appropriate learning experiences for all levels of staff
6. Provides situations in which knowledge is articulated and disseminated to the staff

C. Program Development
   1. Develops the theoretical framework that guides decisions about patient and staff teaching programs
   2. Assesses the continuing education needs and requirements of the staff as reflected in technological developments, changing licensure requirements, standards of nursing practice, and revisions in policies or procedures
   3. Develops learning resource materials and creates programs that are relevant to adult education and facilitate the teaching process for both patients and staff
   4. Develops programs to present subjects in innovative ways and to use appropriately a variety of educational methods
   5. Actively contributes to the growth and the development of the Clinical Nurse IV
      a. Counsels, supports, and assists the Clinical Nurse IV
      b. Participates in the evaluation of the Clinical Nurse IV
   6. Collaborates with other departments to develop and implement intradepartmental teaching programs for patients and staff, thereby integrating the operating rooms with the rest of the hospital
   7. Informs the staff of available continuing education programs
   8. Collaborates with the Nursing Director to develop a budget to support patient and staff teaching programs
   9. Evaluates instruction methods and course content and materials (i.e., films, speakers, skills laboratory)
  10. Submits the annual report that evaluates educational offerings for operating room personnel and forecasts directions for change
  11. Establishes future goals based on the evaluation of yearly activities

D. Students
   1. Collaborates with the faculty to plan student orientation to the unit
   2. Collaborates with the faculty to plan the unit's role in facilitating student objectives
   3. Collaborates with the faculty to assess the learning needs of individual students
   4. Interprets student objectives and expectations for student behaviors to the staff

     5. Participates with the faculty in evaluating the students' clinical experience

III. *Communications*

     1. Promotes an effective communication network within the operating room

     2. Initiates planned change and evaluates the outcomes to improve quality of patient care through conscious, deliberate, and collaborative effort

     3. Communicates rationale, progress, and evaluation of changes to the Administrative Nurse V

     4. Establishes and maintains a communication system with other departments that are used as resources for patient care needs

     5. Provides consultation to the Clinical Nurse IV in conflict resolution

IV. *Evaluation*

     A. Participates in the clinical series reclassification process

     B. Evaluates the clinical competency of personnel and makes recommendations for retention and salary increases

     C. Evaluates personal performance based on attainment of immediate and long-term goals that are congruent with the departmental objectives

V. *Research*

     A. Actively participates in clinical research

       1. Supports and encourages a spirit of inquiry in others

       2. Investigates methods of delivering care

       3. Studies the response to surgical intervention to facilitate planning and implementing new programs

       4. Assists the staff in interpreting and implementing research findings

       5. Uses research findings to modify theory as it relates to clinical practice

     B. Communicates research findings

Using this nontraditional approach to staffing requires reviewing the administrative functions and developing an accompanying administrative series. The administrative series should define roles that require increasing accountability of time, size of clinical staff, and scope of the administrative responsibilities. Figure 4–1 is an example of an organizational chart identifying the ways in which the clinical and the administrative series can interface.

PARAPROFESSIONAL PERSONNEL

Licensed practical/vocational nurses (LPN/LVN) and surgical technologists are trained to function as scrub assistants under the direct supervision of a registered nurse. Current standards of the Joint Commission on Accreditation of Health Care Organizations (JCAHO) permit them to function in the circulating role provided that a registered nurse is immediately available and that the medical record confirms that a qualified registered nurse supervised that activity. In addition to the scrub role, they may be assigned the functions of restocking the operating rooms, outdating sterile supplies, routine cleaning of equipment, and other related housekeeping tasks.

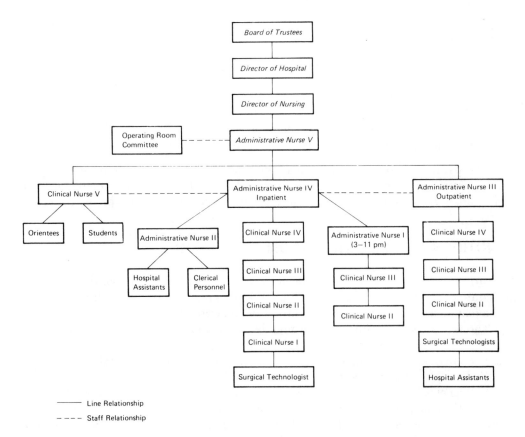

Figure 4-1. Organizational chart.

ANCILLARY POSITIONS

Clerical Personnel

As indicated earlier in this chapter, communications is an important system within the operating rooms. Clerical personnel are the key to this system functioning effectively. In addition, they may be responsible for typing, processing patients' charts, maintaining records, and preparing reports.

Hospital/Nursing Assistant (Orderly)

This group of ancillary personnel is trained to assist the nursing staff with both direct and indirect nursing care activities. In large complex surgical suites, the duties may be defined as restrictive and nonrestrictive. Nonrestrictive duties encompass all the activities occurring outside the surgical suite, such as patient transportation and errands to other departments (e.g., blood blank and bactriology and pathology areas). Duties within the surgical suite may include:

1. Positioning and moving patients
2. Routine housekeeping tasks (e.g., cleaning between surgical cases and cleaning equipment and cupboards)
3. Restocking operating rooms
4. Preparing supplies and instruments for sterilization
5. Operating the sterilizers and the ultrasonic cleaner

The paraprofessional and ancillary personnel are important components in the staffing pattern of the surgical suite (see Figs. 4–2, 4–3). They provide valuable support to the perioperative nurse, and they contribute to the care the surgical patient receives.

FUNCTIONS OF OPERATING ROOM TEAM MEMBERS

The *surgeon* is the individual whose primary responsibility is to perform the operative procedure. The surgeon may assist with the positioning, preparing, and draping; or he or she may delegate this to the first assistant or to perioperative nurses.

The first assistant to the surgeon may be a surgeon, resident, intern, physician's assistant, or nurse. According to the *AORN Journal* of May 1979, "In the absence of a qualified physician the registered nurse with appropriate knowledge and skills is the best qualified nonphysician to act as the first assistant."[2]

In the February 1983 *AORN Journal*, a report of the first assistant survey listed each state and the ruling on whether the RN may perform as first assistant. Seventeen states allowed RNs to act as first assistants, 14 did not, and 20 did not directly address the issue.[3] In the *AORN Journal* of January 1988, the survey was updated and showed that 41 states allowed the RN to first-assist, 3 states clearly do not allow it, and 10 do not address the issue. Of that 10, 2 states have scheduled hearings.[4] These data show that the role of the first assistant is becoming part of the expanded role of perioperative nurses.

In 1984, *AORN* issued a position statement on RN first assistants; a definition of

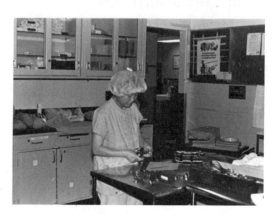

Figure 4–2. Preparing instruments for sterilization.

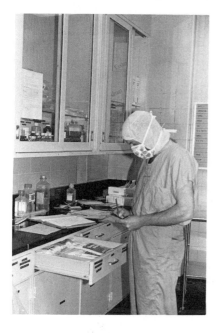

Figure 4-3. Ancillary personnel can be trained to restock the operating rooms.

the role was provided, and the scope of practice defined for individuals performing the role. In addition, the qualifications and the preparation for serving as first assistant were delineated and guidelines for establishing practice privileges were outlined.[5]

> The RN first assistant to the surgeon during a surgical procedure carries out functions that will assist the surgeon in performing a safe operation with optimal results for the patient. The RN first assistant practices perioperative nursing and has acquired the knowledge, skills, and judgment necessary to assist the surgeon, through organized instruction and supervised practice. The RN first assistant practices under the direct supervision of the surgeon during the first assisting phase of the perioperative role. The first assistant does not concurrently function as a scrub nurse. Behaviors unique to the RN first assistant may include:
>
> - Tissue handling
> - Providing exposure using instruments
> - Suturing
> - Providing hemostasis

The statement goes on to indicate that intraoperative practice of the RN first assistant is interdependent with the operating surgeon. Although independent nursing skills and judgment are essential to this practice, the intraoperative activities of the RN first assistant must be directly supervised by the surgeon.[5]

To determine if an RN qualifies as first assistant, a process for verifying her or his credentials must be established by the institution in which the individual will practice. The process of granting practice privileges include mechanisms for[6]:

- assessing individual qualifications for practice
- assessing continuing proficiency
- evaluating performance annually
- assessing compliance with relevant institutional and departmental policies
- defining lines of accountability
- retrieving documentation of participation as first assistant

The *anesthesiologist* is a physician who specializes in administering anesthetic agents. During the surgical procedure, the anesthesiologist administers drugs, fluids, and blood components as required and monitors the patient's vital signs. An anesthetist is a nurse who specializes in anesthesiology.

The *scrub assistant* may be a nurse or a surgical technologist. In 1988, the AORN House of Delegates adopted a resolution regarding the role of the scrub person. This resolution indicated that[6]

> Activities of the role of the scrub person are considered an integral part of perioperative nursing practice: therefore the registered nurse who performs the role of the scrub person is practicing nursing; and that the individual who is not licensed to practice professional nursing and performs the role of the scrub person is doing so as a delegated technical function and under direct supervision of a perioperative nurse.

As does the surgeon, this team member scrubs his or her hands and arms, dons a sterile gown and gloves, and is responsible for setting up and handing sterile supplies and instruments to the surgeon or first assistant. Throughout the surgical procedure, the scrub assistant maintains an accurate account of sponges, needles, and instruments and assures that all team members adhere to the principles of aseptic technique.

Knowledge of anatomy and physiology is essential to the performance of this role, as the scrub assistant can then anticipate the surgeon's needs. This reduces the amount of time required for the procedure.

During the intraoperative phase, the circulating nurse coordinates the activities of the room, implements the nursing care plan, and serves as the patient's advocate. He or she provides emotional support to the patient prior to the anesthesia induction, assists the anesthesiologist with the induction, and throughout the surgical procedure is responsible for monitoring the traffic in the room and maintaining an accurate account of urine and blood loss. Using this information, the anesthesiologist will make decisions regarding the replacement of fluid and electrolytes.

When the procedure is performed under local anesthesia, a second circulating nurse continuously provides emotional support for the patient, administers intravenous narcotics at the surgeon's request, monitors vital signs, and reports abnormalities to the surgeon.

Prior to the completion of the surgical procedure, the circulating nurse completes the documentation, informs the PACU of special needs, and assures that the sponge, needle, and instrument counts are completed.

Postoperatively, the circulating nurse accompanies the patient to the PACU, provides the PACU nurse with a report on the patient's preoperative status and pertinent information about the intraoperative phase, and performs a preliminary evaluation of the patient's postoperative status to determine the outcome of nursing actions.

The preliminary preparation and planning for a surgical procedure may be performed by both the scrub assistant and the circulating nurse. However, from the time the scrub assistant begins the surgical hand scrub to the dressing application, there is a definite line of demarcation between these two roles.

REFERENCES

1. Colavecchio R, Tescher B, Scalzi C. A clinical ladder for nursing practice. *J Nurs Admin.* September–October 1974;54
2. Delegates approve 1st assisting statement, single level for entry. *AORN J.* 1979; 29(6)
3. Survey shows State Board positions on first assistant. *AORN J.* 1983;37(3):428–436
4. RN first assistant 1987 survey update. *AORN J.* 1988;47(1):238–248
5. Task force defines first assisting. *AORN J.* 1984;39(3):404–405
6. House adopts resolution on role of scrub person. *AORN J.* 1988;47(5):1118

PART TWO

Implementation of the Nursing Process

Chapter 5
The Perioperative Role

The perioperative role is based on Schlotfeldt's definition of nursing[1]:

> Nursing is an independent, autonomous, self-regulating profession with the primary function that of helping each person attain his highest possible level of general health. The practice of nursing focuses on assessing people's health status, assets and deviations from health, and on helping sick people to regain health, and the well or near-well to maintain or attain health through selective application of nursing science and use of available nursing strategies

The perioperative role is comprised of nursing activities performed by the professional operating room nurse during the preoperative, intraoperative, and postoperative phases of the surgical patient's experience. Operating room nurses enter the perioperative role at a basic competency level and progress toward an increasing level of excellence (Fig. 5–1).

In the preoperative and postoperative phases, the scope of nursing activities can expand as the nurse performs functions for the patient on the surgical unit and in the home/clinic setting. During the intraoperative phase, nursing activities remain the same. However, as the nurse gains additional abilities in decision making, knowledge, skills, experience, education, and ability, he or she progresses on a continuum to an advanced level of practice.[2] Table 5–1 identifies examples of nursing activities in the three phases of perioperative nursing practice.

Essential to the continuum is implementation of the nursing process and of "The Standards of Perioperative Nursing Practice." Within this framework, the perioperative nurse provides continuity of care by collaborating with the patient about his or her needs and then assisting and supporting the patient to meet those needs.

The nursing process is a systematic approach to nursing practice using problem-solving techniques. It is a dynamic and continuous process that guides nursing actions. The nursing process has four components (Fig. 5–2):

1. Assessment
2. Planning
3. Intervention
4. Evaluation

To implement the nursing process effectively, perioperative nurses should:

1. Base nursing practice on principles and theories of biophysical, physiological, behavioral, and social sciences
2. Extend the geographical boundaries for operating room nursing practice beyond the surgical suite

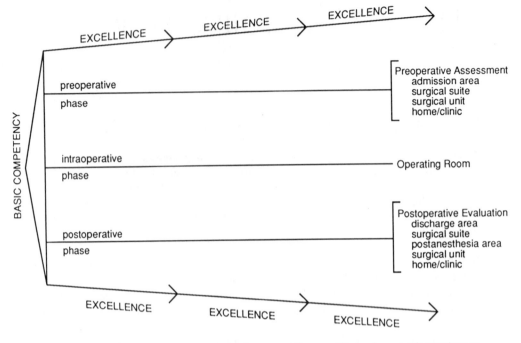

Figure 5-1. Perioperative nursing practice: a continuum. (*From A model for periopera-tive nursing practice. AORN J January 1988;41(1):193, with permission.*)

3. Recognize the need to continuously update knowledge and skills, applying new knowledge generated by research, changes in health care delivery systems, and changes in patient populations
4. Determine the plan of care by considering the patient's needs, the nurse's competence, and the resources available
5. Ensure patient and family participation in identifying needs, assessing the outcome of nursing interventions, and in determining perception of surgery (Fig. 5–3)

The framework of the nursing process was used to develop the "Standards of Perioperative Nursing Practice" (Table 5–2). These standards provide a basic model by which

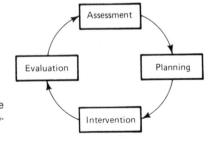

Figure 5-2. Four components of the nursing process. The nursing process is dynamic and continuous. The components are used concurrently and recurrently.

TABLE 5-1. EXAMPLES OF NURSING ACTIVITIES IN PERIOPERATIVE NURSING PRACTICE

Preoperative Phase	Intraoperative Phase	Postoperative Phase

Preoperative assessment
Home/clinic
1. Initiates initial preoperative assessment
2. Plans teaching methods appropriate to patient's needs
3. Involves family in interview
Surgical unit
1. Completes preoperative assessment
2. Coordinates patient teaching with other nursing staff
3. Explains phases in perioperative period and expectations
4. Develops a plan of care
Surgical suite
1. Assesses patient's level of consciousness
2. Reviews chart
3. Identifies patient
4. Verifies surgical site
Planning
1. Determines a plan of care
Psychological support
1. Tells patient what is happening
2. Determines psychological status
3. Gives prior warning of noxious stimuli
4. Communicates patient's emotional status to other appropriate members of the health care team
	Maintenance of safety
	1. Assures that the sponges, needle, and instrument counts are correct
	2. Positions the patient
	  a. Functional alignment
	  b. Exposure of surgical site
	  c. Maintenance of position throughout procedure
	3. Applies grounding device to patient
	4. Provides physical support
	Physiological monitoring
	1. Calculates effects on patient of excessive fluid loss
	2. Distinguishes normal from abnormal cardiopulmonary data
	3. Reports changes in patient's pulse, respirations, temperature, and blood pressure
	Psychological monitoring
	(prior to induction and if patient conscious)
	1. Provides emotional support to patient
	2. Stands near/touches patient during procedures/induction
	3. Continues to assess patient's emotional status
	4. Communicates patient's emotional status to other appropriate members of the health care team
	Nursing management
	1. Provides physical safety for the patient
	2. Maintains aseptic, controlled environment
	3. Effectively manages human resources
		Communication of intraoperative information
		1. Gives patient's name
		2. States type of surgery performed
		3. Provides contributing intraoperative factors (i.e., drain, catheters)
		4. States physical limitations
		5. States impairments resulting from surgery
		6. Reports patient's preoperative level of consciousness
		7. Communicates necessary equipment needs
		Postoperative evaluation
		Recovery area
		1. Determines patient's immediate response to surgical intervention
		Surgical unit
		1. Evaluates effectiveness of nursing care in the OR
		2. Determines patient's level of satisfaction with care given during perioperative period
		3. Evaluates products used on patient in the OR
		4. Determines patient's psychological status
		5. Assists with discharge planning
		Home/clinic
		1. Seeks patient's perception of surgery in terms of the effects of anesthetic agents, impact on body image, distortion, immobilization
		2. Determines family's perceptions of surgery

From A model for perioperative nursing practice, AORN J January 1985; 41(1):189, with permission.

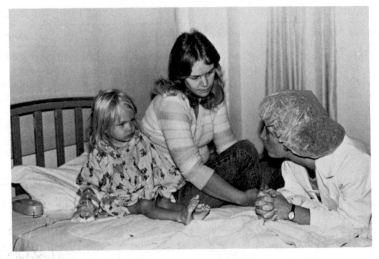

Figure 5-3. Perioperative nurses perform nursing assessments on the surgical unit prior to surgical intervention. This allows the nurse to develop individualized nursing care plans and to answer questions about the surgical experience.

TABLE 5-2. STANDARDS OF PERIOPERATIVE NURSING PRACTICE[a]

Standard I
   The collection of data about the health status of the individual is systematic and continuous. The data are retrievable and communicated to appropriate persons.

Standard II
   Nursing diagnoses are derived from health status data.

Standard III
   The plan of nursing care includes goals derived from the nursing diagnoses.

Standard IV
   The plan for nursing care prescribes nursing actions to achieve the goals.

Standard V
   The plan for nursing care is implemented.

Standard VI
   The plan for nursing care is evaluated.

Standard VII
   Reassessment of the individual, reconsideration of nursing diagnosis, resetting of goals, and modification and implementation of the nursing care plan are a continuous process.

[a]*Revised by the Association of Operating Room Nurses and the Executive Committee of the ANA Division on Medical-Surgical Nursing Practice. Standards of Perioperative Nursing Practice Kansas City, Mo: Association of Operating Room Nurses; 1981. Used with permission.*

the quality of perioperative nursing practice may be measured. Inclusion of the nursing process in the perioperative role expands the focus from task orientation to a dynamic professional specialty using theories and concepts derived from the biologic, natural, and behavioral sciences.

COMPETENCY MODEL

In 1984, using the nursing process as the framework, a committee of AORN members developed a Competency Model that can be used for[3]:

1. Position descriptions
2. Performance appraisals
3. Orientation
4. Staff development
5. Peer review
6. Clinical ladders
7. Course outline for generic curriculum
8. Quality assurance activities by monitoring accountability in the care of the surgical patient.

Eighteen competency statements were placed in a three-part model that can be used as a basis for its implementation. In the model (Table 5–3) the 18 competency statements

TABLE 5–3. COMPETENCY STATEMENTS IN PERIOPERATIVE NURSING

Competency Statements	Measurable Criteria	Examples
Assessment		
I. Competency to assess the physiological health status of the patient.	1. Verifies operative procedure	1.1 Consent form 1.2 Patient's statement 1.3 Surgeon's verification
	2. Notes condition of skin	2.1 Rashes 2.2 Bruises 2.3 Lesions 2.4 Previous incisions
	3. Determines mobility of body parts	3.1 Patient's statement 3.2 Range of motion 3.3 History and physical
	4. Reports deviation of diagnostic studies	4.1 Laboratory values 4.2 X-ray results
	5. Checks vital signs	5.1 Blood pressure 5.2 Temperature 5.3 Pulse 5.4 Respiration

(continued)

TABLE 5-3. CONTINUED

Competency Statements	Measurable Criteria	Examples
	6. Notes abnormalities, injuries, and previous surgery	6.1 Loss of extremity or body part 6.2 Congenital anomalies
	7. Identifies presence of internal and external prostheses/implants	7.1 Pacemakers 7.2 Harrington rods 7.3 Joint prostheses
	8. Notes sensory impairments	8.1 Hearing deficit 8.2 Visual deficit 8.3 Tactile deficit
	9. Assesses cardiovascular status	9.1 Pulse alteration 9.2 Arrhythmias 9.3 Edema 9.4 Electrocardiogram 9.5 Arterial lines
	10. Assesses respiratory status	10.1 Skin color 10.2 Breath sounds 10.3 Arterial blood gases 10.4 Chest tubes
	11. Assesses renal status	11.1 Intake and output 11.2 Urinalysis 11.3 Renal function studies
	12. Notes nutritional status	12.1 Nothing by mouth 12.2 Weight 12.3 Hyperalimentation line
	13. Verifies allergies	13.1 Medication 13.2 Food 13.3 Chemical
	14. Screens for substance abuse	14.1 Skin changes 14.2 Patient's statement 14.3 History and physical
	15. Communicates physiological data relevant to planning patient's discharge	15.1 Home health service 15.2 Community service
	16. Communicates/documents physical health status	16.1 Verbal reports 16.2 Written records
II. Competency to assess the psychosocial health status of the patient/family	1. Elicits perception of surgery	1.1 Patient's statement 1.2 Overreaction
	2. Elicits expectation of care	2.1 Perceived outcomes 2.2 No identified outcomes
	3. Determines coping mechanisms	3.1 Seeking information 3.2 Denial
	4. Determines knowledge level	4.1 Lack of relevant information 4.2 Well-informed

TABLE 5-3. CONTINUED

Competency Statements	Measurable Criteria	Examples
	5. Determines ability to understand	5.1 Language barrier 5.2 Lack of comprehension
	6. Identifies philosophical and religious beliefs	6.1 Blood transfusions 6.2 Sacrament of the sick 6.3 Symbols
	7. Identifies cultural practices	7.1 Disposition of limbs 7.2 Family member in constant attendance
	8. Communicates psychosocial data relevant to planning	8.1 Support group 8.2 Counseling service 8.3 Social work service
	9. Communicates/documents psychosocial status	9.1 Verbal reports 9.2 Written records
III. Competency to formulate nursing diagnosis based on health status data	1. Interprets assessment data	1.1 Selects pertinent data 1.2 Sets priorities for data
	2. Identifies patient problem/nursing diagnosis pertinent to surgical procedure	2.1 Actual patient problems 2.2 Potential patient problems
	3. Supports nursing diagnosis with current scientific knowledge	3.1 Theoretical base 3.2 Rationale for diagnosis
	4. Communicates/documents nursing diagnosis to health care team	4.1 Verbal reports 4.2 Written records
Planning		
IV. Competency to establish patient goals based on nursing diagnosis	1. Develops outcome statements	1.1 Patient is free from infection 72 hours postoperatively 1.2 Maintenance of skin integrity after discharge from OR
	2. Develops goals that are congruent with present and potential physical capabilities and behavioral patterns	2.1 Realistic 2.2 Attainable
	3. Develops criteria for measurement of goals	3.1 Signs and symptoms 3.2 Laboratory data
	4. Sets priorities for goals based on needs	4.1 Mutually set 4.2 Maslow's hierarchy of needs
	5. Communicates/documents goals to appropriate persons	5.1 Verbal reports 5.2 Written records

(continued)

TABLE 5-3. CONTINUED

Competency Statements	Measurable Criteria	Examples
V. Competency to develop a plan of care that prescribes nursing actions to achieve patient goals	1. Identifies nursing activities necessary for expected outcomes	1.1 Specific positioning aids 1.2 Patient teaching
	2. Establishes priorities for nursing actions	2.1 Immediate 2.2 Long term
	3. Organizes nursing activities in logical sequence	3.1 Dispersive pad placement before draping 3.2 Functional suction before induction
	4. Coordinates use of supplies and equipment for intraoperative care	4.1 Instrument availability 4.2 Scheduling conflicts
	5. Coordinates patient care needs with team members and other appropriate departments	5.1 Patient transfer 5.2 Equipment needs
	6. Controls environment	6.1 Temperature 6.2 Sensory stimuli 6.3 Traffic 6.4 Noise level
	7. Assigns activities to personnel based on their qualifications and patient needs	7.1 Categories of personnel 7.2 Demonstrated competencies
	8. Prepares for potential emergencies	8.1 Cardiopulmonary resuscitation certified 8.2 Disaster plan
	9. Participates in planning for discharge	9.1 Patient/family education 9.2 Referral services
	10. Communicates/ documents patient's plan of care	10.1 Verbal reports 10.2 Written reports
Implementation VI. Competency to implement nursing actions in transferring the patient according to the prescribed plan	1. Confirms identity	1.1 Patient's statement 1.2 Identification bracelet
	2. Selects personnel for transportation as determined by need	2.1 Sufficient number 2.2 Patient acuity
	3. Determines appropriate and safe method according to need	3.1 Stretcher/bed 3.2 Support measures
	4. Provides for the emotional needs during transfer	4.1 Comfort measures 4.2 Touch

TABLE 5-3. CONTINUED

Competency Statements	Measurable Criteria	Examples
	5. Communicates/ documents patient's transfer	5.1 Verbal reports 5.2 Written records
VII. Competency to participate in patient/family teaching	1. Identifies teaching needs	1.1 Surgical routines 1.2 Coughing/deep breathing techniques 1.3 Discharge instructions
	2. Assesses readiness to learn	2.1 Attention span 2.2 Anxiety level
	3. Provides instruction based on identified needs	3.1 Postanesthesia recovery routine 3.2 "Splinting" techniques 3.3 Coughing and deep breathing
	4. Determines teaching effectiveness	4.1 Return demonstration 4.2 Patient verbalization
	5. Communicates/ documents patient/family teaching	5.1 Verbal reports 5.2 Written records
VIII. Competency to create and maintain a sterile field	1. Uses principles of aseptic practice in varying situations	1.1 Skin scrub for colostomy 1.2 Clean vs sterile field
	2. Initiates corrective action when breaks in technique occur	2.1 Changing gown and gloves 2.2 Surgical conscience
	3. Inspects sterile items for contamination before opening	3.1 Intact package 3.2 Sterile indicator
	4. Maintains sterility while opening sterile items for procedure	4.1 Delivery to field 4.2 Pouring solutions
	5. Functions within designated dress code	5.1 Hair covered 5.2 Scrub attire
	6. Communicates/ documents maintenance of sterile field	6.1 Verbal reports 6.2 Written records
IX. Competency to provide equipment and supplies based on patient needs	1. Anticipates the need for equipment and supplies	1.1 Electrosurgical equipment 1.2 Prosthetic devices
	2. Selects equipment and supplies in an organized and timely manner	2.1 Preoperative 2.2 Intraoperative
	3. Assures all equipment is functioning before use	3.1 Mechanical equipment checked 3.2 Pressure-powered equipment checked

(continued)

TABLE 5-3. CONTINUED

Competency Statements	Measurable Criteria	Examples
	4. Operates mechanical, electrical, and air-powered equipment according to manufacturer's instructions	4.1 Tourniquet 4.2 Electrosurgical unit
	5. Removes malfunctioning equipment from OR	5.1 Light sources 5.2 OR bed
	6. Assures emergency equipment and supplies are available at all times	6.1 Defibrillator/monitor 6.2 Emergency drug and supply cart
	7. Uses supplies judiciously and in a cost-effective manner	7.1 Lost charge 7.2 Excess suture use
	8. Communicates/documents provision of equipment and supplies	8.1 Verbal reports 8.2 Written records
X. Competency to perform sponge, sharps, and instrument counts	1. Follows established policies and procedures for counts	1.1 Sponges/sharps/instruments 1.2 Hospital's policies and procedures
	2. Initiates corrective actions when counts are incorrect	2.1 Surgeon notification 2.2 Risk management
	3. Communicates/documents results of counts according to facility policy	3.1 Verbal reports 3.2 Written records
XI. Competency to administer drugs and solutions as prescribed	1. Administers medication according to hospital policy	1.1 Administration route 1.2 Dosage 1.3 Patient identification 1.4 Drug reaction 1.5 Complications/contraindications
	2. Communicates/documents administration of drugs and solutions	2.1 Verbal reports 2.2 Written records
XII. Competency to physiologically monitor the patient during surgery	1. Assists/monitors physical symptoms	1.1 Skin color 1.2 Electrocardiogram
	2. Assists/monitors behavioral changes	2.1 Restlessness 2.2 Level of consciousness
	3. Calculates intake and output	3.1 Fluid intake 3.2 Blood loss
	4. Operates monitor equipment according to manufacturer's instruction	4.1 Automatic blood pressure monitor 4.2 Temperature probe
	5. Initiates nursing actions based on interpretation of physiological changes	5.1 Surgeon notification 5.2 Crash cart

TABLE 5-3. CONTINUED

Competency Statements	Measurable Criteria	Examples
	6. Communicates/ documents physiological responses	6.1 Verbal reports 6.2 Written records
XIII. Competency to monitor and control the environment	1. Regulates temperature and humidity as indicated	1.1 Patient need 1.2 Staff need
	2. Adheres to electrical safety policies and procedures	2.1 Hazard identification 2.2 Line isolation monitor
	3. Monitors sensory environment	3.1 Noise levels 3.2 Noxious odors
	4. Maintains traffic patterns	4.1 Hospital's policies and procedures 4.2 Unobstructed corridors
	5. Adheres to OR sanitation policies and procedures	5.1 "Confine and contain" 5.2 Waste disposal
	6. Communicates/ documents environmental controls	6.1 Verbal reports 6.2 Written records
XIV. Competency to respect patient's rights	1. Demonstrates awareness of the individual rights of the patient	1.1 American Hospital Bill of Rights 1.2 American Nurses' Association Code for Nurses
	2. Provides for privacy through maintaining confidentiality	2.1 Communication 2.2 Documentation
	3. Provides for privacy through physical protection	3.1 Examination 3.2 Positioning
	4. Identifies ethnic and spiritual beliefs	4.1 Pastoral counseling 4.2 Communion
	5. Communicates/ documents provisions for patient's rights	5.1 Verbal reports 5.2 Written records
Evaluation		
XV. Competency to perform nursing actions that demonstrate accountability	1. Exercises safe judgment in decision making	1.1 Thorough assessments 1.2 Past experience
	2. Demonstrates flexibility and adaptability to changes in nursing practice	2.1 Change agent 2.2 Professional associations
	3. Responds in a positive manner to constructive criticism	3.1 Self-evaluation 3.2 Peer review
	4. Demonstrates tact and understanding when dealing	4.1 Team negotiation 4.2 Family interaction

(continued)

TABLE 5-3. CONTINUED

Competency Statements	Measurable Criteria	Examples
	with patients, team members, members of other disciplines, and the public	4.3 Consumer awareness
	5. Practices within ethical and legal guidelines	5.1 Nurse Practice Act 5.2 Legal statutes 5.3 American Nurses' Association Code for Nurses
	6. Seeks opportunity for continued learning	6.1 Continuing education 6.2 Inservice education
	7. Communicates/ documents nursing actions	7.1 Verbal reports 7.2 Written records
XVI. Competency to evaluate patient outcomes	1. Develops outcome criteria for goal measurement	1.1 Signs and symptoms 1.2 Laboratory data
	2. Measures degree of goal achievement	2.1 Nurse's observation 2.2 Patient's responses
	3. Communicates/ documents degree of goal achievement	3.1 Verbal reports 3.2 Written records
XVII. Competency to measure effectiveness of nursing care	1. Establishes criteria to measure quality of nursing care	1.1 Nursing audit 1.2 Peer review
	2. Assesses the patient postoperatively	2.1 Patient interview 2.2 Questionnaire 2.3 Physical examination
	3. Compares results of nursing actions to desired patient goals	3.1 Appropriateness of nursing actions 3.2 Realistic goals
	4. Communicates/ documents results of nursing care	4.1 Verbal reports 4.2 Written records
XVIII. Competency to continuously reassess all components of patient care based on new data	1. Reassess health status	1.1 Physiological 1.2 Psychosocial
	2. Refines nursing diagnosis	2.1 Changes in health status
	3. Reestablishes goals	3.1 Changes in signs and symptoms 3.2 Changes in laboratory data
	4. Revises plan of care	4.1 Revised priorities
	5. Implements revised plan of care	5.1 Revise nursing actions
	6. Reevaluates outcomes	6.1 Patient responses 6.2 Outcome criteria
	7. Communicates/ documents reassessment process	7.1 Verbal reports 7.2 Written records

From AORN Standards and Recommended Practices for Perioperative Nursing, 1989. *Denver, Colo: AORN; 1989; 2–4, 2–12, with permission.*

are listed to the far left. Adjacent to the statements, in a middle column, measurable criteria are listed. Measurable criteria are defined as "those expected behaviors or nursing actions that can be used to measure the achievement of the competency statement." To the far right of the model is an example column. These examples are not comprehensive; they serve only to provide suggestions of ways the criteria or expected behaviors can be accomplished and documented.[3]

Basic competencies can be used by all practicing perioperative nurses regardless of the practice setting or job specialty, and can be expected to be attained within a specific time frame such as 6 to 12 months.

PHASES OF THE PERIOPERATIVE ROLE

The preoperative phase begins when the patient is scheduled for surgery and ends at the time of the induction of anesthesia. The intraoperative period starts at that time and ends when the patient is transported to the recovery room or back to the inpatient unit if the recovery room is not required. Finally, the postoperative period extends through the recovery period to a follow-up home or clinic visit.

Preoperative Phase
During the preoperative phase, the perioperative nurse performs a patient assessment to collect data (Fig. 5–4). This assessment, may occur in the preoperative area, the surgical suite, the surgical inpatient unit, the clinic, the physician's office, the patient's home, or on the telephone.

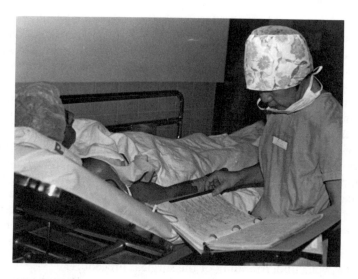

Figure 5–4. Perioperative nurses can collect information about the patient immediately prior to surgical intervention by reviewing the chart and talking with the patient.

If the assessment is performed in the preoperative area or the surgical suite, the information obtained will be limited to the patient's record and to the discussion with the surgeon, the anesthetist, and the patient. The information obtained from the patient is limited due to the premedication and the amount of time available to perform this vital function, whereas, when the preoperative assessment is performed outside the confines of the surgical suite or on the telephone, the nurse has the opportunity not only to collect data about the patient but to provide information about the surgical experience to the patient and family.

The preoperative assessment has three parts:

1. Collection of data
2. Formulation of nursing diagnosis
3. Documentation

Collection of Data. In the first step of preoperative assessment, the perioperative nurse collects baseline data about the patient that will be used to develop an individual care plan. This collection of subjective and objective data will assist later in evaluating the patient's responses to nursing interventions.

The data may be obtained from the following sources:

1. Patient's record
2. Other health team members
3. Patient
   a. Interview
   b. Observation
   c. Examination
4. Patient's family or close friends

If the patient's record is available, the perioperative nurse focuses on the nursing history, medical history (including previous surgical history), laboratory data, diagnostic studies, surgical consent, current medications, allergies, and progress notes (Figure 5–5). The nurse uses this information to establish relationships between the data collected and the proposed surgical procedure.

Discussions with other personnel on the unit, such as the team leader or the primary care nurse, may reveal additional information about the patient and his or her response to hospitalization and the impending surgical procedure.

An interview with the patient and family will allow the nurse to validate and clarify the information obtained from the other sources.

Using appropriate interviewing techniques, the perioperative nurse will assess the patient's perceptions and expectations of the surgical experience. The nurse establishes an environment of trust and support, thereby allowing the patient to express any concerns and questions about the impending surgical procedure. Using open-ended questions facilitates dialogue with patients and their families. Appropriate questions are

- "What is your understanding of the surgical procedure?"
- "You said you were upset about surgery tomorrow. Would you like to tell me about it?"

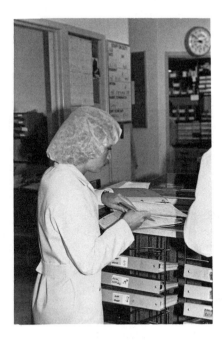

Figure 5-5. Reviewing the chart on the surgical unit provides a more accurate assessment of the patient.

- "I hear frustration in your voice. Would you like to talk about it?"
- "You say you're concerned about your family. What do you mean?"

The questions should be clear, brief, simple, logical, and purposeful and presented on the patient's level of understanding. The nurse must also be alert to nonverbal communication as this will assist in providing necessary information to perform an assessment of the patient's psychosocial behaviors. In addition, nonverbal communication may modify or cancel what the patient is saying and give clues to unexplained emotions. Important areas to observe for nonverbal communication are the following:

- Facial expressions
- Body gestures
- Muscle tension
- Rate of breathing
- Tone of voice

During the preoperative assessment the nurse focuses on the following factors as they relate to the surgical experience:

- Sociocultural status
- Mental–emotional status
- Physical assessment
- Teaching and learning needs

Following is an outline that indicates the factors and areas to be assessed during the preoperative assessment.

Sociocultural Status. The sociocultural assessment includes, but is not limited to, the following factors:

A. Understanding of the language
B. Cultural superstitions associated with illness and specifically with surgical intervention
C. Spiritual requirements
   1. Visit by clergy
   2. Religious mementos
   3. Concerns about death
D. Use or abuse of:

1. Alcohol
2. Drugs
E. Ethnicity
F. Sexuality
G. Occupation
H. Economic concerns
I. Family, friends, significant others
   1. Location
   2. Source of support

The United States is experiencing an influx of refugees from third-world countries, and nursing must give attention to the issues of cultural diversity and its implications for nursing care. In 1978, Madeleine Leininger stated that "human beings are unique because they possess cultural characteristics which shape and guide their behavior in different ways throughout the world."[4]

Definitions important to cross-cultural nursing care are as follows:

Culture. The learned ways of acting and thinking that are transmitted by group members to other group members and which provide for each individual ready-made and tested solutions for vital problems.[5]

   Culture includes diet, language, communication patterns, religion, history, family life process (such as sexuality, child rearing, health care practices, use of birth control, rituals of life and death), social interactive patterns, values, healing beliefs and practices, beliefs about life and death. Culture establishes the rules under which members operate.

Ethnicity. Affiliation due to a shared linguistic, racial and or cultural background.[6]

   Examples of ethnic groups are Germans, Italians, Afro-Americans and Hawaiians.

Subculture. Large aggregations of people who, although members of a larger cultural group, have shared characteristics that are not common to all members of the culture and that enable them to be thought of as a distinguishable subgroup.[7]

   Everyone living in America belongs to the American culture, but they also belong to subcultures. Examples of subcultures are the Amish, Mennonites, and Gypsies.

Ethnic nursing care is the nurse's effective integration of the patient's ethnic cultural background into the nursing process. Table 5–4 will assist the nurse in planning care for the cross-culture patient.

Mental and Emotional Status. Surgical intervention is a stressful experience; therefore, assessment of the mental and emotional status has particular significance for the surgical patient. Identification of the preoperative status establishes an appropriate data base to compare the patient's mental status postoperatively. Areas for assessment are

A. Mental Status
   1. Alert
   2. Drowsy

3. Disoriented
4. Semiconscious
5. Comatose

TABLE 5-4. CULTURAL VARIATIONS RELATED TO HEALTH CARE

Ethnic/Culture Group	Social Network	Nutritional Patterns	Health Beliefs and Practices	Folk Medicine and Healers	Unique Illnesses
Afro-Americans	Strong kinship bonds; several generations may live in one household. Strong religious beliefs. This is an important source of psychological support in dealing with stresses associated with illness	"Soul food" named from a feeling of kinship among the Afro-Americans. Salt pork as a seasoning is key to vegetables, especially black eyed peas, chicken and pork. Food is usually boiled or fried	Relates to Afro-American belief about life and nature of being. Life is a process rather than a state. All things living or dead influence each other. Health is harmony with nature, whereas illness is a state of disharmony. Traditional Afro-Americans view health, mind, body and spirit as one entity	Roots, herbs, potions, oils, powders, tokens and rituals are important. Predominately "self-treatment" is used under the direction of the "old lady" spiritualist, voodoo priest and root doctors	Sickle cell anemia, hypertension, dermatities (keloids, vitiligo), socioenvironmental diseases
Raza/Latina Americans	Close family ties. Courtesy and respect shown toward elderly and adults. Value modesty and privacy. Retain first language and take pride in speaking and reading Spanish	Food is a form of socialization and consists of what they can afford. Usually corn, beans, potatoes, rice, green bananas, and chilies	Family planning is not discussed and birth control is not used. Diseases are related to spiritual punishment, hot/cold imbalances, witchcraft, dislocation of human organs, natural disease and mental/emotional origin. They use herbs and prayers	Use herbs and potions as stimulants. Copper bracelets used to treat rheumatoid arthritis. Folk healers are (Curandero) spiritualist, folk chiropractors, midwives, and herbalist	Anemia in females Parasites, lactose intolerance, lead poisoning, tuberculosis, diabetes, obesity, and high infant mortality related to malnutrition

(continued)

TABLE 5-4. CONTINUED

Ethnic/Culture Group	Social Network	Nutritional Patterns	Health Beliefs and Practices	Folk Medicine and Healers	Unique Illnesses
Filipino Americans	Family has high value. Interdependency among family members stressed. Resources pooled with entire family. Children encouraged to develop modesty, industry and respect toward elderly	Hot and cold concepts influence diets. Mothers believe that what they eat affect their baby's health. Diet is influenced by religion. Rice, fish, and vegetables are staples	Diseases attributed to natural and supernatural causes. Overwork, excessive exposure to cold, heat, rain, anxiety, excessive eating and poor living conditions contribute to illness. Curses come from spirits, dead, witches, evil people	Flushing, heating, and protection are important concepts. Flushing is to rid the body of debris. Heating means that hot and cold in the body must balance. Religious articles are worn to drive away evil forces away	Hyperuricemia, coccidioidomycosis, cardiovascular-renal disease, diabetes mellitus, tuberculosis, and cancer of the liver
American Indian	Extended family very important and has economic as well as a social function Family plays a significant role during illness. Many tribes are matrilineal and this requires that decisions for surgery or treatment be discussed with the elder female family members	Corn, squash and beans. Corn is used in religious ceremonies. Navajo women drink blue cornmeal gruel after childbirth. They believe that it will increase the supply of milk. Food restrictions are frequently followed for 1 year after delivery of a child. Some individuals do not eat certain foods for	Health is defined as a person's state of harmony with nature and the universe. If an individual harms himself, he also harms the earth. Forces that prevent individuals from achieving harmony put them in a vulnerable and unhealthy state. All ailments have a supernatural aspect. Many indi-	There are 6 types of medicine men: 1. Positive role: can transform self into another form 2. Good & evil: can perform negative acts against the enemy 3. Diviner and diagnosticians: can diagnose, define cause, and indicate cure but cannot implement treatment 4. Specialist medi-	High infant mortality Trachoma Tuberculosis Alcoholism Diabetes mellitus Liver disease Heart disease

Group	Family/Social Organization	Diet	Health Beliefs	Health Practices/Healers	Common Health Problems
	cultural and religious reasons	viduals carry objects to guard against witchcraft		cine person: can implement treatment 5. Care for the soul: takes care of the spiritual needs 6. Singers: cures by song and laying on of hands	
Chinese Americans	Close family ties with extended family is very prevalent. Traditionalists have a tendency to cluster around Chinatown. Chinese heritage is preserved. Children are taught to respect elders and have filial piety toward parents. Women are taught to keep their place in the family. They are not an asset but a liability to the family	Rice, tofu, soup, and Chinese vegetables. Food is usually stirfried. Soy sauce and monosodium glutamate are used as condiments	Chinese medicine is based on the theory of Yin/Yang and the 5 elements. Healing is aimed at reestablishing the balance. Health practices emphasize moderation to avoid excesses that bring on illness. The concept of disease is based on wind and poison. Wind enters the body and causes illness. Poison is used to describe disease conditions	Herbalists, acupuncturists, and bone setters are all important. Herbs are used to balance the body and prevent illnesses. Soups and teas are used to increase energy, sedate the "hot" condition and tone the "cold" condition	Lactase intolerance Alcohol intolerance Tuberculosis Dermatitis
Japanese Americans	The individual is seen in relation to the group. The extended family includes the work group, neighbor-	Tea, fish, vegetables beef, pork, and poultry. Soy sauce, monosodium glutamate and miso sauce	Disease is thought to be caused by individual coming into contact with polluting agents such as blood,	Acupuncture, acupressure, massage and moxibustion are used to restore the flow of energy by	Alcohol intolerance Lactase deficiency Hypertension CVA Cancer of the esophagus,

(continued)

101

TABLE 5-4. CONTINUED

Ethnic/Culture Group	Social Network	Nutritional Patterns	Health Beliefs and Practices	Folk Medicine and Healers	Unique Illnesses
	hood and community Behaviors and all aspects of life are interwoven within the group Outsiders are not brought in to help solve problems as the group feels responsible for the members Worship ancestors and think about the past	are used as condiments. Diet is low in total fat, cholesterol, animal protein and sugar; high in CHO and salt. Very rich in linoleic acid	corpses, and skin diseases. Herbal purgatives are used to cleanse the body. Health is achieved through harmony and balance between self and society. Disharmony with society or not taking care of the body results in disease	the use of needles, pressure, or heat at strategic locations along the affected meridians. Natural herbs are also used to help restore equilibrium to the body	stomach, liver and biliary system Ulcers Colitis Psoriasis
South Vietnamese Americans	Strong family centered culture Emphasis on harmony in social relations. Family interests are first over individuals. There is no word for "I" in their language. Kinship system is patrilineal but females are not relegated to a low status, they share in major decisions	Rice and fish cooked in pungent sauce called nuoc-man Vegetables, fruits, spices, noodle soups, sweets made from rice gluten and coconut. Drinking during meals is rare. Naps follow the noon meal	Diseases are caused by natural and physical phenomena Belief that life has been predisposed toward certain events by cosmic forces; therefore, they use astrology and fortune telling to determine these forces. They also believe that mental illnesses are caused by bad spirits that must be exorcised by a sorcerer. Con-	Health depends on maintaining a balance of bodily elements. Cure is dependent on restoring the balance Foods and illness are believed to be related to hot and cold. Women avoid eating some hot and cold foods during pregnancy so the body's balance is not disturbed and they will not be susceptible to illness. They also	Tuberculosis Intestinal parasites Anemia Malnutrition Skin diseases Malaria Hepatitis Dental problems

			cept of Yin/Yang is also important	avoid visiting shrines believed to be inhabited by bad spirits due to affects on the unborn child Healers are generalists or specialists. Generalists have powers from supreme being. They use talismans, magic cloths, prayers and Sino-Vietnamese medical practices. Specialist treat certain ailments and particular patients	
Gypsies	Romany language spoken. Close knit family and ethnic unit. Extended families live together. Marriage between second cousins is ideal. After marriage couple lives with groom's parents. First-born grandson raised by paternal grandparents. Strong wanderlust contributes	Highly seasoned High in salt and sugar Meats high in fat (pork/beef) Tobacco use high	Hospitalization very turbulent—fear of being away from other gypsies. Therefore, members gather to support the sick Hospitals are considered to be polluted Seek "important" (well known) physicians. Distrust in "free" clinics. Family elders may try to shield	Wise female is the elder administrator. Complex set of values containing evil spirits and demons. Special saints are for good luck Traditional remedies are administered with a ceremony and include: • Mold/algae for hemorrhage or epilepsy • Love potions of	Hypertension Diabetes Occlusive coronary or peripheral vascular diseases Elevated triglycerides or cholesterol Obesity

(continued)

TABLE 5-4. CONTINUED

Ethnic/Culture Group	Social Network	Nutritional Patterns	Health Beliefs and Practices	Folk Medicine and Healers	Unique Illnesses
	to lack of formal education Maintain private society with an internal moral code and legal system Home dominated by male. Woman's role to encounter outside world Very distrustful of non-Gypsies (Gaje)		patient from facts of illness. When death occurs they freely scream, pull out clumps of hair and hurl their bodies against the wall and floor. Refuse autopsy Very wary of medical personnel, will change physicians frequently if experience is unfavorable "Crises Care": use emergency facilities freely. Poor preventive or follow-up care Share medications with family Few immunizations or prenatal care Body below waist is considered "polluted," especially women. Menstruating women may not prepare food Upper body is "pure" Measles called "God's Rose"	menstrual blood • Alopecia ointment of hog lard and chrysarobin • Garlic compresses • Tea with crushed strawberries	

B. Orientation to:
   1. Time
   2. Person
   3. Place
C. Level of anxiety
D. Coping mechanisms
   1. Verbal
   2. Nonverbal

E. Concept of body image
   1. Possible rejection due to impending surgery
   2. Relationship with
      1. Family
      2. Friends
      3. Other members of the health care team

Physical Assessment. The physical assessment includes observing the patient's appearance and may require a systematic "hands on" examination. Areas of concern include but are not limited to the following:

A. Mobilty limitations
   1. Skeletal
      a. Limited range of joint motion
      b. Joint replacement
      c. Amputations
      d. Prosthesis
      e. External fixation devices
         1) Casts
         2) Traction
   2. Muscular
      a. Paralysis
      b. Muscle tone
      c. Neurological reflexes
      d. Contractures
B. Sensory impairments (identify bilateral or unilateral)
   1. Acuity of vision
      a. Glasses
      b. Contact lens
      c. Glaucoma
      d. Blind
      e. Unusual discharge
   2. Acuity of hearing
      a. Hearing aid
      b. Lip reading
      c. Sign language
      d. Unusual discharges
   3. Speech patterns
      a. Aphasic
      b. Hoarseness
      c. Tracheostomy
      d. Laryngectomy

   4. Areas of tactile concern
      a. Paranesthesia
      b. Hyperesthesia
      c. Anesthesia
      d. Pain
C. Cardiopulmonary Status: The assessment of the cardiopulmonary status will have specific implications for the cardiovascular patient. However, it has nursing implications for all surgical patients in regard to the transportation and the position of the patient preoperatively and postoperatively.
   1. Vital signs
   2. Labile pressure
   3. Quality of pulses
   4. Quality of breath sounds
   5. Perfusion to extremities
   6. Pacemaker present
   7. Angina
   8. Arrythmias
   9. Cyanosis
   10. Syncope
   11. Edema
   12. Dyspnea
   13. Orthopnea
   14. Cough
       a. Productive
       b. Nonproductive
   15. Smoking history
   16. Respiratory obstruction

   a. Pharyngeal
   b. Pulmonary
  17. Endotracheal tube
  18. Pressure lines
D. Gastrointestinal status
   1. Nausea or vomiting
   2. Gastritis
   3. Nasogastric tube
   4. Gastrostomy
   5. Bowel incontinence
   6. Ileostomy
   7. Colostomy
E. Genitourinary status
   1. Bladder incontinence
   2. Urinary catheter
   3. Suprapubic catheter
   4. Ureteral catheter
   5. Anuria
   6. Oliguria
   7. Kidney transplant
   8. Dialysis
   9. Nephrostomy

  10. Ureterostomy
  11. Ureteral or vaginal discharges
F. Metabolic–endocrine dysfunction
   1. Diabetes
   2. Hypoglycemia
   3. Adrenal
   4. Pituitary
G. Nutritional status
   1. Time of last food or fluid intake
   2. Body structure and size
   3. Dietary customs
   4. Current nutritional status
   5. Fluid and electrolyte status
H. Skin and appendages
   1. Color
   2. Turgor
   3. Temperature
   4. Integrity
   5. Rashes
   6. Abrasions
   7. Bruises
   8. Infection

Teaching and Learning Needs. During the interview with the patient, the perioperative nurse explains the preoperative, intraoperative, and postoperative routines associated with the impending surgical procedure (Table 5–5). In addition, the nurse will assess the following areas:

   1. Patient's understanding of the proposed surgical procedure
   2. Patient's level of comprehension
   3. Patient's ability to verbalize questions, concerns, and needs
   4. Additional teaching and learning needs the patient exhibits

Preoperative teaching of the ambulatory surgery patient is an important factor in the success of these programs. It assists in marketing efforts, as the patient perceives that the facility is concerned about patients' well-being; hence, there is a higher level of compliance with preoperative routines. Preoperative education assists in the management of stress and apprehension that patients and their families may be experiencing. It also provides information regarding postoperative activities and how to cope with potential and actual problems when the patient returns home.

In addition to the one-on-one instruction that occurs, many facilities conduct tours of the unit. Role-playing with pediatric, elderly, and mentally or physically handicapped patients is a very effective method of education. Booklets and audio–visual materials written at the eighth-grade level are also excellent tools to assist with the teaching and learning process of all surgical patients.

Following data collection, the nurse analyzes the data, sorting out the information

TABLE 5-5. GUIDELINES FOR PREOPERATIVE ASSESSMENT

1. Introduce yourself
2. Identify the purpose of the assessment
   a. To obtain information that will be helpful in planning care in the operating room
   b. To answer questions and concerns about the surgical experience
3. Determine the patient's general knowledge of the intended surgery and the need or desire for additional or supplemental information
4. Explain the routine for the day of surgery
   a. Absence of food or fluid
   b. Premedication
   c. Time to arrive at the hospital
   d. Transportation to operating room (i.e., time and mode)
   e. Location and anticipated length of wait prior to being taken into the operating room
   f. Special skin preparations
5. Familiarize the patient with what he or she will see and experience in the operating room.
   a. Operating room lights and table
   b. Accessory equipment
   c. Temperature of the room
   d. Intravenous fluids
   e. Blood pressure cuff
   f. Electrocardiogram monitoring
6. Tell the patient, family, and significant others
   a. Time to arrive at the hospital
   b. Where they should wait during surgery
   c. Restaurant facilities
   d. Anticipated length of time in the operating room and the recovery room
7. Explain the postanesthesia care:
   a. Location of PACU
   b. Purpose of the PACU
   c. Routines of postanesthesia care (i.e., vital signs, checking dressings)
   d. Identify anticipated dressings, drains, catheters, packs, casts, traction
8. Discuss any relevant physical problems with the patients to determine the focus of the intraoperative care plan (visual or hearing alterations, joint, or muscle immobility).
9. Formulate a written assessment and individual nursing care plan.
   a. Discuss relevant information with the unit nurse
   b. Make an entry on the patient's chart that a preoperative assessment was completed
   c. Formulate a nursing diagnosis, identify expected outcome, and prescribe nursing action
10. Other considerations
    a. Establish an atmosphere of confidence and a climate of acceptance
    b. Give the patient ample opportunity to ask questions or verbalize concerns
    c. Be aware of nonverbal communication
    d. Allow the patient to decide if family or significant others should remain during the interview
    e. Avoid conflict or judgement or instilling false encouragement
    f. Determine the patient's comprehension and use appropriate language, avoid jargon
    g. Write individual care plan after leaving patient's room

that is pertinent to the surgical experience. The nurse then formulates a nursing diagnosis based on current scientific nursing knowledge, patient's condition, and anticipated post-operative outcomes.

Formulation of a Nursing Diagnosis. A nursing diagnosis identifies health problems that nurses are qualified and licensed to treat. It is derived from the data collected and forms the basis for developing an individual patient care plan.

Patient problems are classified as actual, potential, and possible. Actual patient problems are related to existing conditions that are currently presenting a difficulty for the surgical patient. Some examples are

1. Deafness
2. Joint immobility
3. Inability to understand the language

Potential patient problems do not actually exist, but are anticipated as a result of surgical intervention. Whenever possible, clarifying phrases beginning with "related to" should be used to explain the reason for the problem. Appropriate nursing actions can modify or diminish the occurrence of potential patient problems. Some examples are

1. Potential disruption of skin integrity related to use of an electrosurgical unit
2. Potential muscular discomfort related to improper positioning
3. Potential anxiety related to fear of surgery and of the unknown

Possible patient problems have a high probability of developing due to existing disease process, diagnosis, or circumstances within the scope of perioperative nursing. Some examples are

1. Possible discomfort during transportation related to emphysema
2. Possible drying of cornea intraoperatively related to absence of tears
3. Possible rejection of body image related to amputation
4. Possible increase in anxiety and depression related to a history of manic-depressive psychosis

The propriety of a nursing diagnosis can be assessed by referring to the list of currently accepted nursing diagnoses (Table 5–6). Additional validation can be achieved by asking the following questions[8]:

- Is the data base sufficient and accurate and developed from some concept of nursing?
- Does the synthesis of the data demonstrate the existence of a pattern?
- Is the nursing diagnosis based on scientific nursing knowledge and clinical expertise?
- Is the nursing diagnosis amenable to independent nursing actions?
- Would other qualified practitioners formulate the same nursing diagnosis based on the data?

Documentation. The third and final step of assessment is documentation. In addition to the nursing diagnosis, it is essential that relevant data obtained from the patient, the

TABLE 5-6. ACCEPTED NURSING DIAGNOSIS

Pattern 1: Exchanging
1.1.2.1	Altered nutrition: more than body requirements
1.1.2.2	Altered nutrition: less than body requirements
1.1.2.3	Altered nutrition: potential for more than body requirements
1.2.1.1	Potential for infection
1.2.2.1	Potential altered body temperature
1.2.2.2	Hypothermia
1.2.2.3	Hyperthermia
1.2.2.4	Ineffective thermoregulation
1.2.3.1	Dysreflexia
1.3.1.1	Constipation
1.3.1.1.1	Perceived constipation
1.3.1.1.2	Colonic constipation
1.3.1.2	Diarrhea
1.3.1.3	Bowel incontinence
1.3.2	Altered patterns of urinary elimination
1.3.2.1.1	Stress incontinence
1.3.2.1.2	Reflex incontinence
1.3.2.1.3	Urge incontinence
1.3.2.1.4	Functional incontinence
1.3.2.1.5	Total incontinence
1.3.2.2	Urinary retention
1.4.1.1	Altered (specify type) tissue perfusion (renal, cerebral, cardiopulmonary, peripheral)
1.4.1.2.1	Fluid volume excess
1.4.1.2.2.1	Fluid volume deficit (1)
1.4.1.2.2.1	Fluid volume deficit (2)
1.4.1.2.2.2	Potential fluid volume deficit
1.4.2.1	Decreased cardiac output
1.5.1.1	Impaired gas exchange
1.5.1.2	Ineffective airway clearance
1.5.1.3	Ineffective breathing pattern
1.6.1	Potential for injury
1.6.1.1	Potential for suffocation
1.6.1.2	Potential for poisoning
1.6.1.3	Potential for trauma
1.6.1.4	Potential for aspiration
1.6.1.5	Potential for disuse syndrome
1.6.2.1	Impaired tissue integrity
1.6.2.1.1	Altered oral mucous membrane
1.6.2.1.2.1	Impaired skin integrity
1.6.2.1.2.2	Potential impaired skin integrity

Pattern 2: Communicating
2.1.1.1	Impaired verbal communication

Pattern 3: Relating
3.1.1	Impaired social interaction
3.1.2	Social isolation
3.2.1	Altered role performance
3.2.1.1.1	Altered parenting
3.2.1.1.2	Potential altered parenting
3.2.1.2.1	Sexual dysfunction
3.2.2	Altered family processes
3.2.3.1	Parental role conflict
3.3	Altered sexuality patterns

Pattern 4: Valuing
4.1.1	Spiritual distress (distress of the human spirit)

(continued)

TABLE 5-6. CONTINUED

Pattern 5: Choosing

5.1.1.1	Ineffective individual coping
5.1.1.1.1	Impaired adjustment
5.1.1.1.2	Defensive coping
5.1.1.1.3	Ineffective denial
5.1.2.1.1	Ineffective family coping: disabling
5.1.2.1.2	Ineffective family coping: compromised
5.1.2.2	Family coping: potential for growth
5.2.1.1	Noncompliance (specify)
5.3.1.1	Decisional conflict (specify)
5.4	Health seeking behaviors (specify)

Pattern 6: Moving

6.1.1.1	Impaired physical mobility
6.1.1.2	Activity intolerance
6.1.1.2.1	Fatigue
6.1.1.3	Potential activity intolerance
6.2.1	Sleep pattern disturbance
6.3.1.1	Diversional activity deficit
6.4.1.1	Impaired home maintenance management
6.4.2	Altered health maintenance
6.5.1	Feeding self-care deficit
6.5.1.1	Impaired swallowing
6.5.1.2	Ineffective breastfeeding
6.5.2	Bathing/hygiene self-care deficit
6.5.3	Dressing/grooming self-care deficit
6.5.4	Toileting self-care deficit
6.6.	Altered growth and development

Pattern 7: Perceiving

7.1.1	Body image disturbance
7.1.2	Self esteem disturbance
7.1.2.1	Chronic low self-esteem
7.1.2.2	Situational low self-esteem
7.1.3	Personal identity disturbance
7.2	Sensory/perceptual alternations (specify) (Visual, auditory, kinesthetic, gustatory, tactile, olfactory)
7.2.1.1	Unilateral neglect
7.3.1.	Hopelessness
7.3.2.	Powerlessness

Pattern 8: Knowing

8.1.1	Knowledge deficit (specify)
8.3	Altered thought processes

Pattern 9: Feeling

9.1.1	Pain
9.1.1.1	Chronic pain
9.2.1.1	Dysfunctional grieving
9.2.1.2	Anticipatory grieving
9.2.2	Potential for violence: self-directed or directed at others
9.2.3	Post-trauma response
9.2.3.1	Rape-trauma syndrome
9.2.3.1.1	Rape-trauma syndrome: compound reaction
9.2.3.1.2	Rape-trauma syndrome: silent reaction
9.3.1	Anxiety
9.3.2	Fear

From the North American Nursing Diagnosis Association, St Louis, MO; 1989, with permission.

record, and other health care team members be recorded to provide a framework for the second step of the nursing process—the planning of patient care.

Documentation is critical in all phases of the perioperative role; therefore, it will be discussed in detail at the end of this chapter.

PLANNING PATIENT CARE BY FORMULATING PATIENT GOALS

Planning of patient care by identifying patient-centered goals for nursing care and then prescribing nursing orders or nursing actions to achieve the goals completes the preoperative phase. During this component of the nursing process, the patient, his or her significant others, and the perioperative nurse collaborate to identify the patient's goals or expected outcomes. The goals are directly related to the nursing diagnosis and are statements of the outcome desired by the patient. They are specific, attainable, and measurable behaviors with a projected schedule for achievement. After the patient's goals are identified, they are assigned priorities.

The patient's goals are identified as short or long term. Short-term goals are either immediate or intermediate. Immediate goals are life-threatening conditions and require immediate nursing actions (for example, maintenance of the airway). Intermediate goals are not life threatening and do not require immediate nursing actions. Examples of these goals are

- Maintain skin integrity
- No muscular discomfort postoperatively

Long-term goals reflect the maximum level of health the patient will be able to achieve and reflect nursing activities that occur over a long period of time. Examples of long-term goals for the surgical patient are

- Establish a positive self-image (e.g., following amputation of a leg, radical mastectomy, laryngectomy)
- Verbalize concerns and feelings regarding change in life-style (e.g., following abdominoperineal resection, coronary artery bypass, gastric resection)

Prescribing Nursing Orders

Prescribing nursing orders or nursing actions consists of identifying the activities within the scope of the nurse's responsibility that will assist the patient to achieve the identified goals. Nursing order are based on current scientific knowledge, reflect consideration of the "Patient's Bill of Rights,"* and are realistic. Nursing orders must be explicit to avoid misinterpretation. They describe specific nursing actions and include information on who is to perform the activities, when the activity is to be performed, and where the activity will occur.

According to the *Standards of Perioperative Nursing Practice*[9]

---

*Statement on the Patient's Bill of Rights, American Hospital Association, November 17, 1972, Chicago, Ill.

The plan includes but is not limited to the following specific nursing activities in the operating room:

1. Assurance of information and supportive preoperative teaching specifically related to the surgical intervention and operating room nursing care
2. Identification of individual
3. Verification of surgical site
4. Verification of operative consent and procedure and reports of essential diagnostic procedures
5. Positioning according to physiological principles
6. Adherence to principles of asepsis
7. Assurance of appropriate and properly functioning equipment and supplies for the individual
8. Provision for comfort measures and supportive care to the individual
9. Environmental monitoring and safety
   a. Temperature range
   b. Humidity range
   c. Electrical safety measures
   d. Physical safety measures
   e. Noise control
   f. Traffic control
   g. Control of contaminants
10. Psychological and physiological monitoring of the individual
11. Evaluation of outcomes in relation to identified nursing activities
12. Communication of intraoperative information to significant others and members of the health care team

Communication of the nursing care plan to the patient, family, significant others, and appropriate health personnel is essential to the successful implementation of the plan. Communication with other health personnel may occur in team conferences, change of shift report, individual communication with the staff assigned to participate in the patient's care, or in written nursing care plans that are available to appropriate staff members (Figs. 5–6, 5–7).

Additional resources that can be used to plan patient care are models of patient care (standard care plans) and surgeon preference cards.

Models of Patient Care (Standard Care Plans)

Models of patient care are defined as a nursing care plan written in advance for groups of patients who have common predictable problems as a result of their diagnosis or condition. The components of model care plans are the same as those of the individual care plan:

- Nursing diagnosis
- Expected outcomes
- Nursing orders
- Schedule for assessing outcomes

Four methods may be used in developing models of patient care for the surgical patient. They are:

UCSF
The Medical Center
at the University of California, San Francisco
San Francisco, California 94143

Address 001 FIRST AVE. S.F.	UNIT NUMBER
Phone 555-1111 Age 70 Sex F Marital Status S Primary Language ENGLISH	PT. NAME
Religion NA Occupation RETIRED	BIRTHDATE
Accompanied By (Name) SELF Relationship	
Waiting Location	LOCATION DATE
Emergency Contact (If Patient Alone) MRS. M. — SISTER Phone 555-1111	Mode of Admission
Person Taking Patient Home MR B. Location SF	Phone 555-1111 Travel Time 15 MIN
Medical Diagnosis CERVICAL CIS.	Intended Surgery CONE BIOPSY

PREOP CHECKLIST

✓ Lab Work
✓ CXR
✓ EKG
✓ Consent for Operation   B
✓ History & Physical
✓ ID Band Checked
✓ Old Chart Available
NA Parent ID Band

NPO Since 0800 → 1 CUP BLACK COFFEE
Allergies NKDA
Last Voided 1330
Dentures/Bridge PARTIAL UPPER
Disposition IN CUP Ξ BELONGINGS
Contacts/Eyeglasses
Disposition IN CASE Ξ BELONGINGS
Other Prostheses ⊘
Disposition

Patient Belongings (eg. garment bag, suitcase, purse, toys, etc)

Items BLUE CLOTHING BAG   Labeled ✓
Valuables Locked ✓   If yes, Receipt # ③
Checklist Completed by B

Nursing Assessment

Temp 37² Pulse 68 Resp. 16 B/P 120/70 Weight 157 LB. | Preop Medications
Current Medications MVI, NAPROSYN, DIAZIDE — TAKEN THIS AM
Previous Medical Illness/Surgery: BACK SURGERY - LUMBAR
1982 & 1988, HEPATITIS A X25YR AGO   IV - #20 ANGIOCATH ⓇHAND
                                    lower   L.R. TKVO BY B
Physical/Sensory Deficits: ARTHRITIS - BACK & HIPS
Mental/Emotional Status ALERT, ANXIOUS

Growth & Development (Pedi) NA
Pt./Family Understanding & Expectations of Surgery PT STATES UNDERSTANDING OF PROCEDURE
Teaching/Learning Needs REINFORCE POST-OP CARE

NURSING CARE PLAN

Nursing Diagnosis	Expected Outcome	Nursing Actions	Post-op Evaluation
① PT UNABLE TO VERBALIZE POST-OP INSTRUCTIONS	PT WILL VERBALIZE POST-OP INSTRUCTIONS	REINFORCE THERE WILL BE ORAL & WRITTEN INSTRUCTIONS POST-OP	No Untoward events
② SEE STANDARD OF CARE FOR PT IN LITHOTOMY POSITION			

B Cuthbertson CB N RN   N. Burns RN ___ RN
11-15-89 Date of Assessment   11/17/89 Date of Evaluation

6/88
685-24

MEDICAL RECORDS COPY

Figure 5-6. Operating room/PAR preoperative assessment - care plan.

PROCEDURE PERFORMED

CONE BIOPSY

Date
11-15-89

POSITION

Supine _____ Prone _____ Lateral (L/R) _____
Lithotomy ✓ Sitting _____ Kraske _____
Positioning Note: FEET IN FOAM BOOTIES
ARMS PADDED ON ARM BOARDS

PREP

Shaved by ~~B~~
Iodine 1% _____ Iodophor Scrub ✓ Solution ✓
Alcohol 70% _____
Other LUGOLS SOLN VAG. PREP

ELECTROSURGICAL UNIT

Ground Site _____
Model _____ Control# _____

TEMPERATURE CONTROL

Model _____ Control# _____
Pt. Temperature Monitored Yes ___ No ___
High _____ Low _____ Postop _____

TOURNIQUET #1	**TOURNIQUET #2**
Location	Location
Pressure	Pressure
Time	Time

URINARY CATHETER

Straight Cath #14 R.R.
Indwelling _____
By ~~B~~
Total Urine Output 100 CC

IMPLANTS (LOT #/SERIAL #)

MEDICATIONS

SPECIMENS

Microbiology Yes ___ No _____ Number _____
Pathology Yes ✓ No _____ Number ③
Other (Describe) _____

DRAINS/PACKS (Type & Location)

EBL 30 CC

DRESSINGS

PERI PAD

PAR Bed # To PAR I VIA GURNEY

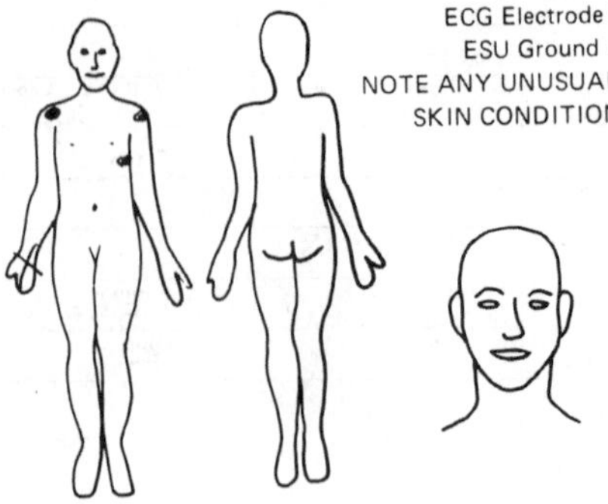

ECG Electrode ●
ESU Ground ■
NOTE ANY UNUSUAL
SKIN CONDITION

PRE-, INTRA- AND POSTOP NOTES

TO OR I VIA GURNEY. TRANSFERRED
TO OR TABLE 5 ASSISTANCE.

POST OP- TRANSFERRED TO GURNEY
C ROLLER
ADMITTED TO PAR I - PERI PAD DRY

RN Signature B Culbertson (B) RN

Pre-Operative Nursing Instructions and Information
given to patient.

on _____ time _____

RN Signature _____

Discharge Information (For patients not admitted to PAR)
MD Order Written _____
Medications _____

Instructions Reviewed/Teaching _____

Wound/Dressing Condition _____

Condition at Discharge _____

Mode of Transportation _____
Name of Escort _____
RN Signature _____

Figure 5-6. Continued.

UCSF
The Medical Center
at the University of California, San Francisco

UNIT NUMBER	75-5654-2
PT. NAME	John Fulton
BIRTHDATE	8/23/57

MEDICAL DIAGNOSIS: Ulcerative Colitis

INTENDED SURGERY: Total Colectomy Ileoanal Anastomosis   **LOCATION** 9L   **DATE** 12/7/89

MEDICAL HISTORY: (INCLUDE PREVIOUS SURGERY)
5 yr. history of abdominal pain, diarrhea, and rectal bleeding.

Fx left humerus (open reduction) 1987

PERTINENT LAB DATA OR PREOPERATIVE DIAGNOSTIC STUDIES:
WNL
Hct 41.0

ALLERGIES: (FOOD, DRUGS, OTHERS)
none

MEDICATIONS: (INCLUDE UNUSUAL DOSES)
Prednisone
Sulfazalamine

SOCIAL HISTORY

AGE 26   SEX ♂   MARITAL STATUS M   RELIGION P   OCCUPATION CPA

LANGUAGE SPOKEN/UNDERSTOOD (INCLUDE NEED FOR TRANSLATOR): English
FAMILY/OTHERS (ESPECIALLY THOSE WHO WILL BE AT HOSPITAL): Wife will wait on 9L.

PHYSICAL ASSESSMENT: (REFER TO "ASSESSMENT FACTOR")
T- 36.5 P- 80 R- 20 B/P- 117/74 HT- 5'10" WT- 165 lbs.
Slight Cushingoid appearance
Decreased R.O.M. left arm.

TEACHING/LEARNING NEEDS
Routine preop teaching done.
Needs: Postop Ileostomy care

MENTAL/EMOTIONAL ASSESSMENT Pleasant, A+O X3, Extremely anxious about entering O.R. awake. Good verbalization of anxieties.

PATIENT'S/FAMILIES UNDERSTANDING/EXPECTATIONS OF SURGERY Pt and wife verbalize understanding of surgery; Optimistic

MODEL OF CARE IMPLEMENTED:
① Pt undergoing General Anesthesia
② Colectomy and Ileoanal

SPECIAL PREPARATION OR TRANSPORTATION
none

INTRAOPERATIVE NURSING CARE PLAN

NURSING DIAGNOSIS	EXPECTED OUTCOME	NURSING ACTIONS	POST-OP EVALUATION
Potential Inability to cope related to fear of being awake in O.R.	Pt will be able to verbalize fears + remaining fear will be minimized	- Speak c Anesth. about preop med. and/or starting induction in preop holding area. - Stay c pt + use touch for reassurance preop	- Appreciates my support preop. Does not remember entering OR. - Feels no pain or discomfort in Lt arm.
Potential pain postop related to improper positioning of injured left arm	- No pain or discomfort in arm in PACU or postop. - Pt will verbalize comfort pre + postop	- Have pt demonstrate comfortable position preop + duplicate position when he's asleep. - Have extra padding available.	- Recovering well - Pt and wife verbalizing optimistic outlook!

Deborah Wagman, R.N.   12/7/89 Date of Assessment

Deborah Wagman, R.N.   12/9/89 Date of Evaluation

Figure 5-7. Operating room/PAR preoperative assessment - care plan.

INTRAOPERATIVE RECORD OF NURSING CARE

PROCEDURES PERFORMED   Total Colectomy, Ileoanal Anastomosis   DATE 12/8/89

POSITION: PRONE   FLANK (L/R)   KRASKE   SITTING   AXILLARY ROLL   SUPINE   LATERAL (L/R)   LOW LITHOTOMY (circled)   *Allen stirrups*   EQUIPMENT USED   OTHER:

PREP: ☑ 1% IODINE   ☐ BETADINE (SCRUB-SOLUTION)   ☐ PREPODYNE (SCRUB-SOLUTION)   ☐ GEL-PREP   ☐ OTHER: SHAVE PREP: BR

ESU GROUND: ☐ BUTTOCK (L-R) ×2   ☑ THIGH OR ANT-POST-MED (LAT circled)   ☐ SHOULDER (L-R)   OTHER: TYPE UNIT CSV II & SERIAL # L-1923 R-1744

TEMP CONTROL UNIT & SERIAL # 2352 Blanketrol   UNIT TEMP. HI 37° LO____   PT. TEMP. HI____ LO____

TOURNIQUET PRESSURE N/A   LOCATION____   TIME____

CROSSCLAMP N/A   VESSEL____   ISCHEMIA TIME____

MEDICATIONS (OTHER THAN THOSE GIVEN BY ANESTHESIA)   TIME 1130   DRUG Epinephrine   DOSE 1:300,000 10 cc   ROUTE Local Infiltration rectum

IMPLANTS/PROSTHETICS: (INDICATE LOT/SERIAL NO.)   N/A

TRANSC O₂ MONITOR
ECG ELECTRODES . . . . ●
ELECTROSURGERY PLATE . . ■
PERIPERAL IV X
ARTERIAL LINE . . . . O
CVP/PAP . . . . Z
LACERATIONS . . . . /
BRUISES . . . . B
gelpads . . . . □

ADDITIONAL PRE-OP INFORMATION (E.G. LOC, DISPOSITION OF PROSTHETICS, EMOTIONAL STATUS)
Drowsy + calm from medication on arrival to O.R. 19
Lt. arm positioned on armboard + padded. Pt. verbalized comfort.
Sequential Compression Stockings applied @ 45mm.

STATUS OF SKIN POSTOP Warm, dry, intact

ADDITIONAL POST-OP INFORMATION. (COMMUNICATIONS TO POST-OP UNIT: [INCL. PRESSURE LINES: VENTILATOR-TYPE, TV, RATE & PT. WEIGHT]; HYPOTHERMIA, ETC.)
PAR BED # 19
- Loop Ileostomy draining into appliance
- Sump drains to intermittent suction
- Epidural cath. in place: Morphine drip in PACU

DISCHARGED VIA GUERNEY, BED, CRIB
OTHER____ TO PACU
ACCOMPANIED BY D. Smith, S.W.

SIGNATURE   Deborah Wagman,   R.N.

URINE OUTPUT (Kind and Amount) 650cc   Clear, yellow
CATHED BY DW   16 Foley (5cc)
EBL/DRAINAGE (Kind and Amount) 800 cc

SPECIMEN TO PATHOLOGY:	YES ☑	NO	NUMBER 3	SPECIMEN TO BACTERIOLOGY	YES	NO ☑	NUMBER

CATH-ETERS/ DRAINS/ PACKS	TYPE	LOCATION
	PENROSE DRAIN	
	R.R. CATHETER	
	SALEM SUMP	1X N.G.
	LATEX MUSHROOM	
	CHEST TUBE	
	HEMOVAC	
	JERGUNSON	
	PACKS (PLAIN, IODOFORM, VASELINE, VAGINAL, OTHER)	
	OTHER	Sump ×2 — Stab wound LLQ

Figure 5-7. Continued.

1. Surgical procedure (i.e., total hip replacement, kidney transplant, abdominal hysterectomy) (Table 5–7)
2. Position of the patient intraoperatively (i.e., lithotomy, lateral, prone) (Table 5–8)
3. Age of patient (Table 5–9)
4. Type of anesthesia (Table 5–10)

The third model, age of the patient, is based on the patient's age and any attendant physiological and psychological needs relevant to planning surgical intervention. By combining the appropriate models of patient care, routine nursing care is determined and a foundation for nursing activities is established. A notation should be made on the patient's chart identifying the models of patient care that were implemented.

Surgeon Preference Cards
Another valuable tool in planning for surgical procedures is the surgeon preference card. This card lists specific requests and preferences for each surgical procedure by each surgeon. The card identifies type of skin preparation, position, method of draping, special supplies, instruments, sutures, and dressing required for a given surgical procedure (Table 5–11). Each card is routinely revised to reflect changes in the surgeon's requests and preferences.

Implementation of the Plan
Implementation of the patient care plan begins when the patient is transported to the operating room and is completed when the patient is transported to the recovery room. The focus of this phase is implementing the nursing orders with consideration of the individual's dignity and desires.

Determination as to who performs the nursing activities depends upon the patient's needs and condition; the complexity of the surgical procedure; and the knowledge, skill, and expertise of the available nursing team members.

Using the plan of care as a guide, the perioperative nurse may supervise others in carrying out the plan or implement the prescribed nursing actions by providing direct care. As a patient advocate, the nurse maintains an awareness of the immediate and long-term implications of the nursing actions being performed. If necessary, the nurse revises the plan to accommodate changes in either the patient's psychological or physiological condition.

The implementation phase is concluded when all the identified nursing actions have been carried out and are documented on the patient's chart.

Evaluation of the Plan
Evaluation of patient care may occur in the recovery room, on the unit, in the clinic, the physician's office, or in the patient's home. Performing the evaluation in areas other than the recovery room allows participation and feedback from the patient, the family, and significant others.

The goals of the postoperative evaluation are to:

1. Assess the quality of care delivered by determining if the nursing activities assisted in solving the identified nursing diagnoses

TABLE 5-7. MODEL OF PATIENT CARE FOR: ABDOMINAL HYSTERECTOMY

Nursing Diagnosis	Expected Outcome	Nursing Orders/Actions	Schedule for Assessment

1. Potential anxiety related to unfamiliar environment and/or impending surgery	1a. Ability to cope with anxiety
	b. Verbalizes basic understanding of surgical procedure
	c. Understand preoperative and postoperative activities
		1a. Assess patient's perception of surgical procedure—note degree of anxiety, denial, depression
		b. Assess support systems
		c. Explain events of day of surgery with rationale
		   1. *Preoperative:* n.p.o., premedication, time of transportation to OR, time of surgery, holding area, shave-prep, OR environment (i.e., lights, equipment), anticipated length of surgery
		   2. *Postoperative:* Recovery room location and activities, anticipated length of stay, pain, pain medication, Foley catheter, dressings, vaginal drainage of blood
		d. Encourage patient to verbalize concerns and questions
		e. Communicate to surgeon any unresolved concerns or questions the patient may have
			Preoperatively
			
			24–48 hours postoperatively

2. Potential musculoskeletal discomfort, nerve damage, or circulatory and respiratory compromise related to improper positioning	2a. No musculoskeletal discomfort b. No nerve damage c. No compromise in circulation or respirations d. Skin integrity maintained	2a. Place safety strap above knees, over blanket b. Pad all boney prominences c. Align extremities anatomically d. Instruct Hospital Assistant to have shoulder braces padded and available e. Provide anesthesiologist with free access to airway and IV lines f. When position of OR table is adjusted, check toes and feet for pressure areas	24–48 hours postoperatively
3. Possible unwarranted anxiety about sexual appeal or activity related to misinformation or superstitions regarding hysterectomy	3. Misinformation and superstitions replaced with accurate information	3a. Provide support and information regarding sexual concerns b. Dispel superstitions and myths about outcome c. Encourage patient to verbalize concerns d. Alert surgeon and other team members to patient's concerns	Preoperatively
4. Potential loss of dignity related to excessive exposure	4. Dignity maintained	4a. Limit exposure of patient only to area needed for surgical procedure	Intraoperatively
5. Potential damage to skin related to pooling of antiseptic solution under the patient	5. No skin damage	5a. When prepping the patient, place towels along patient's trunk to absorb excess solution b. Remove towels when prep is complete	Recovery Room, 24–48 hours postoperatively

(continued)

119

TABLE 5-7. CONTINUED

Nursing Diagnosis	Expected Outcome	Nursing Order/Actions	Schedule for Assessment
6. Potential urinary tract infection related to insertion of Foley catheter	6. No urinary tract infection	6a. Follow procedure for insertion of Foley catheter b. Connect to straight drainage c. At all times, keep urinary drainage bag below level of patient's bladder	24–48 hours postoperatively
7. Potential skin damage related to improper placement of electrosurgical ground plate	7. Skin integrity maintained Absence of: Burns Bruises Blisters Redness	7a. Cover plate evenly with conductive substance b. Place plate as close as possible to incision site c. Check connection of inactive cord to plate and electrosurgical unit d. Set controls to appropriate setting	Recovery Room, 24–48 hours postoperatively
8. Potential foreign body left in patient related to surgical incision	8. Absence of foreign body	8. Instruments, sponges, and needles counted according to procedure	Intraoperatively
9. Potential wound infection related to contamination during intraoperative period	9. Wound free of infection Absence of: Edema Redness Tenderness Heat Pain Exudate	9a. Ensure compliance with principles of asepsis b. Report noncompliance with principles of asepsis on appropriate form	24–48 hours postoperatively

120

Nursing Diagnosis	Expected Outcome	Nursing Interventions	Timing
10. Potential fluid imbalance related to n.p.o. and loss of body fluids	10. Body fluids maintained within normal limits	10a. Monitor urine output b. Estimate blood loss on sponges and in suction c. Communicate to anesthetist d. Check on blood availability	Intraoperatively 24–48 hours postoperatively
11. Potential decrease in body temperature related to surgical exposure	11. Normal body temperature maintained	11a. Limit exposure of patient to area required for surgical procedure b. Place thermal blanket on OR table c. Provide anesthesiologist with blood/fluid warmer as needed d. Place warm blanket on patient at end of procedure	Recovery room
12. Anxiety of significant others related to lack of communication regarding patient's progress	12. Reduce anxiety and/or able to cope with anxiety	12a. Inform patient's significant others when surgery has started b. Inform of any unusual delay c. Inform when patient goes to recovery room	Postoperatively

TABLE 5-8. MODEL OF PATIENT CARE FOR: LITHOTOMY POSITION

Nursing Diagnosis	Expected Outcome	Nursing Orders/Actions	Schedule for Assessment
1. Potential contamination of surgical site related to shedding of epidermis from feet	1a. Shedding of epidermis contained b. No symptoms of wound	1. Place cotton or flannel boots over patient's feet	24–48 hours postoperatively
2. Potential peripheral vascular compromise related to improper positioning of legs	2. No symptoms of peripheral vascular compromise	2a. Apply antiembolectomy stockings as needed b. Position stirrups to prevent excessive pressure on popliteal space	24–48 hours postoperatively
3. Potential musculoskeletal discomfort and/or hip dislocation related to improper position of legs	3a. No musculoskeletal discomfort b. No dislocation of hips	3a. Use two people when positioning legs in stirrups to facilitate simultaneous placement b. Check sacrum and pad with foam if appropriate c. Use two people to remove legs from stirrups	24–48 hours postoperatively
4. Potential nerve damage related to improper positioning of legs or pressure of instruments	4. No nerve damage	4a. Check pressure areas and pad if appropriate b. Position stirrups properly c. Position footboard at right	24–48 hours postoperatively

122

Nursing diagnosis	Goal	Nursing interventions	Time frame
		angle to OR table to serve as work surface for surgeon as needed	
		d. Remind surgeon that instruments should not be placed on the patient	
5. Potential damage to digits when lowering foot of OR table	5. Digits intact	5a. Place arms or armboards positioned parallel to the table when allowed by surgical procedure	Recovery room
		b. Before lowering end of table check location of digits	
6. Potential loss of dignity related to excessive exposure	6. Dignity maintained	6a. Pull shades on doors	Intraoperatively
7. Potential damage to skin related to pooling of antiseptic solution under the patient	7. No skin damage	7a. Place "prep" pad under buttocks prior to prepping	Intraoperatively
		b. Remove "prep" pad when prep is complete and check for wet linen	24–48 hours postoperatively
8. Potential circulatory compromise related to pooling of blood in lumbar region	8. Signs and symptoms of circulatory compromise prevented or controlled	8a. Raise and lower legs slowly with anesthesiologist's knowledge	Intraoperatively

TABLE 5-9. MODEL OF PATIENT CARE FOR 2- TO 3-YEAR-OLD

Nursing Diagnosis	Expected Outcome	Nursing Orders/Actions	Schedule for Assessment
1. Potential anxiety related to fear of separation	1. Minimal anxiety	1a. Request that parents accompany child to the OR b. Encourage child to bring familiar object to the OR (i.e., toy, blanket) c. Communicate level of anxiety to recovery room	Preoperatively
2. Potential fear of being transported in crib	2. Transported to operating room without fear	2a. Allow parents to carry patient b. Instruct hospital assistant to use wagon to transport child	Immediately preoperative
3. Inability to express fears	3. Express fears	3a. Allow child to express feelings (i.e., crying, anger) b. Use terminology and examples child can understand c. Organize activities to be able to stay with patient prior to induction d. Request additional circulator if needed	Preoperatively Postoperatively 24 hours
4. Potential fear of being immobilized related to restraints being applied	4. No feelings of immobility	4a. Hold or touch patient b. Speak softly c. Apply restraints after patient is anesthetized	Intraoperatively
5. Potential loss of dignity related to clothes being removed	5. Preserve dignity	5a. Remove clothes after patient is anesthetized b. Reapply clothes prior to patient going to recovery room	Intraoperatively

6. Potential alteration in body temperature	6. Body temperature maintained within normal limits	6a. Turn temperature of room up to 70° 30 minutes prior to bringing patient into room b. Instruct hospital assistant to place K-Pad on OR bed	Preoperatively
		c. Insert temperature probe and connect to monitor d. Warm solutions for prepping	Intraoperatively
		e. Place warm blankets on child	Postoperatively
		f. Know procedure for malignant hyperpyrexia	Intraoperatively
7. Potential skin burn related to use of electrosurgical unit	7. Integrity of skin maintained: No burns No blisters No redness	7a. Use proper size ground plate b. Cover plate evenly with conductive substance c. Place plate as close as possible to incision site d. Check connections of inactive cord to plate and electrosurgical unit e. Set controls on appropriate setting	Intraoperatively
8. Patient size	8. No delay in surgical procedure	8a. Instruct hospital assistant on appropriate selection of instruments consistent with size of child b. Select supplies consistent with size of child	Preoperatively
9. Potential impaired circulation related to use of restraints	9. Circulation monitored	9a. Wrap arms and legs with Webril prior to applying restraints b. Check circulation in extremities every 30 minutes during procedure	Intraoperatively

(continued)

125

TABLE 5-9. CONTINUED

Nursing Diagnosis	Expected Outcome	Nursing Orders/Actions	Schedule for Assessment
10. Potential imbalance of fluid volume related to n.p.o. and loss of body fluids	10. Body fluids maintained within normal limits	10a. Instruct hospital assistant to obtain sponge scale when setting up OR b. Weigh sponges for blood loss; communicate to anesthetist as they are handed off the field c. Use pediatric suction container d. Monitor amount of irrigating solution used e. Provide 1000 cc bag with Buretrol and minidrip administration set	Preoperatively Intraoperatively
11. Potential musculoskeletal discomfort, nerve damage, or circulatory and respiratory compromise related to improper positioning	11a. No musculoskeletal discomfort b. No nerve damage c. No compromise in circulation or respirations d. Skin integrity maintained	11a. Place safety strap above knees b. Pad all boney prominences c. Align extremities anatomically and support if necessary d. Provide anesthesia with free access to airway and IV lines	24-48 hours Postoperatively

126

12. Anxiety of parents related to separation from the child, unknown diagnosis, or surgical treatment	12a. Ability to verbalize feelings of depression, helplessness, fear, anger b. Ability to verbalize realistic understanding of proposed surgery and activities of day of surgery c. Ability to cope with anxiety	12a. Encourage parents to verbalize concerns and to ask questions b. Assess level of knowledge regarding surgical procedure c. Give clear, succinct information appropriate to the parent's level of education d. Reinforce surgeon's explanation of surgical procedure e. Explain sequence of events on day of surgery (i.e., n.p.o., transportation to OR, recovery room location and length of stay, anticipated catheters, tubes, drains, casts, or dressings) f. Inform parents of waiting area g. Communicate with parents at time of incision and upon completion of surgical intervention h. Explain child's reaction to impending surgical intervention i. Communicate to surgeon any unresolved concerns or questions parents may have	Preoperatively Intraoperatively Preoperatively Preoperatively Postoperatively

TABLE 5–10. OPERATING ROOM MODEL OF PATIENT CARE FOR: LOCAL INFILTRATION

Nursing Diagnosis	Expected Outcome	Nursing Actions	Time Frame for Assessment
1. Potential anxiety related to unfamiliar environment and/or impending surgery	1. Ability to cope with anxiety	1a. Explain preoperative and intraoperative activities b. Encourage patient to verbalize questions and concerns c. Stay with patient and provide non-verbal support d. Provide non-verbal support by touching patient	Preoperatively Intraoperatively 12–24 hours postoperatively
2. Potential fear of pain	2. Pain controlled	2a. Encourage patient to verbalize discomfort b. Discuss with patient availability of pain medication	Intraoperatively
3. Potential altered sensory perceptions related to preoperative medication	3. Able to respond appropriately and to follow directions	3a. Maintain quiet atmosphere b. Post sign on door "Patient Awake" c. Turn off auditory intercom	Intraoperatively 12–24 hours postoperatively
4. Potential loss of dignity related to excessive exposure and lack of personal care	4. Dignity maintained	4a. Limit exposure of patient only to area required for surgical procedure b. Call patient by name c. Only pertinent team members permitted in room	Intraoperatively 12–24 hours postoperatively
5. Possible discomfort related to position	5. Comfortable position	5a. Position patient anatomically b. Flex table slightly at knees to reduce strain on back muscles c. Place pillow under knees d. Pad all bony prominences e. Pad wrists with webril prior to restraints being applied	Intraoperatively 12–24 postoperatively

Problem	Expected Outcome	Nursing Intervention	Timing
		f. Ask patient about position	
6. Potential contamination of wound related to patient inadvertently touching wound	6. No wound contamination	6. Apply padded clover leaf hitch arm restraints	Intraoperatively
7. Potential alteration in body temperature related to temperature of operating room	7. Body temperature maintained within normal limits	7a. Apply warm blankets b. Use warm solutions c. Limit skin exposure to area required for surgical procedure d. Ask patient about body temperature	Intraoperatively
8. Possible adverse reaction to local anesthetic agent	8. Avoid or minimize cardiovascular and respiratory compromise	8a. Two nurses assigned to circulate b. Check chart for allergies c. Obtain baseline vital signs before surgery d. Use electrocardiograph to monitor patient for cardiac arrhythmias e. Monitor and record vital signs as indicated or at least: every 15 minutes before and after medication f. Communicate changes to surgeon	Intraoperatively
9. Potential lack in continuity of care related to patient returning to primary care nurse/inpatient unit	9. Continuity of care maintained	9a. Inform primary care nurse what procedure was performed b. Vital signs c. All medications administered d. Amount of intravenous fluids infused e. Estimated blood loss f. Location of any drains or packs	Immediate postoperative and 12–24 hours postoperative

(continued)

TABLE 5-10. CONTINUED

Nursing Diagnosis	Expected Outcome	Nursing Actions	Time Frame for Assessment
		g. Type of dressing h. How the patient tolerated the procedure	
Ambulatory Patients Only 10. Potential latent adverse reaction or side effects to local anesthesia or surgical procedure	10. Adverse reaction or side effects treated appropriately	10a. Observe patient for minimum of 30 minutes postoperatively prior to discharge b. Alert patient and significant others to signs and symptoms of adverse reaction and how to respond appropriately c. Validate postoperative instructions by requesting verbal feedback d. Give patient and significant others telephone number of operating room surgeon and emergency room. Instruct patient to call regarding any questions or concerns e. Obtain telephone number where patient can be reached for postoperative phone call in 24 hours	Immediate postoperative 24 hours postoperative

TABLE 5-11. SURGEON PREFERENCE CARD

Surgeon: Dr. C. Rocky
Procedure: Abdominoperineal Resection
Skin prep: 1% Iodine
Suture and needles:
Ties: 2-0, 3-0, 4-0, 18″ Silk & Dexon
    2-0, 3-0, 4-0, Silk (D-Tach)
    2-0 Silk 30″
    2-0 Dexon 27″
Pelvic floor: 0 Chromic (T-12)
Colostomy: 4-0 Dexon (CE-4) × 4
Peritoneum: #1 Chromic (T-12)
Fascia: #1 Dexon—Large Mayos
Subcutaneous: 4-0 Dexon (CE-4)
Skin: Stapler or Steristrips
Anus:' #2 Ticron—Retention
Perineum: 0 Dexon—Large Mayo
        4-0 Dexon (CE-4)

Glove size: 8
Patient position: Supine then lithotomy
Drapes: Towels, towel clips
    Lap sheet
    Half sheet
    Perineal sheet
Instruments:
    Basic instrument set
    Major retractor pan
    GI specials
    Israels × 2
    Wertheim clamps × 4
    Peans × 6
    Straight Jones clamps × 4

Supplies:
    Hernia tape × 3
    Wound protector
    Magnetic mat
    Catheter plugs × 2

Drains: Abramson sump × 1
    Penrose drains $\frac{1}{2}$″ × 6

Dressings:
    Telfa, 4× 4s, Benzoin, paper tape, Colostomy Bag, Fluffs, Male patient: Fuller Shield.
    Female patient: T-Binder.

2. Reassess the patient goals that remain unresolved by evaluating the nursing diagnoses, patient's goals, and nursing orders
3. Assess the patient's current status
4. Provide feedback to the patient, family, and significant others regarding goal achievement
5. Address any concern or questions the patient, family, or significant others may have

    In conducting the postoperative evaluation, the nurse examines the patient's record for signs and symptoms; observes the patient; and interviews the primary care nurse, the patient, family and significant others to measure the results of nursing practice. Through direct questioning, the nurse will gain information about his or her nursing practice and the level of goal achievement.

    If patient goals were not achieved, the nurse must question the reason for the lack of attainment. "Were the data collected complete?" "Were the nursing diagnoses appropriate?" "Were the goals realistic?" "Were the appropriate resources available?" The plan must then be revised in collaboration with other health personnel, the patient, family, and significant others. Following the postoperative evaluation, the nurse documents on the patient's chart or care plan the level of goal achievement and any new nursing diagnoses, patient goals, and nursing orders.

Reassessment of the Nursing Process

Reassessment occurs continuously throughout the nursing process (Fig. 5–8). Using scientific knowledge, interpersonal skills, research and past experience, the nurse continuously monitors the patient's response to nursing activities. He or she is alert to changes in the psychological and physiological status of the patient that may require identifying new problems, resetting goals, and modifying the care plan.

As a final step in implementing the perioperative role, the nurse uses introspection to judge the level of his or her practice. By asking the question, "What could I have done to provide more effective and efficient patient care?," the professional perioperative nurse will fulfill his or her commitment to the delivery of individual quality patient care and will be a patient advocate.

Documentation of the Perioperative Role

Documentation of perioperative nursing care is essential to ensure continuity of care and to validate the nursing care rendered. The documentation should include information regarding the status of the patient, what the nurse did for the patient, and the patient's response to that care.

Documentation of the care from the preoperative through the intraoperative and into the postoperative period promotes continuity of care and enhances communications by providing other team members with information about the patient during the perioperative period.

Written records demonstrate responsibility and accountability for nursing practice by identification of the patient's problems and recording the nursing activities implemented and observations of the patient's response. The record provides a comparison of formulated patient objectives to the degree of goal attainment.

Documentation provides a comprehensive method of retrieving information in the event of legal action and for measuring the quality of care delivered in quality assurance programs. In addition, the documentation of perioperative nursing functions provides a data base for research on the perioperative role.

Recording of perioperative nursing care varies from institution to institution and from inpatient to outpatient facilities. Recording may be done on the nurse's notes, the progress notes, or a special form designed to encompass the perioperative role. Documentation forms for ambulatory surgery patients will consist primarily of a checklist that encompasses the preoperative, intraoperative, and postoperative phases of the surgical experience (Figs. 5–6 and 5–7).

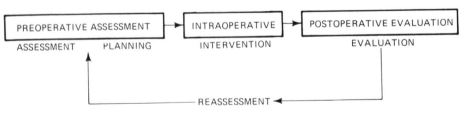

Figure 5-8. Operating room nursing process.

In the traditional narrative, referred to as source-oriented charting, entries are made on the nurse's notes in chronological order. An example of this format is

4/22/81   10AM   Mr. Brown admitted to OR from holding area. Anesthetized on stretcher, turned and transferred to OR table, and placed in prone position. Body rolls placed longitudinally from acromioclavicular joint to the iliac crest. Arms extended upward on arm boards. Pillow placed under feet. Safety strap placed 2 inches above knees. Ground plate for electrosurgical unit 212 placed on left buttock. Skin prepped and painted with iodophor solution.   J. Coleman RN

If the institution uses problem-oriented medical records (POMR), the nurse will document data on the nurse's notes or on the progress notes. Essential to POMR charting is a list of patient problems. Each problem is defined, labeled, and numbered. Narrative notes are recorded in relation to each numbered and titled problem. New problems are numbered and titled and added to the problem list as they are identified by any member of the health care team. An example of POMR charting is

4/22/81   10 AM   #3 Painful right shoulder—instruct transport team to provide adequate support for right shoulder and arm during transportation to operating room. Provide additional support and padding when positioning for surgical procedure. Notify anesthesia and recovery room of positioning requirements.   J. Coleman RN

#6   Shortness of breath—more pronounced when patient is lying flat. Keep head of bed elevated. Notify transport team and recovery room.   J. Coleman RN

The concept of POMR has evolved into the SOAP or SOAPIE models. This six-part model consists of:

1. Subjective data, which involve the health status of the patient and how he or she views it and feels about it
2. Objective data, which include the physical and laboratory findings as well as observations of the patient
3. Assessment, which comprises the formulation of a nursing diagnosis/patient problem, contains a statement of the desired patient outcome, and evaluation criteria to assess degree of goal attainment
4. The Plan, which defines the activities necessary to assist the patient to achieve the desired goal
5. Implementation, which defines how the nursing actions were carried out and by whom
6. The Evaluation statement, which contains the patient's degree of goal attainment as a result of the nursing actions

The SOAPIE system may be written on the nurse's notes or on the progress notes. In some institutions, the nurse's orders are written on a combined physician/nurse's order sheet. An example of the SOAPIE format is

4/22/80 1 PM
S—"I had a stroke last year."

O—Right-sided weakness. Difficulty in moving right arm and leg. Altered sensory perception on right side.

A—Altered sensation on right side to touch and pain. Altered mobility due to left CVA. Safely transported to OR and positioned for surgery by adequate personnel to assist in transfer and positioning; extremities on right side positioned in proper alignment with boney prominences padded. No further nerve damage or areas of ischemia will occur.

P—Obtain additional personnel to assist in transfer from bed to OR stretcher and from Or stretcher to OR table. Provide support to right side while transferring. Use foam padding under heels; pad and protect right arm and elbow with towels when positioning. Support right leg in proper alignment with sandbags.

I—Transferred to OR stretcher without difficulty or untoward incidents by transportation team. Lifted onto OR table with extra support to right side. Foam padding positioned under heels. Towels placed under right arm and elbow. Right leg supported with sandbags in proper alignment.

E—No complaints of discomfort during transfer. No evidence of further damage or ischemia. Body alignment maintained.   J. Coleman RN

In all formats, it is essential that the patient's record reflect the preoperative assessment, the planning carried out by the perioperative nurse, the care delivered by members of the surgical team, and the outcome.

The intraoperative documentation should include but not be limited to the following information[10]:

1. Evidence of continuing assessment and planning during the intraoperative phase
2. Identification of persons providing care, name and title of the person responsible for the entry
3. Evidence of a patient assessment upon arrival to the OR including the level of consciousness, emotional status, and baseline physical data
4. Patient's overall skin condition on arrival and discharge from the OR
5. Presence and disposition of sensory aids and prosthetic devices accompanying the patient to surgery; prosthetic devices are defined as artificial substitutes for body parts, such as an arm, leg, eye, dentures, hearing aid, or wig
6. Position, supports and restraints used during the surgical procedure
7. Area of placement for the dispersive electrode pad and identification of electrosurgical unit and settings
8. Areas of placement of temperature control devices and identification of unit and recording of time and temperature
9. Placement of electrocardiographic or other monitoring electrodes
10. Medications administered or dispensed by the registered nurse
11. Placement of drains, catheters, packings and dressings
12. Area of placement of tourniquet cuff, pressure, time, and identification of unit
13. Urinary output and estimated blood loss, as appropriate
14. Implants (type, size, or other identifying information). Implants are tissue or

inert or radioactive material inserted into a body cavity or grafted onto the tissues of the recipient

15. Occurrence and results of surgical item counts
16. Time of discharge and disposition of patient from the OR, including method of transfer and patient status
17. Wound classification

Using the criteria identified in the expected outcome and in the patient's responses to the nursing activities, the patient's record should reflect an ongoing evaluation of perioperative nursing care and the patient responses to nursing interventions.

REFERENCES

1. Schlotfeldt M. *Planning for progress. Nurs Out.* 1973; 21(12):766–769
2. A model for perioperative nursing practice. *AORN* 1985; 41(1):188
3. *Competency Statements In Perioperative Nursing.* Denver, Colo: Assoc Operating Room Nurses. 1986:2
4. Leininger M. *Transcultural Nursing: Concepts, Theories and Practice.* New York: John Wiley; 1978:8
5. Walter P. *Race and Culture Relations.* New York: McGraw-Hill Inc; 1952:17
6. Werner E. *Cross-Cultural Child Development: A View from the Plant Earth.* Monterey, CA: Brooks/Cole Publishing. 1979:345
7. Saunders L. *Cultural Differences and Medical Care: The Case of the Spanish-Speaking People of the Southwest.* New York: Russell Sage Foundation; 1954:248
8. Radatovichy Price M. Nursing diagnosis: Making a concept come alive. *Am J Nurs.* 1980; 80(4):670
9. *Standards of Perioperative Nursing Practice.* Denver, Colo: Assoc Operating Room Nurses; 1981
10. Recommended practices for documentation of perioperative nursing care. *AORN J. 1987;* 45(3):777

PART THREE

Making Surgery
Safe for the Patient

Chapter 6

Evolution of Asepsis and Microbiology Review

HISTORICAL REVIEW OF ASEPSIS

The history of surgical asepsis is as old as civilization. In the book of Leviticus in the Old Testament, Moses identified quarantine regulations and sanitary practices to be used when disposing of wastes, touching unclean objects, and treating leprosy.

The ancient Egyptians used herbs and drugs as antiseptics in embalming bodies. They also used the fumes of burning chemicals to deodorize and disinfect the environment.

Records indicate that surgery was far more advanced in Babylonia than in any other country. The Code of Hammurabi was established about 1800 BC. The Code was a collection of laws set up to identify legal practices in Babylonia. The code also listed the penalties that had to be paid by unsuccessful surgeons. For example, if the patient lost an eye because of faulty surgery, the surgeon's eye was put out.

History reveals that Greek philosophers contributed the concept of the "doctrine of the four humors." The humors were blood, black bile, yellow bile, and phlegm. They believed that any disturbance of these fluids in the body led to disease. In addition, they held the theory that under favorable conditions, animal and vegetable life might arise spontaneously. Aristotle (384 BC) asserted that "sometimes animals are formed in putrefying soil, sometimes in plants and sometimes in the fluids of other animals."[1]

Hippocrates (460–370 BC) recognized the importance of cleansing his hands prior to performing surgery, and he used boiling water for irrigating wounds. He forbade wounds to be moistened with anything except wine unless the wound was on a joint. "Because dryness is more nearly a condition of health, and moisture more nearly an ally to disease. A wound is moist and healthy tissue is dry."[2]

Marcus Terentius Varro (117–26 BC), one of Caesar's physicians, expanded on his germ theory of disease in *Rerum Rusticarum*. He stated, "Small creatures, invisible to the eye, fill the atmosphere, and breathed through the nose cause dangerous diseases."

Ambroise Paré (1517–1590) was among the first physicians to win recognition as a surgeon. He studied and taught new ideas about wounds and wound healing. He proved that tying blood vessels was a better method of stopping hemorrhages than cauterizing with hot oil or hot iron, and he recognized the importance of keeping wounds clean.

In 1546, Fracastorius published *De Contagione* in which he identified the existence of airborne pestilence. He believed that diseases were spread in three ways: direct contact, touching objects touched by an infected individual, and airborne transmission.

Fracastorius's observations were validated in 1683 when Anton van Leeuwenhoek, a Dutch linen draper, developed the microscope. Through the use of the microscope, bacteria could be studied. The question of spontaneous generation of living things once again became a subject for discussion. This theory persisted until Louis Pasteur (1822–1895), a French chemist, settled the question in 1862.

Pasteur disproved the doctrine of spontaneous generation and proved that fermentation, putrefacation, infection, and souring are caused by the growth of microbes. To these microorganisms he gave the name of "germs." These germs, according to Pasteur, were carried by the air and could be destroyed by heat or other means. On April 30, 1878, members of the *Academie de Médecine* heard Pasteur deliver a lecture on the germ theory[3]:

> If I had the honour of being a surgeon, convinced as I am of the dangers caused by the germs of microbes scattered on the surface of every object, particularly in the hospitals, not only would I use absolutely clean instruments, but, after cleansing my hands with the greatest care and putting them quickly through a flame, I would only make use of charpie, bandages, and sponges which had previously been raised to a heat of 130° C to 150°C; I would only employ water which had been heated to a temperature of 110° C to 120° C. All that is easy in practice, and, in that way, I should still have to fear the germs suspended in the atmosphere surrounding the bed of the patient; but observation shows us every day that the number of these germs is almost insignificant compared to that of those which lie scattered on the surface of objects, or in the cleanest ordinary water.

Historically, physicians had attempted to prevent infections associated with a specific disease such as puerperal fever. As early as 1773 Charles Wite of Manchester, England insisted on strict cleanliness and ventilation of the lying-in room (delivery room).

In 1843, Oliver Wendell Holmes of Boston advised his students and obstetricians who had been working in the dissecting room to wash their hands and change their clothes before attending a confinement.

In 1849, Ignaz Semmelweis of Vienna insisted that all students coming from the postmortem or dissecting rooms wash their hands in a solution of chloride of lime before entering the lying-in wards. The result was dramatic; deaths fell from 15% to 3% and then to 1%.[4]

Pasteur's findings that putrefaction was caused by minute organisms carried by the air motivated an English surgeon, Lord Joseph Lister (1827–1912), to identify implications for surgical infections. Lister's theory was that if he could prevent the airborne organisms from gaining access to the wound, infection would be prevented. Lister wrote[2]:

> But when it had been shown by the researchers of Pasteur that the septic property of the atmosphere depended, not upon the oxygen or any gaseous constituent, but on minute organisms suspended in it, which owed their energy to their vitality, it occurred to me that decomposition of the injured part might be avoided without excluding the air, by applying as a dressing some material capable of destroying the life of the floating particles.

Lister was aware that carbolic acid was being used to combat sewage odors, so he decided to experiment with this agent. He used carbolic acid to soak dressings, sponges, and instruments and to spray the environment (Fig. 6–1).

As a result of these experiments the routine nursing preparations for surgery were as follows[4]:

> No. 8 Ward in which the operation was performed was purified two days previously with sulphur fumes. Subsequently, walls and floors washed with 1:20 carbolic lotion and two carbolic sprays were turned on for two hours immediately previous to the operation. The patient was also prepared for the operation by being dieted on milk for two days previous to operation. All instruments were soaked in 1:20 carbolic lotion and warm 1:40 was used throughout for sponges, etc.

These antiseptic techniques earned Sir Joseph Lister the title of "Father of Antiseptic Surgery."

Further advances in asepsis occurred from 1881 to 82 when Robert Koch, a German bacteriologist, and his assistant, Wolffhügel, introduced methods of steam sterilization and thus surgery took the form of a mixed "antiseptic–aseptic technique."[4]

> The surgeon scrubbed up; towels were treated by steam heat; some instruments were boiled; sharp instruments, such as scissors and scalpels, were still soaked for twenty minutes in carbolic; hands, face, and hair went uncovered; antiseptics such as carbolic and mercuric chloride were freely used.

Around 1890, Ludwig Lautenschlagen, a German pharmacologist, working with Ernst von Bergmann and Ernst Schimmelbusch, both German surgeons, introduced an

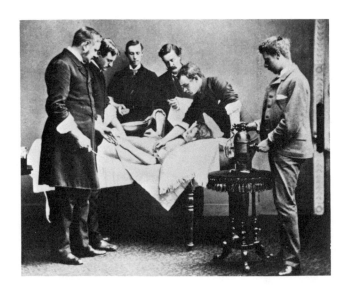

Figure 6-1. Operation during the reign of the Carbolic Spray (1870). The age of gowns, caps, and globes had not dawned. (*The Bettmann Archive.*)

improved apparatus for steam sterilization. This apparatus enabled Bergmann and Schimmelbusch to practice almost pure aseptic technique. This having been achieved, attention was directed at protective coverings for the hands, hair, and face.

A covering for the hands was first suggested by Thomas Watson, a physician in 1843; however, it was not implemented until 1885 when J. von Mikulicz-Radecki wore cotton gloves. The modern "rubber glove" was introduced, but not invented, by William Stewart Halsted of Johns Hopkins Hospital, Baltimore, in 1894.

Halsted also introduced the wearing of caps to cover the hair. Gauze face masks were first worn by either Mikulicz or the French surgeon Paul Berger in 1896 or 1897. Masks did not come into general use for many years, as some surgeons incorrectly believed that silence would be enough to prevent droplet infections. The operating room gown appears to have originated in Italy around the mid-1800s.

Thus, the methods to achieve aseptic technique have evolved since Lister first introduced the use of carbolic acid. However, the basic objective remains unaltered: to prevent infection by eliminating microorganisms.

PRINCIPLES OF BACTERIOLOGY

A basic understanding of bacteriology will aid the perioperative nurse in providing a safe environment where surgical asepsis can be maintained.

Bacteria are single-celled microorganisms that are measured in microns. One bacterium measures 1/25,400 of an inch, 1/1,000 of a millimeter, or 2 microns in length; and 0.5 micron in diameter. Under optimum conditions, bacteria divide on the average of every 20 minutes; therefore, 1 million new cells may be produced in 10 hours from a single bacterium. Disease-producing bacteria are identified as pathogenic.

Bacteria occur in three distinct shapes: cocci, bacilli, and spirilla (Fig. 6–2). Cocci are ball-shaped and are found as a single cell or group of cells. Bacilli are rod-shaped and may occur as a single cell or in chains. Spirilla are corkscrew in shape and always occur as a single cell.

Bacteria are further classified depending upon the reaction of the organism to a gram stain. Distinct physical and chemical differences have been demonstrated between the cell walls of gram-positive and gram-negative bacteria. The cell wall of gram-positive bacteria appears as a single, homogeneous, dense layer, almost twice as thick as

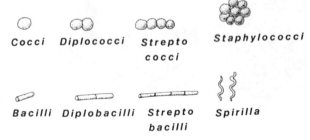

Figure 6–2. Bacteria have three distinct shapes; cocci, bacilli, and spirilla. When they occur in pairs they are called diplococci or diplobacillis. When they form chains, streptococci or streptobacilli. When cocci form irregular clusters, they are called staphylococci.

Cocci   Diplococci   Strepto cocci   Staphylococci

Bacilli   Diplobacilli   Strepto bacilli   Spirilla

the wall of the gram-negative bacteria, whereas the cell wall of the gram-negative organism appears to be composed of several individual layers and is chemically more complex. The reaction of the bacteria to the gram stain has nothing to do with the pathogenicity of the organism, but it is important to the choice of drug therapy.

Bacteria Cell Structure

The cytoplasm of the bacteria cell is surrounded by a thin membrane called the cytoplasmic membrane. The nuclear structures located in the chromatinic area are designated as bacteria chromosomes, nucleoids, and chromatin bodies.

Surrounding the cytoplasmic membrane is the cell wall. The cell wall gives the bacterium its characteristic shape (i.e., cocci, bacilli, spirilla) and like the cytoplasmic membrane is semipermeable (Fig. 6–3).

Many pathogenic bacteria are able to secrete a third layer of material that covers the cell wall and increases the virulence. This layer is known as the capsule or slime layer. The thickness of the capsule varies. In some species of bacteria it can be twice as thick as the cell itself, whereas in others it is hardly detectable. The chemical composition of the capsule is composed of polysaccharides and proteins and sometimes mucinlike material.

The capsule acts as a protective layer that resists the action of certain of the defense mechanisms of the human body such as phagocytosis or the bactericidal activity of body fluids.

The propulsive mechanism of a bacterium is a threadlike appendage called the flagellum. The number of flagella and their position on the bacterium vary with the species. Flagella, however, are not the only means by which bacteria move. Some species

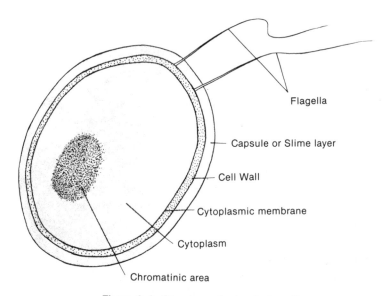

Figure 6-3. Structure of a bacteria cell.

"crawl" over a surface by waves of contraction produced within the protoplasm. Almost all the spiral bacteria and about half the species of bacilli are motile, whereas most cocci are nonmotile.

Bacteria in their active state are known as vegetative. However, there are a few bacteria that have the ability to develop a specialized structure called a spore. When a certain period arrives within the life cycle of these organisms, the vegetative cell disintegrates releasing a highly resistant dehydrated bit of the cell's protoplasm—the spore. A spore is so resistant that it can survive prolonged exposure to drying, heat, chemical disinfectants, and other unfavorable conditions. The protoplasm within a bacterial spore can stay alive for many years. As long as environmental conditions are adverse to the growth of the bacterium, the spore will remain a spore. However, when the proper conditions for growth occur (for example, through introduction of the spore into the human body through a wound), the wall splits, a vegetative cell emerges, and the bacterial cell begins to reproduce. *Clostridium tetani*, which produces tetanus, and *C perfringens*, which results in gas gangrene, are spore-producing bacteria.

FIVE FACTORS THAT FAVOR BACTERIAL GROWTH AND REPRODUCTION

Appropriate Temperature
The optimum temperature for growth and reproduction varies for different bacteria. Thermophilic bacteria function best in 140° to 190° F (60° to 90° C). Mesophilic bacteria find 98.6° F (37° C) optimum, and psychrophilic bacteria function best from 39° to 50° F (4° to 10° C). Most bacteria that are pathogenic to human beings are mesophilic.

Food or Nourishment
Bacteria require nutrients for both protoplasm synthesis and energy.

Proper Moisture
Moisture is important for bacteria to grow and multiply, as water is the means by which dissolved nutrients enter the cells and the wastes leave. The absence of moisture does not, however, necessarily kill microorganisms.

Presence or Absence of Oxygen
Most microorganisms grow best in air containing oxygen. Facultative bacteria can live and reproduce with or without oxygen. Aerobic bacteria must have free oxygen to live, whereas anaerobic organisms can live only in the absence of air.

Appropriate Environmental pH
Most pathogenic bacteria grow best in a neutral pH. However, some will grow and reproduce in an acid pH, and others in a pH as low as 1 or 2.

NORMAL FLORA

Microorganisms that are found inhabiting some areas of the human body are referred to as the normal flora. These organisms do not produce disease unless they are transplanted to an environment in which they grow and cause an infection. For instance, *Escherichia coli* is part of the normal flora of the large intestine. However, if contamination with this organism occurs during a bladder catheterization, a urinary tract infection will result. Staphylococci are part of the normal flora of the skin. However, when the integrity of the skin is disrupted, staphylococci may enter and an infection results.

The type of flora present in various body areas depends upon the temperature, pH, moisture, and available nutrients.

INFECTIOUS PROPERTIES OF BACTERIA

Infection is an undesirable host–parasite relationship. It results when the body or a part of it is invaded by a pathogenic agent that, under favorable conditions, grows and multiplies producing injurious effects.

Pathogens may enter the body through the respiratory tract, the digestive tract, the blood, the genitourinary system, the skin, and the mucous membranes. They leave the body through secretions and excretions from the respiratory tract and through feces, urine, blood, mucous membranes, and infected areas such as wounds and boils.

Pathogens may be transmitted either by direct or indirect contact. Direct transmission occurs when there is body contact with an infected person. Indirect transmission may occur from droplets, dust, water, blood, insects, equipment, hands, and infected persons or carriers.

Many pathogenic bacteria are capable of secreting certain substances that contribute to their virulence. Endotoxins are present inside the bacterial cell and are released only after its death and disintegration. Some of the clinical symptoms attributable to the release of endotoxins into the bloodstream are fever, weakness, lethargy, hypotension, irreversible shock, and death.

Exotoxins are injurious substances that are secreted by the living bacterium and released into the surrounding area. These microorganisms do not have to die in order to release exotoxins. *C. botulinum* that produces food poisoning and *C. tetani* that results in tetanus are two examples of bacteria that produce exotoxins.

In addition, there are several substances secreted by various bacteria that assist in the breakdown of body tissue and the spread of disease within the host. Some of these are hemolysins, leukocidins, hyaluronidase, streptokinase, coagulase, and collagenase.

NONBACTERIAL INFECTIONS

With the expanded use of steroids, immunosuppressive agents, and multiple antibiotic agents, the incidence of fungal and viral infections has been steadily increasing.

Fungi are much larger, considerably more complex, and more highly organized than bacteria. Among pathogenic fungi are certain species of molds and yeast. Yeasts and molds that cause human infections fall into one of two categories. The first includes those organisms that infect only skin, hair, and nails: the dermatophytes. The second includes those that infect deeper organs of the body as well as the skin.

Most of the diseases caused by systemic fungi are very difficult to treat as they do not respond well to antibiotic therapy.

Viruses are much smaller than bacteria as they range in size from 20 to 250 mμ. However, unlike bacteria, viruses multiply only within living cells. Viruses may be present in the air, on surfaces of equipment, or in dirt; but they cannot multiply until they invade living tissue.

One virus that is of concern to the perioperative nurse is the virus that results in infectious and serum hepatitis. The principal mode of transmission of these two diseases is oral or parenteral injection of fecal- or blood-contaminated food or water and bloodstream contact with blood or blood products contaminated with the virus of hepatitus. The hepatitus virus may be present in blood or feces without the existence of previous or current signs and symptoms in the host.

Of primary concern is the virus that causes acquired immune deficiency syndrome (AIDS). This virus weakens and eventually can destroy the body's immune system. The AIDS virus, known as the human immunodeficiency virus (HIV), leaves the body vulnerable to "opportunistic infections" caused by a variety of organisms found in the environment such as *Pneumocystis carinii*.

Malignancies such as Kaposi's sarcoma (KS) and central nervous system lymphoma also develop as the result of AIDS. In addition, it has been demonstrated that the AIDS virus infects cells of the nervous system directly, leading to encephalopathy, meningitis, myelopathy, and peripheral neuropathy.

The HIV is very fragile and normally needs to live inside a human body to survive. The virus requires a direct route from an infected person's blood, semen, or vaginal fluids, into another persons blood stream, through mucous membranes, or via a break in the protective surface of the skin. Contact with unbroken skin is not enough to transmit infection.

Those groups at high risk for AIDS include: homosexual or bisexual men, IV drug abusers, recipients of contaminated blood or blood products, heterosexual partners of HIV-infected persons, and children born to infected mothers. Table 6–1 identifies the types of surgical procedures AIDS patients may require. Viruses pose a hazard to all health care workers unless appropriate procedures are instituted.

BODY'S DEFENSE MECHANISMS

The body's first line of defense against infection is the intact skin and mucous membranes and their secretions. For example, the cilia, located on the mucous membranes of the respiratory tract, assist in moving the microorganisms to the exterior; the acid pH of the mucous secretions of the vagina assists in limiting the growth of microorganisms; the cleansing action of tears assists in removing pathogenic bacteria; and the acid pH plus

TABLE 6-1. SURGICAL PROCEDURES IN AIDS PATIENTS

Diagnostic procedures
  Tissue biopsies
Supportive procedures
  Placement of longterm indwelling intravenous catheters for TPN or antimicrobial therapy
Emergencies
  Intraabdominal complications
    Evaluation of acute abdomen
    Herpes zoster presenting as acute pain days to weeks before appearance of characteristic skin
      lesions
    Inflammation of the adrenals as a result of cytomegalovirus (CMV) infection presenting as ab-
      dominal pain, associated with signs of adrenal insufficiency, such as hypotension and electro-
      lyte imbalance
    CMV infection of the gastrointestinal tract producing chronic colitis which on rare occasions
      may be complicated by toxic megacolon and colonic perforation
    Pancreatitis as the result of infection or treatment courses with pentamidine used for *P. carinii*
      pneumonia (PCP).
    Acute acalculous cholecystitis caused by infection with cryptosporidium or by obstruction of
      biliary drainage related to enlarged lymph nodes
    Hepatitis and hepatic and splenic involvement with opportunistic agents causing abdominal
      pain
    Gastrointestinal bleeding associated with Kaposi's sarcoma (KS) or ulcerative lesions caused
      by candida or herpes simplex virus (HSV) infection
  Pulmonary complications
    Spontaneous pneumothorax requiring emergency chest tube placement, and on rare occasions
      thoracoplasty, which can occur after multiple episodes of PCP or other opportunistic pneumo-
      nias

From Schlamm H, Midvan D. The impact of AIDS on surgery. Surg Prac News. *May 1987; 5.*

the outward flow of urine contribute to the body's defense of preventing the invasion of organisms into the urethra.

Phagocytes provide the second line of defense. Phagocytic cells include leukocytes of the blood, wandering macrophages, and the fixed phagocytes of the reticuloendothelial system.

Leukocytes function by removing debris (including bacteria) by phagocytosis.

Wandering macrophages are another type of phagocytic cell that can pass through tissue space and travel to the site of the injury. They are also capable of phagocytosis.

The reticuloendothelial system is another system of phagocytic cells. These cells are found in the liver, spleen, bone marrow, lungs, and lymph nodes. They function in removing bacteria and other material from the circulating fluids.

The third line of defense present within the body is antibodies, which are formed in response to antigens. Antibodies are found in the gamma globulin and are able to react with the antigen that stimulated their production. Antibodies function in a variety of ways; some react with bacteria making them more susceptible to phagocytosis, whereas others cause lysis of bacterial cells. Antibodies developed in response to viruses neutralize the virus against which they are formed.

INFLAMMATORY RESPONSE

Any surgical incision results in an inflammatory response. Signs of acute inflammation are discoloration, swelling, heat, and pain. The discoloration and the heat are due to the increased blood supply to the "injured" area, resulting in dilated vessels. The swelling results from dilated vessels and the increased pressure from tissue fluids. The pressure on the nerve endings due to the swelling and the incision produce the pain.

If there are no bacteria present, the inflammation goes no farther and healing takes place. If bacteria are present, the tissues provide the necessary environment for an infection to occur. In this case, the leukocytes begin the process of phagocytosis. The exudate around the infected area contains fibrin, and as connective tissue cells multiply, the area becomes walled off. The result is a mass of dead white cells, tissue, blood, tissue fluids, and dead and living bacteria that form pus. The pus and the necrotic tissue within the walled-off area are an abscess.

If the walling-off process is incomplete, large amounts of poisonous products may be absorbed into the bloodstream. If only the toxins are absorbed, the condition is toxemia; if bacteria are also present, it is a septicemia. Bacteria in the bloodstream may localize at points away from the original area, and secondary abscesses result.

CLASSIFICATION OF SURGICAL INFECTIONS

Infections may develop in persons spontaneously either in the home or in the community. As many as 30% to 40% of patients admitted to a surgical service may have developed home-based infections (e.g., acute appendicitis, acute cholecystitis, acute diverticulitis with perforation and peritonitis, foreign bodies, animal bites).[5] Infections in this category are treated effectively with antibiotics.

Infections occurring in patients during their hospitalization are hospital acquired, or nosocomial. They are the result of microbial invasion of the body, most often by antibiotic-resistant and virulent microorganisms of the hospital environment. Invasion may follow surgical intervention; diagnostic procedures such as arteriography; or therapeutic procedures such as bladder catheterization, tracheostomy or IV therapy.

The bacteria most recently concerned with nosocomial infection have been *E. coli*, *Aerobacter aerogenes*, *Proteus*, *Pseudomonas aeruginosa*, *Serratia*, and *Staphylococcus aureus*.[8] Table 6–2 identifies some of the most common bacteria that result in surgical infections.

The risk of surgical infections may be anticipated due to the preoperative status of the wound, the site of the incision, and breaks in aseptic technique that occur intraoperatively. Operative wounds are classified as follows:

Category 1. A *clean wound* is a nontraumatic, uninfected operative wound in which neither the respiratory, alimentary, or genitourinary tracts nor the oropharyngeal cavities are entered. Clean wounds are made under aseptic conditions. They are usually primarily closed without drains. Reported infection rates are 1% to 5%.

TABLE 6-2. COMMON PATHOGENS RESULTING IN INFECTIONS

Bacteria[a]	Normal Flora/Location	Infection	Prevention and/or Control of Infection[b]
I. Aerobic Bacteria			
A. Gram-positive Coccus			
1. *Staphylococcus aureus*	Skin, hair Naso-oro-pharynx	Boils (furuncles) Wound infection Pneumonia Urinary tract infection Septicemia	1) Strict aseptic technique 2) Hand washing 3) Isolation of infected persons 4) Disinfection of all discharges
2. *Streptococcus pyogenes*	Nose Nasopharynx	Cellulitis Puerperal fever Wound infections Urinary tract infection	1) Strict aseptic techniques around wounds 2) Hand washing 3) Disposal of all discharges 4) Environmental sanitation 5) Adequate ventilation with appropriate air changes
3. *S. pneumoniae*	Nose Naso-oro-pharynx	Lobar pneumonia Conjunctivitis Peritonitis Meningitis	1) Exclusion of infected persons or carriers from the surgical suite 2) Strict adherence to aseptic technique 3) Environmental sanitation 4) Hand washing
B. Gram-negative Coccus			
1. *Neisseria gonorrhoeae*	Genitourinary tract Rectum, mouth Eye	Gonorrhea Pelvic inflammatory disease Septicemia Conjunctivitis	1) Environmental sanitation 2) Early diagnosis and treatment including all contacts
2. *Neisseria meningitidis*	Nose Oro-pharynx	Meningitis Pneumonia	1) Identification of carriers 2) Environmental sanitation 3) Strict adherence to aseptic technique 4) Hand washing
C. Gram-negative Bacillus			
1. *Escherichia coli*	Large intestine Perineum	Septicemia Inflammation of the liver and the gallbladder Urinary tract infection Peritonitis	1) Hand washing 2) Strict aseptic technique during bladder catheterization 3) Isolation of bowel contents and in- **(continued)**

149

TABLE 6-2. CONTINUED

Bacteria[a]	Normal Flora/Location	Infection	Prevention and/or Control of Infection[b]
			struments during large bowel resection
2. *Pseudomonas aeruginosa*	Intestinal tract Skin Soil	Wound infections Urinary tract infection Burns	1) Use aseptic technique when handling wounds and burns 2) Proper disposal of contaminated materials 3) Environmental sanitation
3. *Salmonella typhosa*	Intestinal tract	Typhoid Fever	1) Isolation 2) Disinfection of feces and urine 3) Sanitary control of food, water, and sewage disposal 4) Hand washing
4. *S. shigella*	Intestinal tract	Bacillary dysentery or shigellosis Gastroenteritis Septicemia	Same as for *S. typhosa*
5. *Hemophilus influenzae*	Respiratory tract	Bacterial meningitis Acute airway obstruction	1) Disinfection of respiratory secretions
D. Gram-positive Bacillus 1. *Mycobacterium tuberculosis*	Respiratory tract Urine (occasionally) Lymph nodes	Tuberculosis Peritonitis Meningitis Lungs Bone Skin Lymph nodes Intestinal tract Fallopian tubes	1) Early diagnosis and treatment 2) Environmental sanitation 3) Disposal of all discharges from respiratory tract 4) Disinfection and sterilization of contaminated equipment 5) Isolation of individual with active infection
II. Microaerophilic Bacteria A. Gram-positive Coccus 1. *Hemolytic streptococci*, alpha type	Respiratory tract	Abscess in gums or teeth Subacute bacterial endocarditis Meningitis	1) Identification of carriers 2) Adherence to aseptic technique 3) Proper handling of contaminated masks

Organism	Source	Disease	Control
2. *Nonhemolytic*		Endocarditis Urinary tract infection	4) Exclusion of personnel with upper respiratory infection from operating room 5) Hand washing Same as for *Hemolytic* (alpha)

III. Anaerobic Bacteria

A. Gram-positive Coccus

Organism	Source	Disease	Control
1. *Peptococcus*	Respiratory tract	Abscess of skin or of respiratory and intestinal tract	1) Strict aseptic technique
2. *Peptostreptococcus*	Vagina (premenopausal)	Abscess of respiratory and intestinal tract Septic abortions	1) Strict aseptic technique

B. Gram-positive Bacillus

Organism	Source	Disease	Control
1. *C. perfringens* 2. *C. novyi* 3. *C. septicum* 4. *C. histolyticum*	Soil Dust Manure Human feces Vagina	Gas gangrene (rare) Food poisoning (common)	1) Strict aseptic technique 2) Cleansing of all wounds by irrigation with copious amounts of solution to eliminate extraneous material and necrotic tissue
5. *C. tetani*	Soil Dust Feces	Tetanus (lockjaw) Surgical tetanus	1) Tetanus toxoid 2) Tetanus antitoxin 3) Sterilization of all instruments and dressings

C. Gram-negative Bacillus

Organism	Source	Disease	Control
1. *Bacteroids* species	Nasopharynx Intestinal tract Vagina	Wound infections Rectal, Brain Abscess Endocarditis Osteomyelitis	1) Strict aseptic technique 2) Environmental sanitation 3) Hand washing 4) Plaster casts should be bivalved or removed outside the operating room
2. *Fusobacterium*	Nasopharynx Intestinal tract	Anaerobic infections of brain and respiratory tract	1) Strict aseptic technique 2) Good dental hygiene

(continued)

TABLE 6-2. CONTINUED

Bacteria[a]	Normal Flora/Location	Infection	Prevention and/or Control of Infection[b]
		Vincent's angina (trench mouth) Cellulitis	
Nonbacterial Infections			
IV. Fungi A. *Candida albicans*	Respiratory Gastrointestinal Female genital tracts	Moniliasis or thrush	1) Avoid disturbance of normal microbial flora
V. Viruses A. *Hepatitis A*	Water contaminated by human sewage Shellfish from naturally contaminated sources Blood, Urine Food prepared or handled by infectious persons who practice poor hygiene	Infectious hepatitis	1) Sanitary disposal of sewage 2) Use disposable syringes and needles on infected persons 3) Exercise care in handling syringes, needles, and instruments used on infected persons 4) Sanitary food processing 5) Enforce good hygiene with all food-processing personnel (i.e., hand washing) 6) Gamma globulin immunization within 2 weeks
B. *Hepatitis B*	Blood Saliva Other body fluids Feces	Serum hepatitis	1) Hand washing 2) Use disposable presterile needles and syringes whenever possible 3) Nondisposable items must be terminally sterilized or disinfected following use 4) Careful disposal of contaminated syringes, needles, knife blades, and suture needles 5) Wear gloves when handling contaminated items

		6) Scrub nurse must exercise care not to puncture skin with needles or knife blades
		7) Gamma globulin immunization within 7 days
C. Human Immunodeficiency	AIDS Blood Saliva Semen Cerebrospinal fluid Tears	1) Wear gloves when touching blood saliva or mucous membranes
		2) Wear masks and protective eyewear when splashing of blood or saliva is likely
		3) Do not recap needles
		4) Nondisposable items must be terminally sterilized or disinfected following use
		5) Impervious gowns or plastic aprons should be worn during procedures that are likely to generate splashes of blood or body fluid
		6) Careful disposal of contaminated syringes, needles, knife blades, and suture needles
		7) Team members should refrain from all direct patient care when they have exudative lesions or weeping dermatitis
		8) Scrub nurse must exercise care not to puncture own skin with needles or knife blades
		9) Follow institutional policy after any exposure

[a]Bacterial infections may be mixed (e.g., aerobic and anerobic microorganisms, gram-positive and gram-negative microorganisms, and synergistic microorganisms).

[b]Strict handwashing technique is the most important precaution in the prevention and the control of infections.

Category 2. *Clean contaminated wounds* are (1) operative wounds in which the respiratory, alimentary, or genitourinary tract or oropharyngeal cavities are entered without unusual contamination; or (2) wounds that are mechanically drained. Reported infection rates are 3% to 11%.

Category 3. *Heavily contaminated wounds* include open, fresh traumatic wounds; operations with a major break in sterile technique (e.g., open cardiac massage); and incisions encountering acute, nonpurulent inflammation such as cholecystitis; or wounds made in or near contaminated or inflamed skin. Reported infection rates are 10% to 17%.

Category 4. *Dirty or infected wounds* include old traumatic wounds and those involving clinical infection or perforated viscera. The definition of this classification suggests that the organisms causing post-operative infection are present in the operative field before surgical intervention. Infection rates are usually more than 27%.[6]

REFERENCES

1. Perkins JJ. *Principals and Methods of Sterilization in Health Sciences.* Springfield, Illinois: Charles C. Thomas; 1978:4
2. Zimmerman LM, Veith I. *Great Ideas in the History of Surgery.* New York: Dover Publications; 1967:21,464
3. Vallery-Radat R. *The Life of Pasteur.* Trans R.L. Devonshire. New York: Doubleday; 1926:255
4. Cartwright F. *The Development of Modern Surgery.* New York: Thomas Crowell; 1968:48, 63–64, 80
5. Altemeier WA et al. *Manual on Control of Infection in Surgical Patients.* Philadelphia: J.B. Lippincott; 1984:22, 143
6. Fernsebner B. Infection control survey: Identifying compliance with guidelines. *AORN J.* 1986; 43(4):893.

Chapter 7

Limiting Contamination Sources in the Operating Room

SOURCES OF CONTAMINATION IN THE OPERATING ROOM

During the intraoperative phase, the safety of the patient is the primary focus of the perioperative nurse. One of the most important areas related to safety in the operating room is preventing infections by limiting the source of contamination.

The main sources of bacterial contamination are

1. Surgical team
    a. Health and hygiene
    b. Attire
2. Air circulation
3. Environment
    a. Design
    b. Sanitation
    c. Equipment
4. Supplies used during surgical intervention

PREVENTION AND CONTROL OF INFECTION

Surgical Team—Health and Hygiene

As identified earlier, large numbers of potentially pathogenic bacteria are present on the skin and the hair and in the respiratory tract of all persons. Written policies regarding attire and potential health hazards of personnel will assist in minimizing these bacteria as a source of infection to the surgical patient.

All members of the surgical team and other support personnel in the surgical suite should be free of transmissible bacterial infections. Areas of primary concern are upper respiratory tract infections; skin lesions such as carbuncles, furuncles, dermatitis; any unhealed wounds; and infections of the mouth, eyes, or ears. Any personnel exhibiting signs or symptoms in these areas should be excluded from the surgical suite.

Personal hygiene is an important factor in controlling infections. Hair is a source of bioparticulate matter and should be washed at frequent intervals and always after a haircut. A bath or a shower is recommended daily for all operating room personnel.

However, since the shedding of skin debris and microorganisms is the highest right after showering, it is recommended that personnel bathe or shower a few hours prior to changing into operating room attire. Frequent handwashing is one of the most important means of controlling the spread of infections. It must be carried out by all personnel before and after patient contact, even when gloves are used, and after handling equipment or other potentially contaminated items.

Physical examinations should be conducted upon employment and yearly thereafter.

Operating Room Attire

If not completely covered, the hair of the surgical team can be the source of bacteria causing wound infections.[1,2] Therefore, all personnel entering the semirestricted and restricted areas of the surgical suite must wear a head covering over all head and facial hair, including sideburns and neckline hair. Paper tape may be required to cover bushy sideburns.

The scrub cap or surgical hood must be clean and lint free and made of a fabric that meets the "Standard for the Use of Inhalation Anesthetics" of the National Fire Protection Association (NFPA 56A-78). The head covering should be donned before the scrub attire to prevent hair from collecting on the attire.

Reusable head coverings are acceptable, provided they are laundered after each use in the laundry facilities used by the hospital.

Head coverings such as net or crinoline allow dandruff and hair to fall out and, therefore, are not acceptable.

Proper scrub attire is made of a lint free, flame-resistant fabric that meets the NFPA 56A standards. The sleeves of the scrub top must be short enough to allow adequate scrubbing above the elbow (Fig. 7–1). The top should be tucked inside the pants to prevent contamination as personnel move about the suite and to decrease dissemination of bacterial shedding from the thoracic and abdominal skin of the wearer.

Available data indicate that the securing of scrub pants at the ankle significantly reduces the dispersal of bacteria-carrying particles from the skin.[3] Therefore, the pants should have ankle closures.

Panty hose and tights increase bacterial shedding and dispersal. Their use should be discouraged.[4]

Scrub attire should be changed daily or when it becomes visibly soiled or wet.

When donning scrub attire, care must be exercised not to drag the pants along the floor as the floor is the most bacteria-laden area of the operating room environment.

Name tags are included in proper operating room attire and should be worn by all members of the surgical team, support personnel, and visitors in all areas of the surgical suite.

Circulating nurses and anesthesiologists should wear jackets to prevent shedding from bare arms. The jackets should be buttoned to prevent excessive air movements and contamination when moving around the sterile field. Operating room attire should be transported and stored in closed carts to prevent contamination.

Surgical shoes have the potential for becoming contaminated and soaked with blood

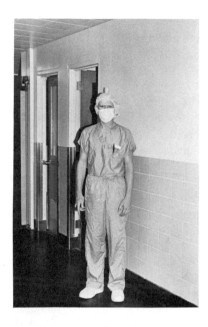

Figure 7-1. Proper operating attire.

or other potentially infectious materials and should be covered with shoe covers when there is a high probability that this may occur. However, they should not be required, as there have not been any controlled clinical studies indicating that they prevent or reduce surgical wound infections. In one study, there was no significant difference in floor contamination when ordinary shoes, clean shoes, or shoe covers were worn.[5]

In another study, Copp and colleagues found that unprotected street shoes transferred a considerable number of bacteria onto a study area in the OR and that this could be reduced by wearing OR-restricted shoes or shoe covers. However, the study did not examine whether the bacteria on street shoes was related directly to wound infections.[6]

Therefore, there is no strong theoretical rationale for their use or indication that the benefits expected from them are cost effective.[7]

If explosive anesthetics are used within the surgical suite, conductive shoe covers must be worn. When applying these shoe covers, the black carbon strip is placed inside the shoe between the sock and in contact with the bottom of the foot. If appropriate measures of conductivity do not occur immediately, a few drops of water in the bottom of the shoe will assist in arriving at the proper measurement. Conductivity should be checked prior to entering the surgical suite and at frequent intervals throughout the day.

When choosing footwear, careful consideration should be given to the kind and type of equipment used in the surgical suite, as well as necessary reaction times. Since most of the equipment is very heavy and emergency situations require quick responses, canvas shoes and clogs are not recommended for use in the surgical suite. Clogs do not provide the necessary ankle support and stability required for efficient and safe functioning within the environment.

Surgical masks are worn at all times in the specified areas of the surgical suite. This area includes the operating room, the substerile area, and the scrub room. Conversation and breathing without a mask results in droplet nuclei entering the air and settling on horizontal surfaces. Given the proper conditions for growth and reproduction, these bacteria multiply, become airborne, and may be deposited on sterile items or in the wound.

Surgical masks are air-purifying devices designed to filter out particulate from the exhaled breath of the wearer and thus protect the patient from the wearer's normal flora. They filter out particles of 5μ or larger with 99% efficiency. Recent studies have shown that potential airborne biohazards may exist in the operating room that could place operating room personnel at risk.[8,9] Infectious agents including bacteria, viruses, and fungi are particulate in nature. An aerosol is particulate formed from the disintegration of solid or liquid material in the matrix of air. Dust, fumes, mists, such as those created by surgical powered tools, and smoke created by lasers, are all types of aerosols. Viruses range in size from 0.003 to 0.05 μm and bacteria range in size from 0.3 to 13.0 μm.[10] Thus, the standard surgical mask does not afford protection when an inhalation risk is perceived. In these situations, a respirator designed to seal to the face and to control the wearer's inhalation exposure to airborne contaminants as small as 0.3 μ should be worn.[11]

When applying the mask, it must be secured in such a way as to prevent venting on the side. The metal strip should be adjusted to conform with the nose. This will assist in proper fitting and in preventing the fogging of eyeglasses. Masks are not to hang around the neck or to be put into a pocket for future use as they harbor bacteria collected from the nasopharyngeal airway and will contaminate the scrub attire.

Surgical masks are disposed of after each surgical procedure. When removing the mask, only the strings are handled. Due to the excessive contamination, care must be exercised not to touch the filter portion of the mask.

Surgical attire should be worn only inside the surgical suite; however, if it becomes necessary to leave the area prior to changing, the head covering should be removed and the scrub attire should be protected by wearing a clean cover gown, tied in the back at the neck and waist. Research has demonstrated that cover gowns provide some protection to certain areas of scrub attire.[12] However, exposure outside the surgical suite does lead to bacterial contamination of scrub suits and personnel must change clothes when they return to the restricted area.

Jumpsuits with shoe coverings and appropriate headgear may be used for individuals if they must enter the semirestricted areas of the surgical suite to perform minor repairs or maintenance (Fig. 7–2). Jumpsuits are not permitted in the restricted areas of the surgical suite.

Jewelry such as rings, watches, and necklaces serve as a reservoir for bacteria and should not be worn in the surgical suite. Earrings that dangle outside the scrub hat may fall into the sterile field; therefore, they should also be prohibited.

Universal Precautions

Medical history and examination cannot reliably identify all patients infected with HIV or other blood-borne pathogens; blood and body-fluid precautions should be consistently used for all patients. This approach, recommended by the Centers for Disease Control, is referred to as universal blood and body-fluid precautions or universal precautions and should be used in the care of all patients, particularly those in emergency situations in

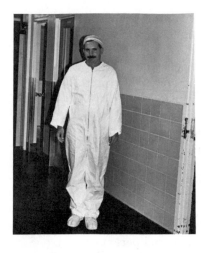

Figure 7-2. Jumpsuit with shoe coverings and appropriate headgear may be used to enter the semirestricted areas of the surgical suite.

which the risk of blood exposure is increased and the infection status of the patient is usually unknown.[13]

1. All personnel should routinely use appropriate barrier precautions to prevent skin and mucous-membrane exposure when contact with blood or other body fluids of any patient is anticipated.
2. Gloves should be worn for touching blood and body fluids, mucous membranes, or nonintact skin of all patients, for handling items or surfaces soiled with blood or body fluids, and for performing venipuncture and other vascular access procedures.
3. Masks and protective eyewear or face shields should be worn during procedures that are likely to generate aerosolization or splashing of fluids.
4. Impervious gowns or plastic aprons should be worn during procedures that are likely to generate splashes of blood or other body fluids.
5. Hands and other skin surfaces should be washed immediately and thoroughly if contaminated with blood or other body fluids. Hands should be washed immediately after gloves are removed.
6. Sharp items (needles, scalpel blades, and other sharp instruments) should be considered potentially infective and should be handled with extraordinary care to prevent accidental injuries.
7. Disposable syringes, needles, scalpel blades, and other sharp items should be placed in puncture-resistant containers located as close as is practical to the area in which they are used. To prevent needle-stick injuries, needles should not be recapped, purposefully bent, broken, removed from disposable syringes, or otherwise manipulated by hand. Disposable syringes and needles are preferred; only needle-locking syringes or one-piece needle–syringe units should be used to aspirate fluids from patients.
8. To minimize the need for emergency mouth-to-mouth resuscitation, mouthpieces, resuscitation bags, and other ventilation devices should be available for use in areas where the need for resuscitation is predictable.

9. Team members who have exudative lesions or weeping dermatitis should refrain from all direct patient care and from handling patient-care equipment until the condition resolves.
10. All specimens of blood, body fluids, or tissue should be put into a container with a secure lid to prevent leaking during transport. Care must be used to prevent contamination of the outside of the container. The use of a self-sealable plastic bag designed with an outside pouch to hold the requisition serves as an excellent method of containing tissue specimens.
11. All soiled linen should be handled as little as possible. It should be placed and transported in bags that prevent leakage.
12. Waste should be disposed of as indicated in Table 7–1.

Air Circulation

There are two sources of airborne organisms that may be present in the operating room: air deliverance to the room through the ventilation system, and personnel.

As mentioned in Chapter 2, an effective ventilation system, properly maintained, can minimize contamination from this source.

Microorganisms collect on horizontal surfaces such as the floor, the countertops, and the equipment. Air turbulence created by excessive numbers of people in the operating room, swinging doors, and shaking of linen may cause these bacteria to settle on the sterile field or in the wound. Education of the staff and a policy regarding the control of traffic and visitors within the operating room will assist in controlling airborne microorganisms.

TABLE 7-1. TYPES OF WASTE DESIGNATED AS INFECTIOUS AND RECOMMENDED DISPOSAL METHODS

Source/Type of Waste	Center for Disease Control		Environmental Protection Agency	
	Infectious Waste	Disposal/ Treatment Method	Infectious Waste	Disposal/ Treatment Method
Microbiological	YES	S,I	YES	S,I,TI,C
Blood and blood products (liquid from suction)	YES	S,I,Sew	YES	S,I,Sew,C
Sharps	YES	S,I	YES	S,I
Pathological (tissue)	YES	I	YES	I,SW,CD

Abbreviations: I, incineration; S, steam sterilization; TI, thermal inactivation; C, chemical disinfection for liquids only; Sew, sanitary sewer; SW, steam sterilization with incineration or grinding; CD, cremation or burial by mortician. Adapted from EPA Guide for Infectious Waste Management, Office of Solid Waste, US Environmental Protection Agency, Washington DC, May 1986, Report No. EPA/530-SW-86-014; and J. S. Garner, M. S. Favero, Infective Waste in Guideline for Handwashing and Hospital Environmental Control, Centers for Disease Control, November 1985.

Environmental Design

As indicated in Chapter 2, the design of the surgical suite and the use of specific building materials will have an impact on the effectiveness of housekeeping procedures.

Cracks and crevices harbor microorganisms and should be eliminated during construction or controlled with proper maintenance. When operating rooms are undergoing renovation or construction, patients must be protected from airborne contaminants. Of prime concern are fungal infections. Spores accumulate with dust and may result in aspergillosis infections. Therefore, it is essential that impervious barriers be constructed between the surgical suite and the construction area to prevent dissemination of dust. Sheet rock walls are preferable to taped plastic drapes that can be pushed aside. Construction materials should be transported during off-hours, and the area thoroughly cleaned prior to the transport of patients through the area.

Sanitation of Equipment and Environment

The environment of the surgical suite cannot be sterilized. However, by appropriate disinfection of floors, furniture, surgical lights, and equipment, the transmission of pathogenic organisms can be prevented.

Responsibility for cleaning the surgical suite may belong to either the housekeeping department or the hospital assistants, or they may share the responsibility. When the responsibility is shared, the hospital assistants are usually responsible for the end-of-procedure cleanup and the housekeeping department for the terminal cleaning.

If any portion of the cleaning responsibilities is delegated to the housekeeping department, it is imperative that the nurse manager and the executive housekeeper together determine the routine procedures to be used in cleaning the surgical suite.

To effectively implement the cleaning program, housekeeping employees and hospital assistants must receive instructions and training on the cleaning procedures required and the rationale for the procedure.

Prior to the first scheduled procedure of the day, all horizontal surfaces including furniture, countertops, equipment, and surgical lights are damp-dusted with a hospital grade disinfectant.

During the surgical procedure, perioperative nurses are responsible for confining and containing the contamination to the area around the sterile field. All surgical procedures are considered to be contaminated. The following techniques are consistent with this concept and will assist in controlling cross-contamination:

1. Sponges should be discarded into a plastic-lined kick bucket.
2. The circulator should use an instrument or disposable gloves when counting sponges or needles and when receiving any item passed from the sterile field.
3. If an area becomes contaminated by organic debris (such as blood) during the procedure, the area should immediately be cleaned using a tuberculocidal hospital grade disinfectant or a 1:10 dilution of household bleach, prepared daily. This will prevent the tracking of organic debris throughout the surgical suite.
4. Surgical instruments that fall on the floor should be picked up by the circulator, wearing disposable gloves, and placed in a pan containing a hospital grade disin-

fectant until the case is completed. This will prevent organic debris from drying and becoming airborne.

If the instrument is needed to complete the surgical procedure, it should be washed in the substerile area prior to being sterilized.

At the conclusion of the surgical procedure, the scrub assistant is responsible for the following areas:

1. Removing the linen from the patient and placing it in an impervious laundry bag
2. Removing all gross blood and other debris from the surgical instruments. All instruments are disassembled and box locks or hinges are opened before being placed in perforated trays for processing in the washer–sterilizer. Separating delicate and special instruments by placing them in a separate pan will provide additional protection and thus prolong the life of these instruments

    If a washer–sterilizer is not available, one of the following alternate procedures can be carried out after instruments are carefully washed and rinsed:

    a. Place the instruments in a perforated tray and autoclave at 270°F (132°C) for 3 minutes or at 250°F (121°C) for 15 to 20 minutes, or
    b. Instruments may be collected in a watertight basin, transferred to a pressure steam sterilizer, and covered with a 2% solution of trisodium phosphate. Sterilize for 30 minutes at 270°F (132°C) or 45 minutes at 250°F (121°C) to 254°F (124°C). Use fast exhaust[14]
3. Irrigating suction tips with clean water prior to being disconnected
4. Disposing all knife blades and needles in a puncture-resistant container so they will not serve as a potential source of injury and contamination to support personnel

    Knowledge of how the trash is disposed of (i.e., use of compactor, incineration, or disposal in the environment such as landfill) and local regulations will influence the procedure used in disposing of all items from the operating room
5. Discarding all disposable items in impervious containers
6. Placing all linen items, whether soiled or not, in an impervious hamper bag to be laundered
7. Suctioning all solutions out of the basins, and drying the items for terminal sterilization
8. Disposable suction tubing is recommended due to the difficulty encountered in cleaning the lumen of the reusable suction tubing. The suction tubing should be disconnected from the wall by the circulator to avoid contamination of the wall outlet. The contents of the suction container should be disposed of during the flushing of a hopper. The addition of a commercial garbage disposal to the hopper will aid in disposing of blood clots and bone chips

    If a hopper is not available, the suction contents should be decontaminated with a proper disinfectant before disposal.[14]

    If glass suction bottles are used, they must be washed and terminally sterilized after each case.
9. Cleaning items requiring gas sterilization and then wiping with a hospital-grade

disinfectant prior to being transported to the workroom or central supply department for reprocessing.

10. The scrub assistant then removes his or her gown and gloves and closes the case cart or covers the table contents by touching the clean ends of the table drape. The table or cart is then removed from the operating room.

Instrument Processing. The potential hazard of direct contact with the virus of serum hepatitis or AIDS is ever present in handling contaminated surgical instruments. Therefore, instruments must be terminally washed and sterilized by one of the methods previously discussed before they are sorted for storage or returned to sets.

The most commonly used method of mechanical cleaning is the instrument washer–sterilizer (Fig. 7–3). For the washer–sterilizer to perform at maximum effectiveness, however, organic debris must not be permitted to dry in the serrations, box locks, and ratchets of the instruments. To achieve this, the instruments must be wiped, rinsed, or soaked during the surgical procedure. Soaking instruments such as intestinal clamps, rongeurs, and bone rasps in cold water immediately after use will facilitate the cleaning process.

In addition, prior to being processed in the washer–sterilizer, some instruments may require a preliminary soaking in warm water with a detergent/disinfecting solution in the decontamination area of the workroom or central supply department. If it is necessary to use a brush in the cleaning of these instruments, the brush must be kept below the level of the water to prevent the dissemination of microorganisms through the release

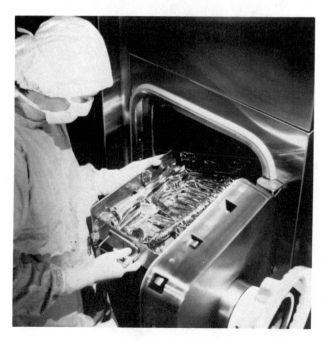

Figure 7–3. Loading a washer sterilizer with all instruments open or on a stringer. (*Courtesy American Sterilizer Company, Erie, Pennsylvania.*)

of aerosols and droplets. Personnel should wear a plastic apron, protective eyewear, gloves, and a mask when performing this task.

The washing process in the washer–sterilizer is accomplished by means of a vigorously agitated detergent bath, which is the result of a combination of high-velocity jet streams of steam and air that develop a violent underwater turbulence (Fig. 7–4). During the washing phase, the water temperature rises to 63° to 68° C (145° to 155°F). The detergent solution disengages the blood, grease, and tissue debris from the instruments and carries the soil to the surface. As the heated water expands in the chamber, the level rises, and the released soil and scum overflow into the waste line. The automatic program control then activates the steam inlet and water outlet valves. Steam is admitted into the top of the chamber, forcing the wash water out through the bottom drain. Steam under pressure floods the chambers, and the temperature of 132°C (270°F) is maintained for not less than 3 minutes. Then the steam is exhausted through an automatic condenser exhaust and an audible signal indicates that the washer–sterilizer is ready for unloading.[15]

If a washer–sterilizer is not available, instruments should be soaked in warm water with a moderately alkaline low-sudsing detergent, thoroughly cleaned, and then rinsed

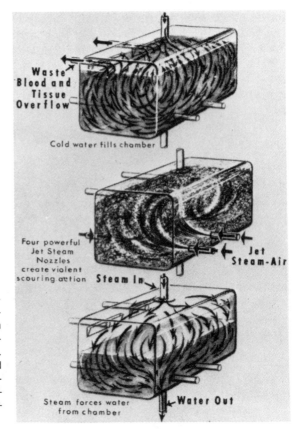

Figure 7-4. Cleaning of instruments is accomplished by means of vigorously agitated detergent bath. Combination of high velocity jet streams of steam and air develop violent underwater turbulence. (*From John J. Perkins.* Principles and Methods of Sterilization in Health Sciences, *Second Edition. Springfield, Illinois: Charles C. Thomas; 1978, with permission.*)

with hot water. Rinsing with hot water is essential because the residual heat will assist in the instruments drying. Moisture remaining on instruments may result in rust and discoloration.

When spots, stains, or areas of discoloration appear on instruments, it may be the result of the wrong detergent, too much detergent, the mineral content of the water, laundry residue from cloth wrappers, or chemicals released from paper wrappers.[15]

Following terminal decontamination, the instruments may be placed in the ultrasonic cleaner.

Ultrasonic Cleaning of Instruments. The ultrasonic cleaner assists in maintaining surgical instruments in proper working condition by removing debris from the box locks and the serrations. It should be used as the final step in the processing of instruments. Dissimilar metals, such as copper, brass, and stainless steel, should not be combined in the ultrasonic unit, as the cleaning of dissimilar metals causes ion transfer resulting in etching and pitting. Chrome-plated instruments should not be placed in the ultrasonic cleaner, as they may be damaged by mechanical vibrations, which cause flaking.[16]

Ultrasonic is the term used to describe a vibrating wave of frequency above that of the upper frequency limit of the human ear; it generally embraces all frequencies above 15,000 cycles per second. The ultrasonic cleaner cleans instruments through a process called cavitation.

Cavitation occurs when sound waves are passed through water, creating within it cavities ranging in size from submicroscopic to very large. These minute bubbles expand until they are unstable, and then they collapse. The implosion (bursting inward) generates minute vacuum areas on the instruments responsible for the cleaning process. During cavitation, the binder that causes adherence of the organic debris to the instrument is dislodged, dispersed, or dissolved. Some of the debris rises to the surface of the solution, while the heavier debris settles to the bottom of the tank.

Following the cleaning process, the instruments must be rinsed under pressure to remove residual debris and any detergent remaining on them. The instruments are then dried at a temperature of 88°C (190°F).

The ultrasonic cleaner does not decontaminate or sterilize and must not be used as a substitute for the washer–sterilizer. If instruments are not decontaminated prior to being placed in the ultrasonic cleaner, the solution will serve as a reservoir for microorganisms with subsequent cross-contamination occurring.

A simple method of measuring the effectiveness of the ultrasonic cleaner consists of rubbing pencil lead into the porous surface of a ceramic ring. The ceramic ring is then placed with the porous side up in a tray, and the ultrasonic cleaner is turned on for 1 minute. If more than 75% of the lead is removed, the cleaner is functioning appropriately.

Lubricating Instruments. Detergents used in the washer–sterilizer and the ultrasonic cleaner remove the lubricant from stainless steel. Therefore, the instruments should be lubricated with an antimicrobial water-soluble lubricant and drained. For maximum efficacy, the lubricating solution must not be rinsed or wiped off the instruments.[17]

The lubricant provides a protective coating for the instruments, reducing rusting, staining, and corrosion; it improves instrument function, reduces the growth of bacteria, and allows penetration of steam. In addition, there is a reduction in the amount of organic debris that adheres to the stainless steel when the instruments are used in subsequent procedures, making them easier to clean.[17]

The lubricant must be water-soluble to allow steam penetration, have a neutral pH, and contain high amounts of surfactants to dissolve the protein material in box locks.

Inspecting and Sorting Instruments. After the instruments are processed, they should be sorted and inspected prior to being stored or placed in sets. Each instrument should be examined for cleanliness and proper working condition. Hinged instruments should be checked for stiffness and alignment of jaws and teeth. Sharp instruments such as scissors and chisels should be checked for sharpness, dents, or chips; and plated instruments should be observed for chips, sharp edges, and worn spots. Any defective instruments should be removed from circulation and repaired at the first sign of damage or malfunctioning.

Stiff instruments should not be oiled, as steam sterilization will not penetrate the oil effectively. Stiff instruments frequently are due to the accumulation of foreign matter in the box lock. Stiffness usually does not occur in instruments processed routinely in the ultrasonic cleaner. To relieve stiffness, a small amount of a water-soluble grinding compound, available from instrument manufacturers, may be worked into the box lock by opening and closing the instrument several times. This will assist the instrument in regaining smooth functioning.

For those instruments that do require lubrication, such as air drills, silicone oil compounds or oil in water preparations that do not inhibit sterilization by autoclaving are available for use by the manufacturer.

Supplies Used During Surgical Intervention

As discussed in Chapter 6, intact skin provides an excellent barrier to microbial invasion. Any break in the skin such as a surgical incision results in a potential port of entry for microorganisms. Therefore, any item that comes in contact with the surgical incision must be sterile. An item is considered to be sterile when there is an absence of living microorganisms.

Aseptic technique is the method by which contamination with microorganisms is prevented. Thus, it is essential that the perioperative nurse know and implement these principles of aseptic technique.

Principles of Aseptic Technique

All Items Used Within a Sterile Field Must Be Sterile. A sterile field is created by placing a sterile towel or sheet over an unsterile surface. The sterile field is maintained by never allowing an unsterile item to come in contact with that field. Once a sterile drape is placed in position, it cannot be moved or shifted.

Sterile items are stored in clean areas free from moisture and must remain sterile until they are opened for use. Before opening a sterile package, the circulator must check the integrity of the package, the expiration date, and the appearance of the sterilizer-indicating tape.

Before removing items from the autoclave, the graph must be checked to ascertain that the proper temperature was achieved for the appropriate amount of time.

If there is any doubt about the sterility of an item, the item is considered unsterile.

The Edges of Sterile Containers Are Not Considered Sterile Once the Package is Opened.

The boundaries between sterile and unsterile are often not easily identified, and the perioperative nurse must exercise professional judgment in making these determinations.

When opening large items such as a linen pack, the item should be placed on a flat surface with the end flaps extended. The outer wrapper is then cuffed so the circulating nurse avoids contact with the sterile contents by keeping all fingers under the cuff. To open the opposite side of the pack, the circulator must move to the other side of the table. If the wrapper is used to drape the table, the margin begins at the table edge.

In opening smaller items, the ends of the flaps are secured in the hand so they do not flip back and contaminate the contents or the sterile individual (Fig. 7–5). A 1-inch safety margin is considered standard on package wrappers.

On peel-back packages, the inner edge of the heat seal is the sterile boundary. The scrub nurse must remove items from these packages by lifting them straight up and not allowing the contents to slide over the edge. Sharp or heavy objects should always be presented to the scrub nurse or opened on a separate surface. Sterile items should not be "tossed" onto a sterile field.

When the cap is removed from a sterile liquid, it is considered contaminated and may not be replaced on the bottle. The contents of the bottle must be used or discarded. When pouring from a bottle, the solution is poured in a steady stream so it does not splash out of the container (Fig. 7–6). In addition, care must be exercised to prevent the solution from running over the unsterile part of the bottle, dripping onto the sterile field, and contaminating it.

To receive solutions, the scrub nurse moves the container to the table's edge or holds the receptacle so the circulator does not reach over the sterile field.

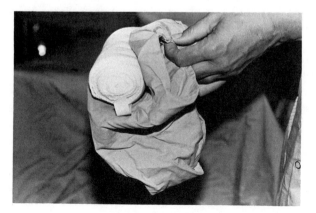

Figure 7-5. To prevent contamination the ends of the flap are secured in the hand so they do not flip back and contaminate the contents of the package.

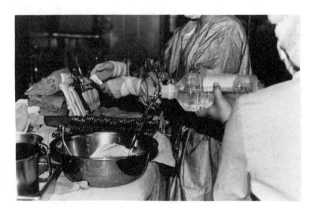

Figure 7-6. The receptacle is moved to the edge of the table and the solution is poured in a steady stream.

Gowns Are Considered Sterile in Front From Shoulder to Table Level. The Sleeves Are Sterile to 2 Inches Above the Elbow, to the Stockinette Cuff. Wraparound gowns that cover the back may be sterile when they are first put on. However, since the back of the gown cannot be continuously observed, sterility cannot be assured. Therefore, the back is not considered to be sterile. The stockinette cuff is not considered to be sterile, as it is a moisture-collection area and not an effective microbial barrier. Therefore, it should be covered by sterile gloves at all times.

Gloved hands should be kept in sight and at or above the waist level. The arms should not be folded with the hands tucked in the axillary region as they may become contaminated with perspiration.

Scrub nurses should avoid changing levels from footstools to floor and should not sit or lean against an unsterile surface. The only time sitting is acceptable is when the surgical procedure is performed from the sitting position.

Draped Tables Are Sterile Only at Table Level. The sterile field on the back table or a "prep" table is limited to the top of the table. Any item falling over the edge is considered contaminated and cannot be brought back into the sterile field.

The same principle applies to the draped patient; however, the boundaries are less distinct. The perioperative nurse must exercise astute observation and professional judgment when interpreting sterile areas versus unsterile areas on the draped patient.

Sterile Persons and Items Contact Only Sterile Areas; Unsterile Persons and Items Contact only Unsterile Areas. The sterile members of the surgical team contact only sterile areas and sterile items. The unsterile members should not touch the sterile field, reach over it, or permit unsterile items to come in contact with it. When opening a sterile item, the hands of the circulator should be positioned to avoid accidental contact with the scrub nurse or the sterile field. This safety margin can be created by using a cuff created by the sterile wrapper or by using an instrument as an extension of the hand. A sterile instrument may be used for one transfer and is then considered contaminated.

When opening a sterile package, the scrub nurse opens the near side first (so the gown is protected) and the far side last, whereas the circulator opens the far side first and the near side last to prevent reaching over a sterile field.

Movement Within or Around a Sterile Field Must Not Cause Contamination of the Sterile Field. Sterile team members stay close to the sterile field; they do not wander about the room or leave the room while in sterile attire. When sterile persons change positions, they move back to back or face to face, maintaining a safe distance from each other and the sterile field.

Unsterile team members circulate around the sterile area but do not come in direct contact with it. When passing a sterile field, unsterile persons should maintain at least 1 foot of distance, always facing the sterile field and never walking between two sterile fields.

A Sterile Barrier That Has Been Permeated Must Be Considered Contaminated. The integrity of drapes and gowns must be inspected before use and continuously during surgical intervention. When liquids soak through linen from the sterile to the unsterile surface, "strikethrough" occurs. When this occurs, the barrier must be replaced or reinforced. Nonwoven and certain treated woven materials are more resistant to strikethrough. However, under abrasive conditions or prolonged exposure, strikethrough will occur in all materials.

Any sterile item that becomes damp or wet is considered contaminated. When items are removed from the autoclave, they must be permitted to dry before being placed on a cold surface. This prevents the condensation of steam, which would contaminate the item.

When a sharp instrument, such as a towel clip, perforates the sterile surface of the barrier, the points of the towel clips are contaminated and the towel clip may not be relocated.

Items of Doubtful Sterility Are Considered Unsterile. When a sterile item wrapped in a pervious wrapper, such as muslin, is dropped on the floor, contaminated air may enter the package from the force of the fall. Therefore, these items should be considered unsterile.

When dropped, items packaged in impervious wrappers are less likely to become contaminated. If the integrity of the package is maintained, the item can be considered sterile and safe for immediate use.

Sterile fields are set up immediately prior to surgical intervention and must never be left unguarded. They should not be set up and then covered for later use as it is impossible to remove the cover sheet without contaminating the field. If a surgical case is canceled or delayed, the field is considered contaminated and a new setup is prepared.

The use of "splash basins" to rinse gloved hands is not acceptable. It is difficult to maintain the sterility of these basins, as they provide a potential breeding ground for the microorganisms that have been removed from the gloves.[18,19]

All members of the surgical team must be aware of aseptic technique. As the patient's advocate, perioperative nurses must constantly be aware of what is occurring in and around the sterile field. They, as well as other members of the team, must be willing to take the risk of pointing out known or suspected violations of sterile technique and then initiating corrective action. To perform this role effectively, perioperative nurses must exercise professional judgment and a thorough knowledge of the application of these principles.

End-of-Case Cleanup

The method of choice used in cleaning the floor between surgical procedures is the built-in central wet vacuum pickup system, the use of which requires plugging a hose-and-wand into a wall outlet. A central system is quiet and eliminates any possibility of bacteria contaminating the air, as well as much of the equipment setup, and reduces cleanup time.

In the absence of a central wet vacuum pickup system, a portable wet vacuum machine (Fig. 7–7), with a bacterial filter, combined with a pump-type garden spray can for dispensing a detergent disinfectant can achieve the desired results.

If a wet vacuum system is unavailable, a two-bucket technique with detergent germicide in both buckets can be used. If this technique is used, the mophead must be laundered and sterilized prior to being used in the surgical suite. A clean mophead must be used for each room, and the buckets cleaned prior to reuse.

Brooms should not be used in the surgical suite due to the air turbulence created.

All personnel involved in cleaning within the surgical suite must wear disposable gloves and protective eyewear as personal safety measures and to assist in preventing cross-contamination.

The end-of-the-case cleanup should consist of the following steps:

1. All horizontal surfaces of furniture, equipment, and countertops are cleaned with a detergent germicide.
2. Walls and doors are spot-cleaned.

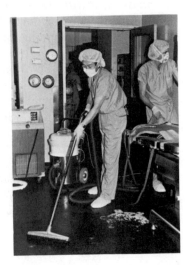

Figure 7–7. The method of choice used in cleaning the floor between surgical procedures is the wet vacuum pickup.

3. To avoid cracking the heat filters, the surgical light is cleaned after it is cooled. It is cleaned with a detergent disinfectant as recommended by the manufacturer. Some disinfectants leave a residue and will reduce the amount of light available for use.
4. The operating room table is cleaned with a detergent disinfectant. Since organic debris tends to accumulate where the sections of the table come together and under the mattress pad, all surfaces must be exposed and cleaned.
5. All equipment used for the surgical procedure is wiped with a detergent disinfectant and returned to the proper storage area.
6. After the floor is sprayed or wet down with the detergent disinfectant, the furniture is moved to one side of the room. Moving the operating room table and other equipment through the solution serves as a method of decontaminating the castors. The floor is then cleaned by one of the previously discussed methods.
7. The linen and trash bags are closed and then moved to the appropriate area for disposal.

During the day, the hallways and the substerile and scrub rooms should be mopped with a detergent disinfectant. The frequency will be determined by the activity of the surgical suite (i.e., the number of surgical cases and personnel).

Doormats placed at the entrance to the surgical suite, with either a tacky surface or soaked in a strong antiseptic solution, are not effective in reducing bacterial population.

A series of tests have shown that doormats with tacky surfaces placed at the entrance to the surgical suite exerted no demonstrable effect on the bacterial population of cart wheels or shoes which had traversed this mat. In other cases in which the mat had been traversed previously, the second set of wheels or shoes were shown to have picked up bacteria deposited during the preceding trip. Similarly—mats soaked with a strong antiseptic solution may have been self-sterilizing, though this did not affect the bacterial count of cart wheels or shoe soles which traversed them. The antiseptic solutions require a contact time of at least 30 seconds.[20]

Terminal Cleaning—Daily
At the completion of the day's surgical schedule, all operating rooms and scrub and substerile areas are terminally cleaned. Terminal cleaning consists of using a chemical disinfectant and mechanical friction to make sure:

1. Surgical lights including the tracks are clean
2. All other fixed and ceiling-mounted equipment are washed
3. All furniture including the wheels and the castors are washed
4. The face plate of all vents are wiped
5. Doors of cabinets and operating room doors around handles and push plates are wiped
6. All horizontal surfaces including tops of counters, autoclaves, solution warmers, and other fixed or recessed shelves are wiped
7. Floors are machine scrubbed, and the solution is picked up with a wet vacuum or a clean mop that has been sterilized. The mop is used for only one room.

Solution should be allowed to remain wet on the floor for at least 5 to 10 minutes

8. Kick buckets are washed and sterilized
9. Scrub sinks are washed, and the spray heads of the faucets removed for sterilization
10. Soap dispensers should be washed and sterilized prior to being refilled
11. All support areas in the surgical suite should be scrubbed daily. In the sterile storage area, care must be taken not to contaminate any sterile items
12. Transportation and utility carts are cleaned with a detergent disinfectant after each use. The terminal cleaning includes the wheels and the castors

Weekly Cleaning

1. All shelves in cabinets are cleaned with a detergent disinfectant.
2. Air-conditioning grills and ducts are vacuumed.
3. Transportation and utility carts are steam cleaned.

Following the terminal cleaning, all cleaning equipment is disassembled, cleaned with a detergent disinfectant, and dried to prevent the growth of microorganisms.

Evaluating the efficacy of the cleaning procedures may be accomplished by using rodac plates. The bacteriologic count on the unused surface of the floor 12 hours after cleaning and disinfecting should be less than 5 organisms per square centimeter. If the count is above this, the cleaning procedure should be reviewed and the equipment observed for appropriate maintenance.

REFERENCES

1. Dineen P, Drusin L. Epidemics of post-operative wound infections associated with hair carriers. *Lancet.* 1973; (2):1157–1159
2. Black W, Bannerman C, Black D. Carriage of potentially pathogenic bacteria in the hair. *Br J Surg.* 1974; 61(9):735–738
3. Dankert J, Zijlstra J, Lubberding H. A garment for us in the operating theatre: The effect upon bacterial shedding. *J Hyg.* (Cambridge) 1979; 82:7–14
4. Mitchell NJ, Gamble DR. Clothing design for operating room personnel. *Lancet.* 1974; 2:1133
5. Hambraeous A, Malmborg A. The influence of different footwear on floor contamination. *Scand J Infect Dis.* 1979; 11(3):243–246
6. Copp G, Slezak L, Dudley N, Malhot C. Footwear practices and OR contamination. *Nurs Res.* 1987; 36(6):366–369
7. Garner J. Guidelines for prevention of surgical wound infection 1985. *Guidelines for the Prevention and Control of Nosocomial Infections.* Atlanta, Ga: Communicable Disease Center; 1985:6
8. Oosterhuis J, Verschueren R, Eibergen R, Oldhoff J. The viability of cells in the waste products of CO_2 laser evaporation of Cloudman mouse melanomas. *Cancer.* 1982; 49:61–67
9. Walker N et al. Possible hazards from irradiation with the carbon dioxide lasers. *Laser Surg Med.* June 1986; 6(1):84–86

10. Hinds W. *Aerosol Technology*. New York: John Wiley; 1982:8
11. Heinsohn P. Surgical masks versus respiratory protection in the healthcare setting. Unpublished paper; 1989
12. Copp G, Malhot C, Zalar M et al. Covergowns and the control of OR contamination. *Nurs Res*. 1986; 35(5):267
13. Recommendations for prevention of HIV transmission in health care settings. *CDC Morbidity and Mortality Weekly Report*. 1984; 36(25):5
14. Recommended practices operating room environmental sanitation. *AORN J*. 1989; 49(3):856–863
15. Perkins J. *Principles and Methods of Sterilization in Health Sciences*. Springfield, Illinois: Charles C. Thomas; 1982:241
16. Recommended practices for care of instruments, scopes and powered surgical instruments. *AORN J*. 1988; 47(2):560
17. Underwood L. Care and handling of instruments. *Hosp Topics*. 1979; 61:46
18. Ginsberg F. Eliminating bird baths: Questions and answers. *Mod Hosp*. 1971; 132
19. Baird R et al. Splash basin contamination in orthopaedic surgery. *Clin Orthopaed*. 1984; 187:129–133
20. Altemeier WA et al. *Manual on Control of Infection in Surgical Patients*. Philadelphia: J. B. Lippincott; 1976:23

Chapter 8

Sterilization and Disinfection

STERILIZATION—WHAT IT IS

Sterilization is the process by which items are rendered free of microorganisms, including spores. However, the term *sterile* is not absolute because microorganisms die logarithmically. The logarithmic order of death implies that the same percentage of living bacteria die each minute. This means that complete sterilization is never attained. For example, assume that an item is contaminated with 1 million cells (10^6). After 1 minute of a given sterilizing procedure, 90% or 900,000 cells would be killed and 100,000 would survive. After the second minute, 90,000 would be killed and 10,000 would survive. After the third minute, there would be 1000 survivors.[1]

The rate at which bacteria die is expressed as the D value. The D value refers to the decimal reduction time (DRT). This is the time required at any constant temperature to destroy 90% of the population of organisms, or the time required for the survivor curve to traverse one log cycle.

The number of actual or suspected organisms located on an item is referred to as the bioburden and affects the sterilization cycle. For example, the automated steam-sterilizing cycle is set to kill a total of 10^6 microbes per item sterilized. Therefore, an item with more than 10^6 bioburden cannot be sterilized in one cycle of the sterilizer without the exposure period being increased.

An item cleaned properly in a clean environment by personnel with clean hands will have a bacterial count of less than 10^6. Thus, these items can be sterilized in the routine manner. Since absolute sterility cannot be achieved, the goal is to reduce the number of microbes to the lowest number possible.

In a healthy individual, 1 million bacteria or 10^6 are necessary for most infections to occur. However, some exceptions do occur. For example, it takes only one myobacterium tuberculosis to reach the lung and cause tuberculosis. The number of organisms needed to cause an infection is also dependent on the virulence of the microbe and the susceptibility of the host.[1] Fewer organisms are needed to cause an infection when the patient is in a compromised state (such as the debilitated patient on immunotherapy or chemotherapy and the very old or very young patient).

Sterilization may be achieved by chemical or physical agents. The chemical agents that are used are ethylene oxide (ETO) and activated glutaraldehyde. The physical methods are ionizing radiation, dry heat, and saturated steam under pressure. The degree of sterilization achieved by any of these methods is directly related to the preparation and the packaging of the supplies.

PREPARATION OF MATERIALS FOR STERILIZATION

In preparing articles for sterilization, one must adhere to the following guidelines:

1. All articles must be clean and dry. Any debris such as grease, dirt, or blood will inhibit the contact by the sterilizing agent and prevent sterilization or will cause the item to require a longer exposure time.

2. The sterilizing agent must contact all surfaces of an item. As a result, the box locks or hinges on all instruments should be opened and detachable parts disassembled. Instruments can be strung on pins or racks. Rubber bands should not be used to hold instruments together. Trays with perforated bottoms should be used to allow adequate circulation of the sterilizing agent. To assure adequate drying the maximum weight of an instrument tray is 16 pounds. Instruments packaged individually should have the tips protected to avoid damage and possible perforation of the packages.

3. To adequately steam-sterilize items with a lumen, such as rubber tubing and needles, the lumen must be flushed with distilled water (Fig. 8–1). The water will become steam as the temperature rises, and the air will be displaced; thus, sterilization of the lumen will occur. The tubing should be packaged in such a way that kinks are avoided.

4. Linen wrappers and drapes should be freshly laundered to avoid superheating. Superheating occurs when dehydrated fabrics are subjected to steam sterilization. In superheating, the temperature of the fabric exceeds that of the surrounding steam, rising as much as 8° to 11°C (15° to 20°F) higher than the temperature of the steam in the sterilizer. When this occurs, it exerts a destructive effect on the strength of the cloth fibers, which hastens fabric deterioration.[2] If not stored in an area of low humidity, freshly laundered fabrics will be in a relatively normal state of hydration prior to sterilization and thus superheating will not occur. All new linen must be washed prior to use to remove sizing and to hydrate.

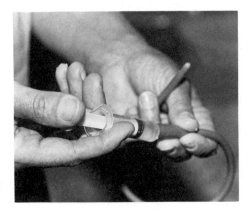

Figure 8–1. All items with a lumen must be flushed with distilled water prior to steam sterilization.

Prior to sterilization, linen wrappers and drapes must be carefully inspected for defects, lint, and stains. To assist in locating the defects, the inspection is conducted over an illuminated glass tabletop. When holes are found, they are repaired with the use of vulcanized heat-sealed patches. To assure sterilization, the patched surface area of the item should be less than 20% of the total area. The decision as to the size of the patch (1" × 1" or 3" × 3") should be made on the basis of appearance and the ease-of-handling characteristics of the fabric.[3] During the inspection, careful attention should be given to the amount of lint on the fabrics. Linting occurs due to thread wear and a breakdown of the fabric as a result of repeated processing. Lint serves as a vehicle for the transfer of organisms from one location to another and must be reduced to a minimum on all linen used in the surgical suite.

Linen items should be fan-folded or rolled loosely, and alternate layers should be crossed to allow penetration of the sterilizing agent.

Linen packs must be limited to 30 cm × 30 cm × 50 cm (12" × 12" × 20") and weigh not more than 5.5 kg (12 lbs).

5. Rubber sheeting should not be folded or rolled tightly, as steam does not penetrate rubber. It should be covered with a piece of linen or gauze and then rolled loosely.

6. Wood should not be steam-sterilized as lignocellulose resin (lignin) is driven out of the wood by heat. This resin may condense onto other items in the autoclave; and if these items come into contact with tissues, a reaction may result.

PACKAGING MATERIALS

The objective of packaging is to keep items sterile following the sterilization process until they are opened and aseptically delivered to the sterile field. Sterile packaging should be suitable for the sterilization method used. It must allow adequate steam penetration if used in steam sterilization. If used in gas sterilization, it must allow adequate penetration and release of the ethylene oxide gas and moisture. The material must be impervious to microorganisms of 0.5 μ in diameter, be moisture resistant and economical, and be able to withstand 40 lbs. of pressure per square inch. Materials used for in-hospital packaging are flexible and memory-free to allow aseptic presentation of the contents. The materials do not pile or delaminate, and the package does not reseal once it is opened.[4] All materials used for packaging must be free of toxic ingredients and nonfast dyes.

Materials available for packaging are woven materials made of various grades and weaves of cotton (with and without special waterproofing treatment), two-way crepe paper, paper, plastic, nonwoven fabrics, and a variety of paper and plastic combinations.

Muslin is suitable for steam, dry heat, and ethylene oxide sterilization. It is reusable, memory-free, flexible, and easy to use. When 140-thread-count muslin is used, the wrapper must consist of four thicknesses or two double wrappers. One double muslin wrapper is two thicknesses of 140-thread-count muslin sewn together at the edges. The 140-

thread-count muslin does not serve as a moisture barrier, and therefore the use of this fabric as a packaging material should be limited.

The 280-thread-count muslin has twice as many threads per square inch as the 140-count muslin and as a result one thickness of 280 is equal to a 140 double wrapper. Many of the 280-thread-count wrappers receive a special moisture-resistant treatment. As a result, they are an improved barrier to microbial and moisture strikethrough. This fabric is more costly than the 140-count muslin, but the advantages compensate for the increased cost. The moisture-resistant properties are usually retained for 90 to 100 washings. When this fabric is used, an accurate method of counting the washings is essential. The manufacturer can provide a grid that is marked each time the item is processed. When the designated number of washings is arrived at, the item must no longer be used in surgery.

Woven wrappers are manufactured in a variety of sizes, and it is important that the correct size be used for all items. Wrappers that are too small will not adequately cover and protect the items, and too large a wrapper will be bulky and difficult to handle when opening the item. When wrapping items in woven material, they are wrapped sequentially in the two wrappers with all corners of the wrapper folded in. A small cuff on the first fold of the fabric over the contents provides a safety margin when opening the item. Pressure-sensitive tape should be used to secure the packages as it indicates that the item has been exposed to the sterilization cycle.

After laundering, linens to be sterilized should be stored at a temperature of 65° to 72°F (18° to 22°C) and at a relative humidity of 35% to 75%.

Canvas or other heavy woven fabrics are not suitable for sterilization as the thread weave does not allow penetration of the steam or the gas.

Paper

There are a variety of paper products (such as two-way crepe paper, parchment, and glassine) available for sterilization. Paper has a memory. As a result, when opening a package, the ends may flip back onto the item and contaminate the contents. Paper is not as durable as muslin or plastic. It punctures easily, and it is difficult to see pinholes or tears. Paper pouches and envelopes are usually sealed with tape. In removing the tape the paper frequently tears, and it is difficult to deliver an item from a pouch or envelope without contamination.

Plastic Films

Plastic films have gained increased popularity as a packaging material. They are pliable, durable, and impervious to dust and may be heat sealed. The contents of a plastic film package are easily visible. Some plastic films are impenetrable to steam; however, polypropylene (1 to 3 mils thickness) is acceptable for steam sterilization.

Polypropylene (1 to 3 mils) is available in rolls, bags, or pouches that are presealed on three sides; after the open side is heat-sealed, the package may be opened as a peel-back package (Fig. 8–2). When using a heat seal, it is advisable to use a double seal as this offers an extra margin of safety. Plastic films should be spot-checked for pinholes.

Polyethylene is used for dust covers on muslin or paper-wrapped packages. Dust covers, applied immediately after sterilization, prolong the shelf life of the item.

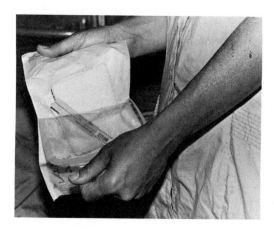

Figure 8-2. Peel back packages allow aseptic presentation of sterile items.

Nylon film is not acceptable for any sterilization process. In gas sterilization, nylon does not allow the gas to penetrate. In steam sterilization, the moisture cannot escape from the package and as a result the package remains wet.

Nonwoven Fabrics

Processed cellulose fibers, either alone or in combination with reinforcements of rayon or nylon, are manufactured as a nonwoven disposable wrapper. Nonwoven fabrics are tear resistant, lint free, flexible, and handle like muslin. Depending upon the process used in manufacturing, they range from water-resistant to water-repellent.

Nonwoven fabrics are available in three strengths. The light-weight strength is comparable to 140-thread-count muslin and requires 4 thicknesses for sterilization. The medium thickness is equal to one double muslin wrapper and requires two wrappers for sterilization. The heavy-duty weight fabric is used to manufacture surgical drapes and is available for instrument pans, basin sets, and large linen packs.

When used for basin and instrument sets, the condensation that occurs on metal during the steam-sterilization process may not be completely evaporated during the drying process. Damp or wet packages may result, and may not be noticed until the items are opened. Using one absorbent towel in the bottom of the instrument tray or between the basins and a second towel under the pans between the wrapper and the pans will alleviate this problem by absorbing the moisture. The towels will also serve as a cushion and will be added protection against the wrapper tearing.

Nonwoven fabrics are expensive as they are a one-use item. Incineration of nonwoven fabrics may come under increasing anti-air pollution regulations of the Environmental Protection Agency.

Plastic and Paper Combination

There are a variety of plastic and paper combinations available that may be used for either gas or steam sterilization. The paper allows the sterilizing agent to penetrate, and the plastic side allows the contents to be visible. Air must be evacuated from these packages prior to sealing to prevent rupture during sterilization. Using one package for both steam and gas alleviates the need to have multiple items in inventory.

Sterilization Containers

Rigid sterilization containers are beginning to take the place of wrappers, and they increase the physical protection to the instruments sterilized in this manner. These containers are made of heat-resistant plastics, stainless steel, and anodized aluminum. Perforations in the lid and the bottom surface are covered with steam-permeable, high-efficiency bacterial filters. The filters most commonly used are nonwoven and disposable.

Gravity-flow and high-vacuum steam or ethylene oxide sterilizers provide an adequate method for sterile processing when the containers are properly positioned for penetration of the steam. Flash sterilization is not currently recommended for sterilization of instruments in closed containers.

The use of one type or color of container for steam and another one for gas sterilization may reduce the number of errors that occur in sterilizing the items by the wrong method, and thus reduce repair and replacement costs.

Container system filters must remain intact, and valves and gaskets remain sealed following sterilization. Failure to do so will result in contamination of the contents.

Sterilization of Implants

Implants require special handling before and during sterilization. Therefore, it is important that these packages be clearly labeled so that they can be appropriately processed. Implantable items should be sterilized with a biologic indicator, and the item should not be implanted until the indicator has a negative reading, usually 48 hours after sterilization. If the implantable item cannot be presterilized with the biologic indicator, the item should be sterilized unwrapped in the equivalent of a full-cycle steam sterilization and not flash sterilized. Included in this cycle should be a biologic indicator that is read at the appropriate time interval after sterilization. If the indicator is found to be positive, the surgeon should be notified immediately.[5]

Time and Temperature Profile for Packaging Material

Steam sterilizers are set by the manufacturer for the time and temperature profile for steam penetration to the center of a test pack of 140-thread-count muslin. Manufacturers of all other packaging material should be requested to supply data indicating that their product has an equivalent time and temperature profile for steam sterilization.

Labeling

All items should be labeled as to the contents, the initials of the individual packaging the item, the date of sterilization, the date of expiration, and a lot-control number. The lot-control number indicates the sterilizer used and the cycle or load number. This facilitates the identification and the retrieval of supplies if the biologic monitor or mechanical control chart demonstrates improper function during the sterilization cycle.

Shelf Life

Shelf life is the length of time a package may be considered sterile. Shelf time is considered to be event-related rather than time-related and depends on many factors:

1. Type of material used for packaging
2. Number of thicknesses used
3. Number of times a package is handled before use
4. Storage on open or closed shelves
5. Condition of the storage area (i.e., cleanliness, temperature, humidity)
6. Type of seal on the package (i.e., heat or tape)
7. Use of dust covers and method of seal

A heat seal is a more secure method of closure and extends the shelf life.

The suggested shelf life for various materials (using closed cabinets) is as follows:

Item	Expiration
Linen (140-thread-count, 4 thicknesses) (280-thread-count, 2 thicknesses)	7 weeks
Linen-wrapped items, heat-sealed in dust covers after sterilization	9 months
Linen-wrapped items, tape-sealed in dust covers after sterilization	3 months
Paper	8 weeks
Plastic–paper combination, heat-sealed	1 year
Plastic films, tape-sealed	3 months
Plastic films, heat-sealed	1 year
Nonwoven fabrics	30 days

Appropriate rotation of supplies should reduce the number of items that require reprocessing.

Steam Sterilization

Historical Development. The research of Robert Koch, a German bacteriologist (1843–1910), on the disinfecting properties of steam and hot air marks the beginning of the science of disinfection and sterilization. Koch demonstrated that moist heat was a more effective method of sterilization than dry heat because of its greater penetrating powers.

In 1881, Koch and his associates developed the first nonpressure flowing-steam sterilizer (Fig. 8–3). It consisted of a metal cylinder in which water was heated through the bottom by a gas flame. The steam that resulted sterilized the items placed on shelves above the water.

In 1885, Schimmelbusch used the first steam sterilizer for the sterilization of surgical dressings, and in 1888, Hugo Davidsohn first demonstrated the use of boiling water as a method of sterilizing surgical instruments.

Other advances in the development of sterilization were made by Von Esmarch and Max Rubner. Von Esmarch emphasized the importance of using saturated steam

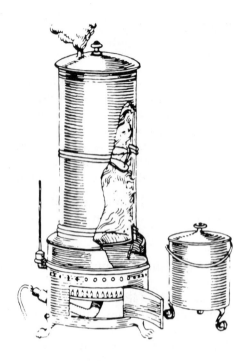

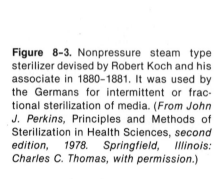

Figure 8-3. Nonpressure steam type sterilizer devised by Robert Koch and his associate in 1880–1881. It was used by the Germans for intermittent or fractional sterilization of media. (*From John J. Perkins,* Principles and Methods of Sterilization in Health Sciences, *second edition, 1978. Springfield, Illinois: Charles C. Thomas, with permission.*)

containing the maximum amount of water vapor in steam sterilization. Max Rubner demonstrated that the bacterial effect of steam is diminished in proportion to the amount of air present in the sterilizer.

In 1888, the Kny-Scheerer Company of New York produced the first steam sterilizer with a steam-tight radial-locking-arm door (Fig. 8–4).

The effects of formaldehyde gas as a disinfectant were identified in 1888. J. J. Kinyoun, an American biologist, discovered that greater penetration of formaldehyde could be achieved if the process was combined with steam.

During the early 1900s, sterilizers were designed for operation by a vacuum system of control. This system consisted of partial evacuation of air from the sterilizing chamber obtained by means of a steam ejection or vacuum attachment. The purpose of the evacuation was to assist in the displacement or removal of air from the chamber to ensure penetration of the items by the steam.[5]

In 1915, the gravity process of eliminating air from the chamber of the sterilizer was introduced through the efforts of W. B. Underwood. This sterilizer used the concept that, as pressure was built up in the chamber from the incoming steam, it would force air out through a drain located in the front and the bottom of the chamber. The drain emptied into a pail on the floor. The efficacy of this sterilizer was entirely dependent upon the individual operating the equipment (Fig. 8–5).

In 1933, the American Sterilizer Company introduced the first pressure steam sterilizer with a thermometer located in the discharge outlet at the bottom of the chamber (Fig. 8–6). The addition of the thermometer refined the process of sterilization and led to the development of high-vacuum, high-temperature steam sterilizers.

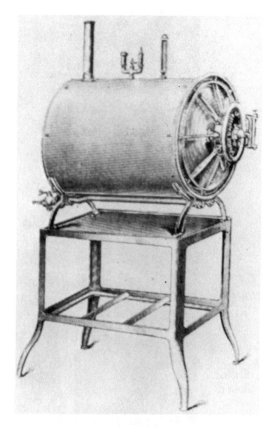

Figure 8-4. Early type of horizontal pressure sterilizer known as Kay-Sprague Steam Sterilizer. This type was steam jacketed and water from which steam was generated was contained in the jacket to which steam was applied directly. No precise system of air elimination was provided. A pressure gauge was furnished, but no thermometer. The door was one of the first equipped with radial arms for locking. (*From John J. Perkins,* Principles and Methods of Sterilization in Health Sciences, *second edition, 1978. Springfield, Illinois: Charles C. Thomas, with permission.*)

Saturated Steam Under Pressure

Moist heat in the form of saturated steam under pressure is the most economical, efficient, and rapid method of sterilization. It destroys all resistant bacterial spores and leaves no toxic residue. The components necessary for sterilization to occur by this method are heat, steam, pressure, and time. Heat independent of the other agents will destroy microorganisms; however, with the addition of moisture (steam) the time required for microbial destruction is reduced. The addition of pressure causes the steam to rise to a higher temperature. For example, in steam sterilization water is heated to boiling, 100°C (212°F), and is then converted to steam. As the pressure increases, the temperature is elevated (i.e., 15 lbs of pressure at 250°F, 27 lbs of pressure at 270°F, and 30 lbs of pressure at 274°F). The time required to kill microbes varies with the size and the physical characteristics of the items being sterilized, the type of sterilizer, cycle design, bioburden and packaging.

Death of microorganisms by moist heat is the result of denaturation and coagulation of the protein within the bacterial cells. Steam at the proper temperature for the proper amount of time must penetrate every fiber and all surfaces of the items for sterilization to occur. Therefore, it is essential that all air be eliminated from the chamber as air blocks the steam from penetrating the items to be sterilized.

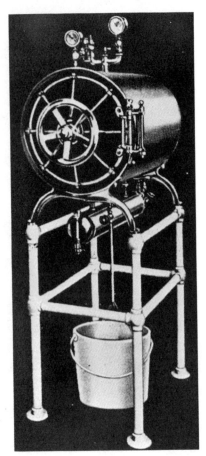

Figure 8–5. Typical pressure steam sterilizer of 1915, newly developed principle of gravity air discharge from chamber— first approach to modern temperature-controlled sterilizer. (*From John J. Perkins,* Principles and Methods of Steriliza- tion in Health Sciences, *second edition, 1978. Springfield, Illinois: Charles C. Thomas, with permission.*)

Two types of steam sterilizers available in most hospitals are the gravity displace- ment sterilizer and the prevacuum or high-vacuum sterilizer (Fig. 8–7).

Sterilizers are constructed of a rectangular or round chamber surrounded by an outer shell. The space between the two forms a jacket. Steam fills the jacket that sur- rounds the chamber. The material used in the construction is void of crevices and is resistant to the corrosive and erosive action of steam and water and other solutions. A safety steam-lock door is located at the front of the chamber.

When the door of the sterilizer is closed, the steam enters the inner chamber of the sterilizer at the back near the top and is deflected upward. By gravity the air goes to the bottom of the chamber and is forced out through a discharge outlet at the bottom front. The discharge outlet has a screen that serves as a filter to prevent lint and sediment from entering the waste line (Fig. 8–8). The temperature gauge for the chamber is located in the air discharge line, below the screen, as this is the coldest point in the chamber. When the proper temperature has been reached, the sterilization cycle begins. When the proper time has elapsed, the steam is exhausted from the chamber and the cycle is completed.

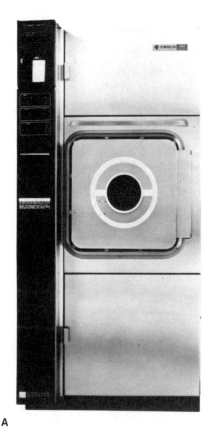

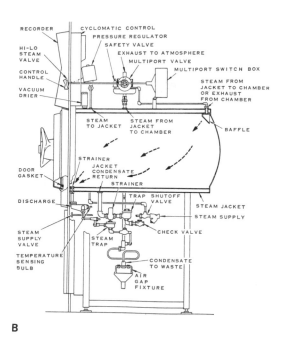

Figure 8-6. A. Modern sterilizer features automatic processing as microcomputer control. This sterilizer provides a printout of cycle parameters. **B.** Longitudinal cross section of sterilizer. (*Courtesy American Sterilizer Company, Erie, Pennsylvania.*)

Gravity displacement sterilizers are operated at 250°F, 270°F, or 274°F. The entire length of the cycle depends on the size and the physical characteristics of the item being sterilized. The heat-up time is the amount of time required to reach the holding time and temperature and is dependent on the density and the physical characteristics of the pack or the items being sterilized. A large pack (12″ × 12″ × 20″, maximum weight 12 lbs) usually requires 30 minutes to reach the holding temperature. The holding temperature is the amount of time required to kill the microbes at the center of the pack. The come-down time includes a drying period; again, this will vary with the density of the pack. The operator sets the holding time and temperature on the automated steam sterilizer. Before removing items from the steam sterilizer, the graph must always be checked for the appropriate time and temperature. Table 8–1 indicates the exposure period for items frequently sterilized in gravity displacement sterilizers. The exposure period represents the sum of the heat-up time, the minimum standard holding time, and a prescribed factor of safety.

Flash sterilization (270°F for 3 minutes) is recommended only when time does not

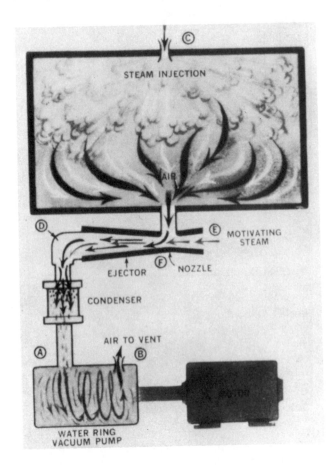

Figure 8-7. Schematic diagram to show one method of operation of a prevacuum sterilizer when simultaneous vacuum and steam injection are employed to rid the chamber and load of air. (*From John J. Perkins,* Principles and Methods of Sterilization in Health Sciences, *second edition, 1978. Springfield, Illinois: Charles C. Thomas, with permission.*)

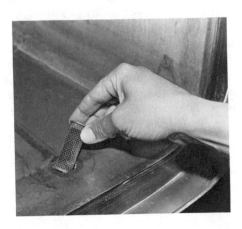

Figure 8-8. The strainer is removed and cleaned so that openings are kept free of lint and sediment.

TABLE 8-1. EXPOSURE PERIODS FOR STERILIZATION IN GRAVITY DISPLACEMENT STERILIZERS

Article	Minimum Time Required in Minutes	
	250–254° F (121–123° C)	*270° F[a] (132° C)*
Brushes, in dispensers, in cans, or individually wrapped	30	15
Dressings, wrapped in paper or muslin	30	15
Glassware, empty, inverted	15	3
Instruments, metal only, any number (unwrapped)[b]	15	3
Instruments, metal, combined with suture, tubing, or other porous materials (unwrapped)[b]	20	10
Instruments, metal only, in covered and/or padded tray[b]	20	10
Instruments, metal, combined with other materials (in covered and/or padded tray)[b]	30	15
Instruments wrapped in double thickness muslin[b]	30	15
Linen, packs (maximum size 12″ × 12″ × 20″ and weight 12 pounds)	30	
Needles, individually packaged in glass tubes or paper, lumen moist	30	15
Needles, unwrapped (lumen moist)	15	3
Rubber catheters, drains, tubing, etc. (lumen moist), unwrapped	20	10
Rubber catheters, drains, tubing, etc., individually packaged in muslin or paper (lumen moist)	30	15
Treatment trays, wrapped in muslin or paper	30	
Utensils, unwrapped, on edge	15	3
Utensils, wrapped in muslin or paper, on edge	20	10
Syringes, unassembled, individually packaged in muslin or paper	30	15
Syringes, unassembled, unwrapped	15	3
Sutures, silk, cotton, or nylon wrapped in paper or muslin	30	15
Solutions	**Slow Exhaust**	
75 ml–250 ml	20	
500 ml–1000 ml	30	
1500 ml–2000 ml	40	

[a]Frequently referred to as "Flash Sterilizer."
[b]Maximum weight of each instrument tray is 16 lbs.

permit sterilization by the preferred wrapped method. Speed works against reliability of sterilization. It reduces the margin of safety, the ability to accommodate operator error, increases the possibility of trapped air, and requires a high degree of reliability in the sterilizer.[6]

Prevacuum or High-Vacuum Sterilizer. The prevacuum or high-vacuum sterilizer differs from the gravity displacement sterilizer in the manner in which air is eliminated from the chamber and the load. As the air is evacuated, "conditioning steam" is injected into the chamber, thus diffusing the air in the space surrounding the items. Conditioning the load assures fast heating to the sterilizing temperatures. At the completion of the steam cycle, a vacuum cycle exhausts steam from the chamber and air is admitted through a bacteria-retentive filter to relieve the vacuum, to return the chamber to atmospheric pressure, to remove moisture, and to cool the load. The prevacuum sterilizer operates at 270°F.

Steam under pressure may not be used on heat-sensitive items, oils, ointments, and powders.

The steam sterilizer must be loaded to allow the passage of steam through the load from the top of the chamber at the back toward the front to the discharge line. This requires that the sterilizer not be overloaded as this would inhibit complete permeation of the materials with the moisture and the heat of the steam.

Flat-bottom trays, such as mayo trays, and large linen packs should be placed on edge in the vertical position. Large packs should be placed on the bottom shelf of the loading car with smaller items on the shelf above. When placing two layers of packages on one shelf, the upper layer should be placed crosswise on the lower layer. When porous and nonporous items are in the same load, the nonporous items should be placed on the bottom shelf to prevent the condensation from dripping onto the surface of the porous items.

All utensils are placed on edge so that if they contained water it would flow out. When utensils are nested, they should be separated with an absorbent towel or other wicking material to facilitate the passage of steam to all surfaces and also the adequate drying of the items. Instrument trays with mesh bottoms may be placed flat on the shelves as the steam and the moisture can adequately circulate through the tray.

Solutions must be sterilized separately and the sterilizer set on "slow exhaust" to prevent the solution from boiling over.

When the sterilization cycle is completed, the door should be opened and the contents be permitted to dry for 20 to 30 minutes. Placing warm, moist articles on a metal surface will cause condensation to form with possible penetration of the wrapper and subsequent contamination of the articles.

Routine Maintenance of Steam Sterilizers. Weekly, the inside of sterilizers, the loading cars, and perforated shelves should be washed with a mild detergent solution, such as Calgonite, and then rinsed with water. This is to prevent the buildup of residue from the steam line on items being sterilized. Abrasive cleaning compounds, steel wool, or wire brushes must not be used on the interior surfaces as they may corrode and scratch the surface.

During the weekly cleaning, the strainer located at the front of the autoclave should be removed and 1 quart of hot water containing 1 ounce of trisodium phosphate should be flushed down the drain line. This should be followed with 1 quart of hot tap water. This weekly flushing of the discharge system will keep the drainline free of clogging substances, such as grease and resins. If these are allowed to accumulate, there may be some retardation of the discharge of air and condensation from the chamber.

This strainer should be removed daily and cleaned so the pores are free from lint and sediment.

Dry-heat Sterilization

Dry-heat sterilization is used only when direct contact of the material with saturated steam is impractical or unattainable. In this method of sterilization organisms are destroyed by oxidation. This requires high temperatures and long exposure periods. Dry heat is used effectively on anhydrous oils, greases, powders, and other substances that would be damaged by steam or that are insoluble in water and therefore not permeated by moist heat. Since dry heat does not exert a corrosive effect on sharp instruments or erode ground glass, it can be used on cutting instruments, needles, and syringes.

The equipment used for dry-heat sterilization consists of a well-insulated oven, heated by electricity, with a fan inside to circulate the air to effect better heat distribution.

The effectiveness of dry heat depends on the penetration of heat through the object to be sterilized. Thus, the nature of the material, the method of preparation and packaging, and the loading of the sterilizer are important factors in determining the time and the temperature. The following time–temperature ratios are considered reliable for dry-heat sterilization (note that times given do not include heat-up time):

356°F (180°C)	30 minutes
340°F (170°C)	1 hour
320°F (160°C)	2 hours
285°F (140°C)	3 hours
250°F (121°C)	6 hours

Ionizing Radiation

Some items purchased from manufacturers as sterile items are sterilized by ionizing radiation. The principal types of radiation plants are the cobalt 60 gamma ray emitters and high-energy electron accelerators. The most commonly used type is the cobalt 60 as it produces gamma rays capable of penetrating bulk objects such as cartons ready for shipment.

Currently, ionizing radiation is used only by industry due to the high initial cost and the size of the facility required. Sterilization by this method is reliable, requires less energy, and is relatively inexpensive to maintain.

Chemical Sterilization—Ethylene Oxide

Ethylene oxide (ETO) was discovered and discussed by C. A. Wurtz in 1859 as a room fumigant. In 1929, H. Schrader and E. Bossert discovered that ethylene oxide possessed bactericidal properties, and in 1956, ETO was first used in hospitals as a sterilizing agent.

Ethylene oxide is currently the most acceptable and effective chemical sterilizing agent for heat- and moisture-sensitive items. It is noncorrosive and completely penetrates all porous material. Ethylene oxide is a highly toxic substance, and all ETO sterilizer and aeration equipment should be exhaust-ventilated to the outside of the building away from pedestrian traffic, other work areas, and air intake vents. Symptoms of ethylene oxide exposure are nausea, vomiting, headache, irritation of the respiratory passage and eyes, drowsiness, weakness, and lack of coordination.

In 1984, the Occupational Safety and Health Administration (OSHA) established a permissible limit for occupational exposure to ETO at one part per one million parts of air (1 ppm). This was determined as a time-weighted average exposure over an 8-hour period. In 1988, OSHA established an additional limit for exposure to ETO as 5 ppm averaged over a sampling period of 15 minutes.[7] To achieve this excursion level, institutions may need to implement the following engineering controls:

1. Implement a postvacuum purge at the end of the sterilization cycle
2. Install a local exhaust above the sterilizer chamber door
3. Implement an exhaust system to the outside of the building
4. Locate the sterilization area in an isolated area under negative pressure
5. Implement 6 to 10 air exchanges per hour in the sterilization area
6. Install conveyors from the sterilizer chamber to the aeration area[8]

To monitor compliance with the OSHA regulations, employers are required to perform breathing zone sampling by a method that is accurate to a confidence level of 95% for airborn concentrations of ETO at the excursion level of 5 ppm. Samplings should represent 15-minute exposures associated with job tasks that are most likely to produce exposures above the excursion level in each area, for each job classification, and for each shift. Monitoring of the individual who would be most likely to receive the greatest exposure is sufficient to meet the regulation.[8] The frequency of monitoring will depend on the results obtained. There are six possible combinations of time-weighted-average and short-term exposures that will dictate monitoring needs (Table 8–2).

Activities such as changing ETO tanks and cleaning the sterilizers may result in short-term, high exposures and the employees performing these tasks should wear respirators for additional protection.[2]

Ethylene oxide's bactericidal action is due to an irreversible alkylation. ETO chemically interferes with the nucleic acids and alters the metabolic and reproductive processes of the microbial cell resulting in inactivation or death of the cell. The rate at which the destruction of the organisms occurs appears to be related to the rate of diffusion of the gas through the cell wall and the availability or accessibility of the cell's nucleic acid to react with ethylene oxide.[2]

Ethylene oxide is commercially available as a highly flammable liquid, explosive in air. For this reason, ETO is mixed with carbon dioxide or fluorocarbons (Freon) to reduce its explosive and flammable potential.

The process of sterilization with ethylene oxide is more complicated than with steam

TABLE 8-2. ETHYLENE OXIDE EXPOSURE REQUIRING MONITORING

Exposure	Required Monitoring
Below the action level at or below the excursion level	No monitoring required
Below the action level and above the excursion level	No time-weighted-average monitoring required; monitor short-term exposures four times per year
At or above the action level, at or below the time weighted average, and at or below the excursion level	Monitor time-weighted-average exposures two times per year
At or above the action level, at or below the time weighted average, and above the excursion level	Monitor time-weighted-average exposures two times per year, and monitor short-term exposures four times per year
Above the time weighted average and at or below the excursion level	Monitor time-weighted-average exposures four times per year
Above the time weighted average and above the excursion level	Monitor time-weighted-average and short-term exposures four times per year.

Time weighted average = 1 ppm averaged during an 8-hour period
Excursion level = 5 ppm averaged during a 15-minute sampling period
From Occupational exposure to ethylene oxide, final standard. Fed Reg. *April 6, 1988, with permission*

or dry heat. In addition to the time and the temperature required for steam and dry heat, the concentration of ETO and moisture are important to gas sterilization.

Temperature ranges from 120° to 140°F (49° to 60°C) are most frequently used in ETO sterilizers. The temperature is an important factor in the sterilizing efficiency of ethylene oxide as it affects the destruction of microorganisms by enhancing the penetration of ETO through the cell wall. An increase in temperature results in the required exposure time being decreased.

The appropriate concentration of ETO is essential in gas sterilization. The recommended concentration is 450 mg/L. Higher concentrations up to 1000 mg/L may be used, and exposure periods are then reduced to about one half. Concentrations greater than 1000 mg/L do not appreciably affect exposure times.

Moisture is important to the sterilizing efficiency of ethylene oxide. The optimum humidity levels are 20% to 40%. A humidity level lower than 20% and higher than 65% reduces the sterilizing properties of ETO.[2] The moisture content of microbial cells is also important in gas sterilization as dry or dessicated organisms are more resistant to the penetration of ETO. To avoid dehydration of organisms, the relative humidity in the area where the items are packaged for sterilization should be maintained at 50% or more.

The amount of time required for gas sterilization is related directly to the temperature, the bioburden, the moisture content, and the porosity of the item; the packaging material; and the concentration of the gas. Adherence to the manufacturer's guidelines in operating the gas sterilizer is imperative to the effectiveness and the efficiency of this method of sterilization.

Ethylene oxide can be used to sterilize telescopic instruments, plastic items, rubber items, delicate instruments, cameras, sutures, electrical cords, pumps, and motors. Exposure of glass vials of solution will result in only the outside of the vial being sterile as ethylene oxide does not penetrate glass.

Ethylene oxide may not be used on some acrylic plastic materials, medications, and pharmaceuticals as it will alter the chemical composition.

Preparation of Items for Gas Sterilization. Prior to packaging, all items must be clean and dry. Wet items will remain wet, and the water may unite with ethylene oxide to form ethylene glycol and ethylene chlorohydrin. These substances are not eliminated by aeration and may result in toxic reactions in patients and personnel.

In loading the gas sterilizer, an attempt should be made to sterilize full loads of items having common aeration times (Fig. 8–9). The sterilizer must be loaded so the gas can circulate freely to penetrate the entire load. Items should be loaded so they do not trap air, pool water, nor contact the chamber wall. Overloading should be avoided. Items should be placed in baskets or on the cart so the operator does not come in contact with the packages when the load is transferred from the sterilizer to the aerator.

Aeration. The sterilizer door should be opened approximately 6 inches as soon as possible after completion of the cycle and left open for 15 minutes to allow most of the residual ETO to dissipate from the chamber and exit via the exhaust system. During this time, personnel should not be near the sterilizer.

Following this period, the cart or baskets should be transported to either a mechanical aerator or to a room designated as the aeration area. The cart should be pulled from the front as this places the employee upwind from the hazardous material. Metal and glass that are unwrapped do not require aeration; all other items must be aerated. Since the residual gas can cause burns if it is in contact with the skin, special gloves for han-

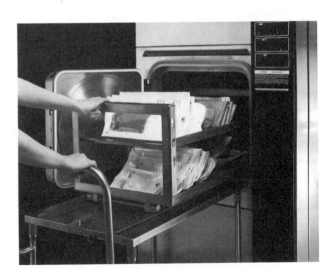

Figure 8-9. Loading the gas sterilizer so the gas can circulate freely to penetrate the entire load. (*Courtesy American Sterilizer Co., Erie, Pennsylvania.*)

dling ETO items must be worn. If protective cotton or rubber gloves are worn, they should be placed in the aerator after use to reduce environmental contamination.

The specific aeration time depends upon the composition and the porosity of the sterilized items, the type of ETO sterilization used, the packaging material, the intended use of the item, the temperature of the aerator, and the air flow rate. Specific aeration recommendations should be obtained in writing from manufacturers on all items requiring gas sterilization. In the absence of such recommendations the guidelines in Table 8–3 may be used.

If ambient aeration is used, the ventilation in the room must be maintained at a negative pressure and ventilated outside the building. Access to the room should be restricted to persons needed to operate the area, and storage of other supplies in this area is prohibited. Inappropriate aeration of items sterilized by ethylene oxide has resulted in the following outcomes: facial burns from anesthesia face masks, laryngotracheal inflammation from endotracheal tubes, and blood hemolysis from tubing used in hemodialysis and cardiopulmonary bypass.

Ethylene oxide should not be used on any item that can be steam sterilized.

Liquid Chemical Sterilization

A solution of 2% activated aqueous glutaraldehyde is the most commonly used liquid chemosterilizer. It is noncorrosive and nonstaining and safe for all instruments that can be immersed in a chemical solution. Glutaraldehyde may be used on heat-sensitive items when ethylene oxide is not available. It is most frequently used on cystoscopes and bronchoscopes because it does not damage lenses or the cement of lensed instruments. Glutaraldehyde kills vegetative microorganisms in 5 minutes, tubercle bacilli in 10 minutes, and spores in 10 hours. Items totally immersed in glutaraldehyde for 10 minutes are disinfected. Sterilization takes 10 hours.

When using a liquid chemosterilizer, the item must be clean and dry before being immersed in the solution. Wet items will dilute the concentration of the sterilant. All surfaces of the item must be in contact with the sterilant. After items are removed from the liquid sterilant, they should be thoroughly rinsed with sterile distilled water to avoid tissue damage.

Most cold sterilizing solutions are effective for a specific period of time and there are no biologic indicators for liquid sterilization or disinfection. Therefore, it is essential that the manufacturer's instructions be followed when preparing the solution and in calculating the expiration date.

In the evaluation of liquid chemosterilizers, only those products that indicate on the product label that they are registered as a sterilant by the United States Environmental Protection Agency should be considered as a sterilizing agent.

TABLE 8-3. MECHANICAL AERATION CABINET

Air Changes Per Hour	Temperature	Time
4	50° C (122° F)	12 hours
4	60° C (140° F)	8 hours
12–25	Room temperature 18–22° C (65–72° F)	7 days

Monitoring the Sterilization Process

A chemical indicator is placed in the center of each package prior to sterilization. The chemical indicator is a paper treated with a sensitive dye or chemical that changes color or its physical status when conditions for sterilization have occurred. The conditions for steam sterilization are time, temperature, and moisture. For gas sterilization, the conditions are time, humidity, gas concentration, and temperature. A pellet in a glass tube may be used as an indication for steam sterilization. This indicator is not as reliable, as the pellet melts in response to time and temperature.

The chemical indicators do not prove that sterilization has been achieved, only that the items have been exposed to the physical conditions within the sterilizing chamber. When sterile packages are opened, the scrub assistant should check the indicator prior to handling the item or to placing it on the sterile field to assure that these conditions were met.

Pressure-sensitive tape on the outside of the package indicates that the items have been exposed to the physical conditions of the sterilization cycle. There are two types of tape, one for steam and the other for gas. Pressure-sensitive tape may change in color if stored in an area of high temperature and high humidity.

In all high-vacuum sterilizers the Bowie-Dick test should be conducted on the first sterilization cycle of the day or at a designated time each day if the sterilizer is used 24 hours a day. The test pack should not be processed with other items. To perform the test four pieces of autoclave tape, 8 inches long, are crisscrossed on a cotton huckaback towel; towels are then folded and stacked one on top of another until the stack measures 10 to 11 inches (25 to 28 cm). The pack is then wrapped and placed in the lower front area of the sterilizer, and the cycle is run. The Bowie-Dick test is designed to monitor the efficiency of the vacuum system of a prevacuum steam sterilizer by detecting air leaks and residual air. Uniform color changes on the autoclave tape indicate the complete elimination of air from the test pack. If the steam supply to the sterilizer was turned off, a minimum of 30 minutes is required between turning on the steam and running the test pack.

A mechanically controlled time–temperature chart is maintained on each steam sterilizer. This graph indicates and records the same temperature as that shown by the indicating thermometer located in the discharge system of the sterilizing chamber. It also records the load number, and the duration of each exposure. If the exposure periods are greater or less than prescribed, or if the temperature was not reached, there is a record of the errors. This provides evidence upon which to act in correcting discrepancies. The graph should be checked after each sterilization cycle and should be changed daily or more often as required by the manufacturer's instructions.

Mechanically controlled charts are not available on all ethylene oxide sterilizers. When they are present, they should be changed daily and used as a reference during and after the cycle to check the effectiveness of the unit.

Biologic monitoring is the only method that provides positive assurance that sterilization was achieved. There are commercially available biological indicators using dry spores that are highly resistant to gas or steam sterilization. *Bacillus stearothermophilus* is used for steam sterilizers and *Bacillus subtilis* for ethylene oxide and dry-heat sterilizers. The spores are available in ampules, capsules, or strips. Each of the biologic control units contain a strip to be sterilized and a control strip not to be sterilized. Two biologic indicators and one internal chemical indicator, separated from each other by one towel, are placed in the center of a pack that consists of 3 muslin surgeon gowns, 12 towels, 30 4 × 4-inch gauze sponges, 5 12 × 12-inch lap sponges, and one muslin drape sheet. The biologic test pack is placed near the bottom front of the steam sterilizer or in the middle section of the gas sterilizer. When the cycle is complete, the test indicator is removed from the pack and sent with the control indicator to the bacteriology laboratory.

Self-contained biologic indicators are available to monitor flash sterilizers. They contain both the dry spore strip and the growth medium and can be incubated in the surgical suite.

Biologic testing is performed weekly on steam and dry-heat sterilizers. Each cycle of ethylene oxide sterilizers should contain a biologic monitor. Whenever possible, the gas-sterilized items should not be used until the results of the bacterial monitoring process are known.

If the results of the bacterial monitoring are positive, the sterilizer is taken out of service until it is inspected by a qualified individual, the sterilizer retested, and negative results obtained. All items processed during the interval of time from when the biologic monitoring was performed to when the positive results were obtained are considered unsterile. They should be retrieved and reprocessed.

The effectiveness of the aeration chambers can be monitored by using a rubber or plastic device that absorbs ethylene oxide. When the device absorbs the gas, it changes color; when the indicator is placed in an aerator, the color will fade to indicate that safe levels of ethylene oxide have been reached. There are two types of indicators, one for polyvinyl chloride items (as these items require the longest aeration) and one for all the other items.

Preventive maintenance should be performed quarterly by a qualified individual. The efficiency and the accuracy of gauges, charts, steam lines, and drains should be tested on a regular schedule. Following any repairs and after the steam supply has been turned on for at least 30 minutes, a test pack with biologic indicators should be run and negative results obtained before the sterilizer is used for regular service.

Records are kept on all sterilizers and retained for the period of time indicated by the state's statute of limitations. A sterilizer record system contains the following:

1. Sterilizer identification number
2. Date
3. Cycle numbers
4. Contents of each lot
5. Duration and temperature of sterilizing phase (recording chart)
6. Identification of the operator
7. Results of biologic tests
8. Bowie-Dick test results on high-vacuum sterilizers
9. Record of repairs
10. Record of preventive maintenance

Commercially Packaged Sterile Items

There are many items commercially available to hospitals that are marketed as *presterile*. Before purchasing these items, it is important to carefully examine the package. The

TABLE 8-4. COMMONLY USED CHEMICAL DISINFECTANTS

Agent	Microorganism Destroyed and Time Required " = Minutes	Mechanisms of Action	Practical Use	Usefulness		Precautions
				Disinfectant	Antiseptic	
Mercurials	Weak bacteriostat	Oxidation combines with proteins	None	None	Poor	Unpleasant odor, tissue reactions on skin and mucous membrane; personnel must wear gloves when using agent.
Phenolic Compounds	Bactericidal—10" Pseudomonacidal—10" Fungicidal—10" Tuberculocidal—20"	Surface active—disrupts membrane Inactivates enzymes Denaturation of proteins	Walls, furniture, floors, equipment	Good	Poor	
Quartenary Ammonium Compounds ("Quats")	Bactericidal—10" Pseudomonacidal—10" Fungicidal—10"	Surface active—disrupts cell membrane Inactivation of enzymes Denaturation of proteins	Limited hospital use as these do not destroy gram negative pathogens and tubercle bacilli	Fair	Fair	Neutralized by soap; active agent is absorbed by gauze and fabrics thus reducing strength.
Chlorine Compounds	Most gram-negative bacteria pseudomonas Virucidal	Oxidation of enzymes	Spot cleaning of floors and furniture	Good	Fair	Inactive in presence of organic debris, unpleasant odor, corrosive to metal.
Iodine Compounds (Iodine + detergents = Iodophors)	Bactericidal—10" Pseudomonacidal—10" Fungicidal—10" Tuberculocidal—20" with minimum concentration of 450 ppm of iodine	Oxidation of essential enzymes	Dark-colored floors, furniture, walls	Good	Good	Iodine stains fabrics and tissues; may corrode instruments. Inactivated by organic debris.

196

Agent	Mechanism of Action	Antimicrobial Activity	Uses			Comments
Alcohol (usually isopropyl and ethyl alcohol 70%–90% by volume)	Denaturation of proteins	Bactericidal—10″ Pseudomonacidal—10″ Fungicidal—10″ Tuberculocidal—15″	Spot cleaning Damp dusting equipment	Good	Very Good	Inactivated by organic debris; becomes ineffective when it evaporates. Dissolves cement mounting on lensed instruments and fogs lenses, blanches floor tile.
Formaldehyde Aqueous Formalin 4% or 10%	Coagulation of proteins	Bactericidal—5″ Pseudomonacidal—5″ Fungicidal—5″ Tuberculocidal—15″ Virucidal—15″	Lensed instruments	Fair	None	Irritating fumes, toxic to tissue, rubber and porous material absorb the agent.
Alcohol Formalin (8% formaldehyde and 70% isopropyl alcohol)	Coagulation of proteins	Tuberculocidal—10″ Virucidal—10″ Sporicidal—12 Hours	Instruments	Good	None	Dissolves cement mounting on lensed instruments; toxic to tissue, irritating fumes.
Glutaraldehyde	Denaturation of protein	Vegetative microorganisms—5″ Tubercle bacilli—10″ Spores—10 hours	Disinfection of instruments in 10″. Useful for lensed instruments Effective liquid chemosterilizer in 10 hours.	Good	None	Unpleasant odor, tissue reaction may occur; instruments must be rinsed well in distilled water.

package should have wide margins that allow easy hand gripping when opening the package. The package must be the appropriate size; too small a package may result in the item falling out of the package when it is opened, and too large a package will take up excessive storage space. The outer edges of the package must not touch the sterile product, and the nurse must have complete control of the product at all times during the opening process.

Manufacturers of presterile supplies culture and quarantine the items until the results of the cultures validate the sterility. These supplies are packaged with inner and outer envelopes that are mechanically sealed. This method of packaging makes it almost impossible for normal biologic contaminants to gain access to the interior of the package. The sterility should be maintained as long as the package remains intact. However, as identified previously in this chapter, sterility is event-related. Therefore, the conditions of storage, the amount of handling, and the type of packaging material will affect the sterility. Nurse managers should emphasize the importance of rotating presterile supplies. Supply levels should be evaluated routinely and adjusted according to the changes in the surgical case load.

DISINFECTANTS

Disinfection is the process by which pathogenic agents or disease-producing microbes, excluding bacterial spores, are destroyed by either physical or chemical means. Disinfectants are liquid chemical compounds used on inanimate objects such as furniture, floors, walls, equipment, and some heat-sensitive items. An antiseptic is a chemical substance that prevents growth either by inhibiting or destroying microorganisms. These agents are used primarily for topical application to the skin and the mucous membrane. There are some chemical compounds that may be used as both disinfectants and antiseptics.

Disinfectants and antiseptics are identified as bacteriostatic or bactericidal. Agents that are bacteriostatic act by inhibiting growth. However, when the agent is removed, the cells will resume normal multiplication. Bactericidal agents kill bacteria. Sporicides, virucides, and fungicides are agents that kill spores, viruses, or fungi, respectively. Microorganisms differ in their resistance to chemicals. Most vegetative bacteria are susceptible to chemical compounds, tubercle bacilli and nonlipid viruses are significantly more resistant, and bacterial spores are highly resistant.

For disinfectants or antiseptics to affect microorganisms, they must act on some vital part of the cell. Some agents alter the cytoplasmic membrane. This membrane is easily injured by substances that reduce surface tension. Other chemical agents can react directly with certain enzymes, the nucleus, or structural proteins such as the cell wall. Certain chemical compounds are effective against one type of organism and not another.

Several important factors to be considered in using the disinfection process are the following:

1. Number of microorganisms
2. Amount and kind of organic debris
3. Concentration of the disinfectant
4. Temperature of the solution

The larger the number of organisms contaminating the skin or inanimate object, the longer it takes for the germicide to destroy them. Organic matter such as blood, feces, and tissue inhibits the efficiency of the germicide by absorbing the germicide molecules and inactivating them. The proper concentration of the disinfectant will depend on the material to be disinfected and the manufacturer's guidelines. Higher concentrations will affect the bactericidal activity. Most chemical compounds will be bacteriostatic in low-level concentrations and become bactericidal in high-level concentrations. An increase in temperature will accelerate the rate of the chemical reaction. Table 8–4 identifies some of the commonly used chemical disinfectants.

REFERENCES

1. Litsky BY. Microbiology of sterilization. *AORN J.* 1977; 26(2):334
2. Perkins JJ. *Principles and Methods of Sterilization in Health Sciences.* Springfield, Ill: Charles C. Thomas; 1982:33, 213
3. Greene VW, Borlaug GM, Nelson E. Effects of patching on sterilization of surgical textiles. *AORN J.* 1981; 33(7):1260
4. Recommended Practices for Selection and use of Packaging Materials. Denver: AORN; 1988; 48(5):961–968
5. Garner J, Favero M. Guidelines for Handwashing and Hospital Environmental Control 1985. Atlanta, Ga: Centers for Disease Control; 1985:11
6. In Hospital Sterility Assurance—Current Perspectives, Flash Sterilization. Arlington, Va: Association for the Advancement of Medical Instrumentation; 1982:63
7. Occupational exposure to ethylene oxide final standard. *Fed Reg.* 1988; 53(66):11414
8. Occupational exposure to ethylene oxide. *Fed Reg.* 1983; 48(78):17285

PART FOUR

Intraoperative Care
of the Surgical Patient

Chapter 9

Preparation of the Patient and Surgical Team Members

ADMISSION OF THE PATIENT TO THE SURGICAL SUITE

The information obtained by the perioperative nurse during the preoperative assessment with regard to appropriate method or mode of transportation; unusual patient problems such as impaired mobility; alterations in sensory perceptions, or emotional status; and any individual patient requests such as wearing a prosthesis to the surgical suite should be conveyed to the individual responsible for transporting the patient to the surgical suite.

As indicated in Chapter 5 in the model care plan for the 2- to 3-year-old (Table 5–9), children should be allowed and encouraged to bring a favorite toy or security blanket to the surgical suite to assist in minimizing their anxiety.

The stretcher used to transport presurgical patients is equipped with side rails, a safety strap, and an IV pole, and should have the capability of being placed in Trendelenburg's position.

In some institutions, the primary care nurse will accompany the patient to the surgical suite or the holding area and will give a report to the perioperative nurse (Fig. 9–1).

The operating room nurse greets the patient by identifying herself or himself and then identifies the patient by asking the patient, "What is your name?" This precludes errors that may occur when a patient is asked, "Are you Mrs. Brown?" Patients who have received a premedication may be drowsy or disoriented and may respond inappropriately to this form of questioning. The patient's name is verified with the identification bracelet and the chart using the patient's name and patient identification number. Correct identification is everyone's responsibility, and it should not be assumed that someone else has correctly identified the patient.

Following the identification process, the perioperative nurse will check the chart and the preoperative check list for completeness. The preoperative checklist (Fig. 9–2) enhances the admission process since it identifies, according to hospital policy, the information required on all presurgical patients. This form is completed by the unit nurse prior to the patient's transport to the surgical suite and is then verified by the operating room nurse when admitting the patient to the surgical suite. Specific areas that must be checked are as follows:

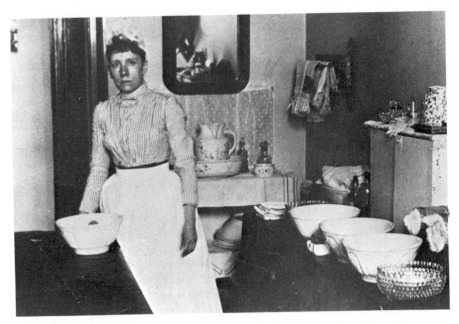

Figure 9-1. Setting up for an operation, Bellevue Hospital, 1885. (*The Bettmann Archive.*)

1. Patient's identification band checked against chart, addressograph card, and name on surgical schedule
2. Allergies
3. Laboratory results as determined by hospital policy (these usually include hemoglobin, hematocrit, urine analysis, chest x-ray, and electrocardiogram on patients over 40 years of age)
4. Physician's history and physical examination completed and recorded on the chart
5. The last time the patient had anything to eat or drink
6. Prosthetic devices such as eyeglasses, contact lenses, artificial hair or eyelashes, dentures, hearing aid, and other implants such as pacemakers, intraocular lens, total joints replaced, etc.
7. Preoperative medication given and charted and effects noted by the unit nurse; the perioperative nurse should also observe the patient for signs and symptoms of any adverse affects of the preoperative medication
8. Specific preoperative orders such as a surgical shave, a plaster cast that is to be bivalved or removed, and medications such as eye drops that need to be administered
9. The consent for surgery form must be signed, witnessed, and dated; the operative permit must agree with the site and the side as listed on the surgical schedule; perioperative nurses should be familiar with state and hospital requirements regarding who may sign the consent and who may witness the consent

Instructions:
1. Sign initials and name - top left corner.
2. Complete Pre-Operative Teaching checklist on reverse side.
3. If necessary, circle, ✓, or write in response. (NA=not applicable). Write comments on line to right.
4. Initial each item after completion.
5. Circled items are to be completed for both adult and pediatric patients.

UNIT NUMBER

PT. NAME

BIRTHDATE

INITIALS	NAME

LOCATION   DATE

INITIALS OF FLOOR NURSE | INITIALS PRE-OP/HOLDING AREA NURSE | INITIALS OF OR NURSE

Chart Information
1. Isolation type: _____ Precautions: _____
2. Allergies: ☐ NKA ☐ YES (list) _____ Chart flagged: ☐Yes
3. Mental and physical disabilities: ☐ No ☐ Yes (list) _____
4. Primary language: ☐ English ☐ Other _____ Interpreter ☐Obtained ☐Ordered
5. Old charts are required to be sent to the OR: (specify how many volumes are sent) _____

Procedures Completed
1. NPO since: _____ 2.☐ Voided at _____ ☐ Catheterized on-call at _____
3. Prep completed on floor as per medical order _____
4. Neuro prep orders written _____
5. Prep completed in Holding/Pre-Op Area by: (signature) _____
6. Pre-Op Meds given: _____
7. Pre-Op teaching completed: (see back of form) _____
8. Weight: (to be done on cardiac, major abdominal/vascular and pediatric patients) _____ Kg

Patient Assessment
1. Identification band checked against chart & addressograph card: (location of band) _____
2. Allergy band on patient: ☐ NKA ☐ Yes (location of allergy band) _____
3. Pressure Sore Risk Assessment Score: _____ Describe precautions taken if applicable _____
4. Pre-Op mental status: (describe) _____
5. Eyeglasses, lenses, make-up, wigs, dentures, hearing aid or other prosthesis removed: ☐ N/A ☐ YES (note disposition and exceptions) _____
6. Rings taped, other valuables removed: ☐ N/A ☐ YES (note disposition) _____
7. Garments removed: ☐ N/A ☐ YES (belongings record complete) _____

Chart Complete
1. ☐ UA _____ ☐ Hgb & HCT _____ reports in chart: (must be within 1 week)
2. ☐ CXR _____ ☐ EKG _____ reports in chart if ordered.
3. Informed consent progress notes written by Physician.
4. Necessary forms complete and in chart: (check those included) ___NURSING HISTORY AND ASSESSMENT
   ___NURSES NOTES ___FLOWSHEET ___I & O ___V.S. ___Hx & P.E. BY M.D.
   ___MEDICATION SHEET ___EFFECTS OF PRE-OP MED CHARTED ___SIGNED/DATED/WITNESSED CONSENT

___N/A Pediatrics Only (all items above also required)
1. Description of security blanket or toy with patient (ID Band on toy) _____

___N/A SCN/ICN Requirements (circled items above also required)
1. Record results of diagnostic work:
   A. CBC: Hct _____ Hgb _____ WBC _____ Platelets _____ E. Lytes: _____
   B. Hct from ICN: _____   F. Calcium: _____
   C. ABG: _____   G. Glucose Heelstick: _____
   D. PT & PTT: _____   H. UA: _____
2. Ventilation: ET Size _____ ; placement _____ ; FIO2 _____ ; f _____ ; PIP _____ ; PEEP _____
3. Temperature immediately prior to departure _____ 4. Weight _____ 5. Available Blood _____
6. Baptized (if requested) ☐Yes ☐No 7. Visit by parents ☐Yes ☐No
8. Pictures taken ☐Yes ☐No 9.Equipment protocol complete _____
10. External heat source applied ☐Yes ☐No Type _____

Patient sent to OR by: _____ Title _____
Patient received in Holding/Pre-Op Area by: _____ Title _____
Patient received in OR by: _____ Title _____

Figure 9–2A. Perioperative checklist. (*From the University of California, San Francisco, Calif., with permission.*)

PRE-OPERATIVE TEACHING CHECKLIST

Instructions:
1. Sign name and initials on reverse side.
2. In initial column, initial those items you explain. If CCTV is used or material is not applicable (NA), circle appropriate items and initial.
3. Where necessary, place a "√" to indicate specific items discussed. If appropriate, fill in item 7.
4. For each item covered, circle Y (yes), N (no) or NA to indicate whether patient/family understand information.
5. Briefly describe the patients' reaction.

Initials of teacher and/or nurse who assessed level of understanding if CCTV was used (Circle if CCTV or NA)	Verbalizes and/or demonstrates understanding of:	THE PATIENT, CHILD, AND/OR PARENT:
	Y N	1. IDENTIFIES SURGICAL PROCEDURE AND REASONS NEEDED.
		2. VIEWED PRE-OPERATIVE TEACHING PROGRAM (CCTV) ADULT _____ PEDIATRIC _____ CRITICAL CARE _____ DATE _____
CCTV:		3. IS INFORMED OF RELEVANT PRE-OPERATIVE PROCEDURES
	Y NA N	A. NPO
	Y NA N	B. PREPS
	Y NA N	C. MEDICATIONS
	Y NA N	D. INFORMATION FOR SIGNIFICANT OTHERS (e.g. waiting room, visiting on op day)
CCTV:		4. IS INFORMED OF RELEVANT POST-OP PROCEDURES/EQUIPMENT
	Y NA N	A. PAR
	Y NA N	B. PAIN/MEDICATIONS
	Y NA N	C. PHYSICAL APPEARANCE ON RETURN FROM PAR
	Y NA N	D. TUBES: IV _____ ; Foley _____ ; NG _____ ; _____ ; _____
	Y NA N	E. INCISION(S)/DRESSING(S)
	Y NA N	F. RT: C,T,DB _____ ; ICSP Pre-op vol. _____ ; CPT _____ ; O_2 _____ ; Suction _____
	Y NA N	G. MEDICATIONS (Specify)
	Y NA N	H. DIET
	Y NA N	I. ACTIVITY (Include possible use of restraints if necessary)
	Y NA N	J. OTHER
NA: CCTV:		5. IS INFORMED OF CRITICAL CARE PROCEDURES (e.g. ICU, CCU, CVS, NICU, PICU, ICN)
	Y NA N	A. VISITING POLICY
	Y NA N	B. VENTILATION (Include monitors & alarms)
	Y NA N	C. INTRAVASCULAR LINES
	Y NA N	D. AVAILABILITY OF A NURSE
NA: CCTV:		6. IS INFORMED OF PEDIATRIC PROCEDURES
	Y NA N	A. REWARMING AFTER SURGERY
		B. PUPPET THERAPY
		7. MISCELLANEOUS
		A.
		B.
		C.

Reaction to teaching/comments:

Initials _____ Date _____

Figure 9–2B. Perioperative teaching checklist. (*From the University of California, San Francisco, Calif., with permission.*)

An informed consent is necessary for any elective surgical procedure or diagnostic study. The consent is usually obtained by the responsible physician either through a verbal discussion, a verbal and written discussion, or with the use of an audio cassette and a verbal discussion. The informed consent consists of the nature of the treatment and the risks, complications, and expected benefits of the treatment. In addition, the alternative forms of treatment are discussed. The informed consent is valid until the procedure has been performed or at such a time as there are changes in the circumstances or in the procedure to be performed. For example, if a patient signs a consent for a specific operation but the diagnostic studies indicate that another procedure should be performed, a new consent must be obtained.

An informed consent is not necessary where emergency treatment is required to prevent deterioration of the patient's condition.

Generally, any competent adult more than 18 years of age may consent to his or her own treatment. Incompetent adults must have a conservator, identified by the courts, who may give consent for medical treatment.

Minor patients may consent to surgical treatment procedures or diagnostic studies if they are

1. Fifteen years of age, living apart from parents or guardian, and managing his or her own financial affairs
2. On active duty with the United States Armed Forces
3. Pregnant
4. Married, whether or not the marriage has been terminated by dissolution

The signing of the consent may be witnessed by any employee of the facility. The witness on the permit does not have any responsibility for informing the patient about the treatment. The witness only validates that the patient signed the permit.

If the patient is physically unable to write his or her name, a mark must be obtained. The individual securing the permit signs the patient's name, and then the patient puts his or her "X" beneath it. In this situation, two people should witness the consent.

Consents by telephone or telegraph may be necessary if the person having legal capacity to consent for the patient is not available. The telephone consent should be witnessed and a signed record made by the person obtaining the consent that denotes the exact time and nature of the consent. The witness should countersign and date the request. During the telephone conversation, the individual giving consent should be instructed to send a confirmation by telegram or letter confirming the oral consent.

Following the admission procedure, the patient may have an IV inserted, a surgical shave performed, or a cast bivalved or removed. The cast saw should not be used in the operating room as the plaster dust may become airborne and contaminate the sterile field. During these activities, the perioperative nurse provides support for the patient by explaining all the procedures and the reason they are necessary. The noise in the environment should be kept to a minimum, and the patient should never be left unattended. When these preoperative routines are completed and the operating room is prepared for the surgical procedure, the patient is transported into the operating room.

PREPARATION OF SKIN

The purpose of the surgical scrub and preoperative skin preparation of patients is to reduce the number of microorganisms to a minimum. Chemical disinfection of the skin is called degermation.

The skin is composed of two layers: epidermis and dermis. The epidermis is constantly worn away and replaced with cells from the dermis. The thickness of the dermis varies in different parts of the body. For example, it is thicker on the soles of the feet and the palms than on the eyelids or the forehead. The dermis is composed of blood vessels, lymphatics, nerves, the secreting portions of the sebaceous glands and the sweat glands, and hair follicles (Fig. 9–3).

The bacteria of the skin are identified as transients and residents. The transient microorganisms are held in place by sweat, oil, and grime. They can easily be removed with soap and water aided by mechanical scrubbing.

The resident bacteria adhere to epithelial cells and extend downward between the cells into the hair follicles and the glands. Among the common resident bacteria are *epidermis*, aerobic and anaerobic diphtheroid bacilli, aerobic spore-forming bacilli, aerobic and anaerobic streptococci of several types, and gram-negative rods of intestinal organisms.[1]

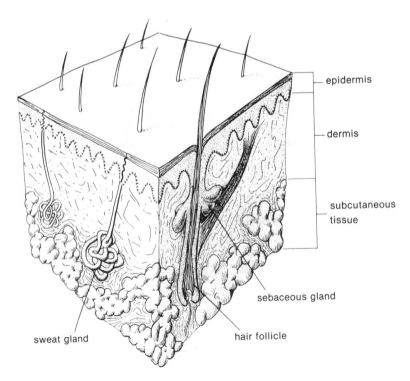

epidermis

dermis

subcutaneous tissue

sebaceous gland

sweat gland

hair follicle

Figure 9–3. A section of human skin.

The resident flora are modified by the presence of hair; folded skin surfaces; excessive secretions of sweat and sebaceous glands; proximity to mouth, nose, anal, or genital regions; and the nature and the condition of the clothing worn.

The antiseptic agents used in skin preparation and the surgical scrub reduce the transient organisms, but they do not penetrate deeply into the dermis. The mechanical action of scrubbing and the rinsing with water are important factors in degerming the deeper layers of the dermis, but a portion of these resident flora remain. When surgical gloves are applied, the diminished resident flora is replenished from the deeper skin layers. Therefore, care must be exercised to avoid glove punctures and to change gloves immediately if punctures do occur. The knife, needle, or instrument causing the puncture should be removed from the sterile field.

The objectives of the surgical scrub and skin preparation of patients are to[2,3]:

1. Remove soil and transient microbes from the skin
2. Reduce the resident microbial count to a minimum
3. Inhibit rapid rebound growth of microbes

Soaps and Detergents

Soaps reduce surface tension; therefore dirt, oil, and microbes are enmeshed in the soap lather and are removed through the washing process.

Detergents also reduce surface tension. They appear to exert their antiseptic effect by disrupting membranes and denaturing proteins. Those possessing a positive charge are called cationic detergents, and those having a negative charge are known as anionic detergents. Soaps and detergents can be combined with antimicrobial agents to form antiseptics used in preoperative skin preparation or surgical scrubs.

Antiseptic Agents. An antimicrobial soap or detergent should meet the following criteria:

1. Act rapidly
2. Not require cumulative action
3. A broad spectrum of activity in the reduction of transient and resident microflora
4. Minimal harsh effects on the skin
5. Inhibition of rapid rebound growth of microbes
6. Nontoxicity

The antiseptic of choice is an iodophor, polyvinylpyrrolidone and iodine (PVP-iodine), combined with a detergent. PVP-iodine is germicidal against fungi, spores, viruses, and both gram-positive and gram-negative bacteria. The germicidal action may remain for up to 8 hours.

Chlorhexidine gluconate offers a broad spectrum bactericidal action. It is effective against gram-positive and gram-negative microorganisms. Residues tend to accumulate on the skin with repeated use and produce a prolonged effect for up to 4 hours.

Hexachlorophene, 3%, combined with a soap, is a bacteriostatic agent active against gram-positive organisms but has only minimal activity against gram-negative microorganisms. It is not sporicidal or tuberculocidal and requires a cumulative action to obtain its maximum effectiveness.

The Federal Drug Administration (FDA) has limited the use of hexachlorophene, except by a physician's prescription, due to the serious toxic hazards that may accompany its continued use. Research findings indicated that the use of hexachlorophene in bathing newborns could result in absorption of some of the disinfectant into their circulation, resulting in permanent brain damage.

With these findings and the predominance of gram-negative nosocomial infection, hexachlorophene, 3%, should have very limited use as an antiseptic agent.

Ethyl alcohol, 70%, may be used as a degerming agent. It is effective on M. *tuberculosis* and vegetative forms of other bacteria, but it does not destroy spores. Other disinfectants are sometimes dissolved in alcohol resulting in a tincture with added disinfectant properties as well as increased grease solvency.

Iodine, 1%, is an effective germicidal agent as it kills bacteria, fungi, viruses, and spores. However, it is limited in its use as it stains fabric and causes skin burns and tissue irritation.

On some selected surgical procedures, such as plastic surgery, a defatting agent, Freon TF, is used. Freon TF emulsifies the residue from soaps and removes any remaining skin oils. This allows the surgeon to make identifying marks without the lines being distorted by the skin oils.[4]

Receptacles used to dispense antiseptics should be cleaned and sterilized weekly to prevent the growth of resistant microorganisms.

Preoperative Skin Preparation of Patients

Preoperative skin preparation of patients may consist of four steps:

1. A shower or bath prior to the patient leaving for the surgical suite
2. Removal of hair by shaving or using a depilatory cream
3. Mechanical scrubbing with an antimicrobial solution
4. Application of an antiseptic agent

Removal of hair from the operative site is not necessary unless it interferes with the surgical procedure. Children, and the head and neck of female patients rarely require hair removal. Some surgeons advocate that removal of the hair is necessary to assure cleanliness of the site and to prevent hair from gaining access into the wound where it would act as a foreign body or carrier of bacteria.

When shaving is the method of choice for removing hair, it should be performed not more than 2 hours prior to the surgical procedure, as there is evidence that the length of time between the shave and the operation is critical and has a direct effect on the infection rate. Shaving destroys some of the natural integumentary defenses and may produce multiple superficial lesions containing exuded tissue fluids that favor or contain bacterial growth.[5] One study showed that the postoperative infection rate was 3.1% when the shave was done immediately prior to surgery, 7.1% when it was done up to 24 hours prior to surgery, and 20% when the shave was done more than 24 hours before surgery.[6]

The area to be shaved is determined by the site of the incision and the nature of the operation. A wide area around the incision is usually prepared to allow for extension of the incision and placement of any tubes and drains. In orthopedics, the area prepared usually includes the joint above and the joint below the area of the incision.

Unusual circumstances, such as traumatic injuries, may require that the patient be shaved in the operating room. However, this should not occur routinely, as loose hair may be deposited in the wound. An area outside the operating room, such as the preoperative area, is preferable, provided that it affords privacy and adequate lighting.

The wet method of shaving is mandatory, as it facilitates hair removal, minimizes skin trauma, and prevents dry hair and debris from becoming airborne. To avoid soiling the linen and the patient's gown, waterproof pads or towels should be placed under the area to be shaved. The razor should be disposable or one that can be terminally sterilized following the procedure.

Plastic disposable gloves, soap, and warm water are used. The skin is lathered well with gauze sponges or a disposable scrub sponge, the skin is held taut with one hand, and the hair is shaved in the direction that it grows. Hair should be removed periodically from the razor by rinsing it in the water. Extreme care must be exercised to avoid cutting the skin and in shaving the area over a boney prominence.

Cotton-tipped applicators may be used to clean the umbilicus, scrub brushes are effective in cleaning hands and feet, and a disposable nail cleaner may be used to clean under the nails. When shaving the head, electric hair clippers are effective.

When the shave is completed, the area is rinsed well with water to remove loose hair and soap residues. The area is then dried. Adhesive tape will aid in the removal of any hair adhering to the skin or the linen.

Items used in shaving are either disposed of or cleaned and terminally sterilized. This includes the head on the electric hair clippers. The clipper head is removed from the body, washed under running water, and autoclaved. The body of the clippers should be wiped with a disinfectant.

Hands should be washed immediately after the procedure to avoid cross-contamination (Table 9–1).

The use of depilatory creams, provided the patient is not sensitive to them, is a safer method of removing hair. One study determined that patients who were shaved had an infection rate of 5.6%, whereas patients who were not, or patients on whom depilatory creams were used had an infection rate of 0.6%.[6] Another study showed similar results; patients who were shaved had an infection rate of 2.3%, and patients who were not had an infection rate of 0.9%.[7]

The depilatory is applied to the skin according to the manufacturer's directions for a specified time and then wiped off, and the skin is thoroughly rinsed and dried.

A manual containing routine preoperative skin preparations and approved by the surgeon facilitates the shaving process and serves as a guideline in choosing the appropriate skin preparation according to the surgical procedure (Fig. 9–4).

The mechanical scrubbing usually occurs after the patient is anesthetized and positioned on the operating room table. The pooling of solutions under the patient may result in a skin burn or irritation due to the chemical action of the laundry detergent and the antimicrobial scrub solution. This is prevented by using waterproof pads or additional linen that is discarded at the end of the scrub procedure. Recent research has

TABLE 9-1. MODEL OF PATIENT CARE FOR PREOPERATIVE SHAVE PREPARATION

Nursing Diagnosis	Expected Outcome	Nursing Actions	Schedule for Assessment
1. Potential inappropriate preoperative shave performed on patient	1. Appropriate shave performed	1a. Check patient's identification band with chart b. Confirm site and side of surgical procedure by comparing consent and OR schedule c. Check physician's orders for type of shave or check standard skin preparation manual	1. Preoperatively
2. Potential infection related to cross-contamination	2. No infection related to cross-contamination	2a. Wash hands prior to contact with patient b. Wear plastic disposable gloves while performing shave c. Wash hands at end of the procedure	2. 24-48 hours postoperatively
3. Potential anxiety related to having body shaved	3a. Ability to cope with anxiety b. Ability to verbalize questions and concerns	3a. Explain procedure to patient in a reassuring professional manner b. Answer questions and concerns using terminology the patient understands	3. During shave procedure
4. Potential loss of dignity related to excessive exposure	4. Dignity maintained	4a. Limit exposure of patient only to area needed for adequate shave b. Provide for privacy while performing the shave	4. During shave procedure

5. Possible discomfort from the procedure	5. Minimal discomfort	5a. Maintain proper body alignment b. Use additional supports if indicated c. Place extra linen or waterproof pad under and around area to be shaved d. Use warm water e. Use wet method of shaving f. Shave hair in direction it grows g. After completion of prep check with patient to ascertain that he or she is: Comfortable Warm Dry	5. During shave procedure and immediately following the procedure
6. Potential abrasions and rashes related to shave procedures	6. Skin integrity maintained	6a. Provide for adequate lighting b. Check area to be shaved for any abnormal skin conditions (i.e., lesions, allergies, irritations); if present check with surgeon before proceeding with shave c. Maintain an awareness of skin irregularities such as warts and moles d. Maintain an awareness of the anatomical area to be prepped, exercising special precautions on boney prominences e. Alert surgeon to any untoward affects of the shave following the procedure	6. Immediately following the shave

213

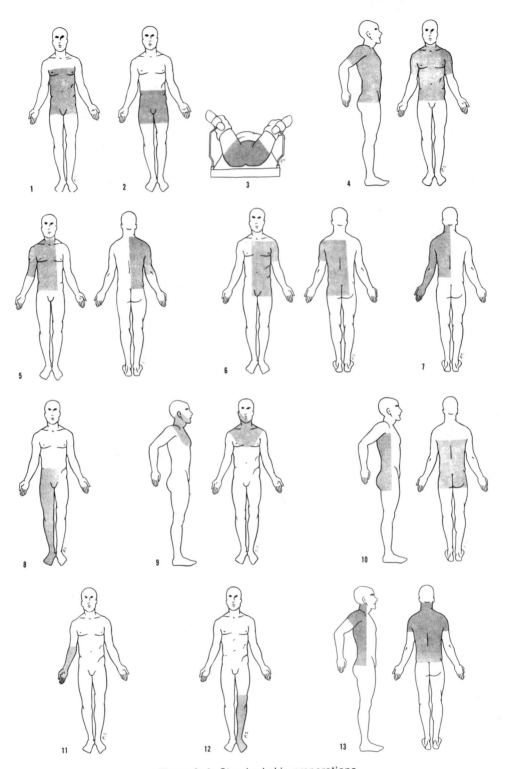

Figure 9-4. Standard skin preparations.

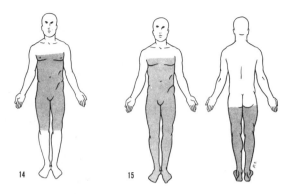

Procedure	Figure #	Procedure	Figure #
Abdominal hysterectomy	1	Graft—skin	Check chart
Abdominal perineal resec-			for orders
tion	1, 3	Hand surgery	11
Adrenalectomy	1	Hernia, inguinal	2
Adrenalectomy—posterior		Hip total joint	8
approach	10	Laminectomy cervical	13
Amputation—leg	8	Laminectomy lumbar	10
Ankle	12	Laparotomy	1
Aortic aneurysmectomy	14	Laryngectomy	9
Aortic valve	4	Mandibular resection	9
Appendectomy	1	Mastectomy	5
Arm—forearm	7	Mediastinal exploration	4
Axillary dissection	5	Mitral valve	4
Brachial duct cyst	9	Nephrectomy	6
Carotid artery	9	Porto-caval shunt	14
Cholecystectomy	1	Rectal fistulectomy	3
Coronary artery bypass	15	Shoulder surgery	7
Crainotomy	Check chart	Sympathectomy lumbar	6
	for orders	Thyroidectomy	9
Esophageal diverticulec-		Thoractomy	6
tomy	9	Vaginal hysterectomy	3
Esophagotomy	9	Varicose vein ligation	
Foot surgery	12	(unilateral)	8

Figure 9-4. Continued.

indicated that prewarming skin cleansing agents to 40°C reduces patient temperature loss significantly but does not deactivate the solutions.[8]

A sterile tray is used, and the operative site is scrubbed with 4 × 4 sponges and an antimicrobial scrub solution. The routine procedure is to begin at the site of the incision, exerting firm pressure and circular strokes, and then proceed to the periphery (Fig. 9–5). The sponge is then discarded, and a fresh sponge is used. The soiled sponge is never brought back over the area previously scrubbed. The area is then rinsed and dried.

If the site to be scrubbed contains a contaminated area such as an external stoma, the area should be sealed off with a plastic drape or scrubbed last.

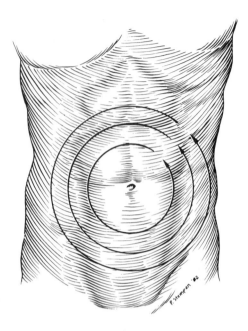

Figure 9-5. The scrub begins at the site of the incision and proceeds to the periphery.

As part of the skin preparation, traumatic wounds may require irrigation of the wound to dislodge and rinse out debris. The amount of irrigation will depend on the site and the size of the wound.

Following the mechanical scrub, an antiseptic agent may be applied. These agents leave an antimicrobial residue on the skin that prevents microbial growth during surgery, and should be allowed to dry before drapes are applied.

Surgical Hand Scrub

The surgical hand scrub is performed prior to donning a sterile gown and gloves. The hand scrub does not render the skin sterile, but if effectively performed it does reduce the number of microorganisms (Fig. 9–6). Therefore, if gloves are perforated during the surgical procedure, the number of microorganisms released into the wound will be reduced.

The surgical hand scrub is accomplished with the use of a reusable or disposable scrub brush or sponge. Studies indicate that there is no difference in the removal of microbes between reusable and disposable brushes[9] and that the brush offers no advantage over the sponge.[10]

If reusable brushes are used, they must be sterilized in a container that permits removal of a single brush without contaminating the other brushes. The decision to use a reusable or a disposable scrub brush should be based on economic factors. Included in the cost analysis should be the amount of labor required to clean and process the reusable brushes.

Nail cleaners should be metal or plastic and must be sterilized between uses. Orangewood sticks are not acceptable as they cannot be sterilized.

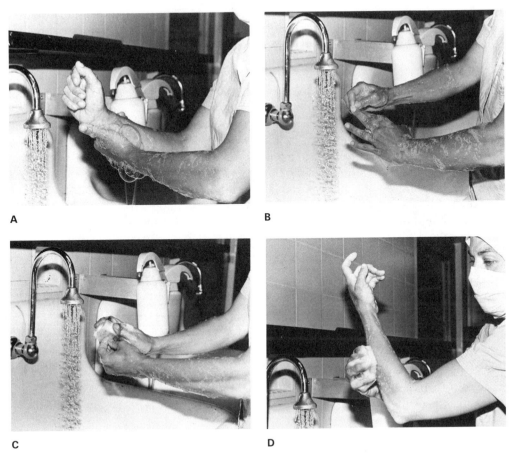

Figure 9-6. Surgical scrub technique. **A.** Hands and arms are lathered to 2 inches above elbow. **B.** Clean the nails and the subungal area with a nail cleaner. **C.** Hold the brush perpendicular to the nails and scrub the fingertips. **D.** Using a circular motion, scrub all sides of the forearm to 2 inches above the elbow.

Some disposable brushes are impregnated with an antimicrobial scrub agent. As indicated previously in this chapter, the antimicrobial scrub solution of choice is an iodophor. Hexachlorophene should be used only by those members of the surgical team allergic to the iodophors.

The two methods used in surgical hand scrubs are the time method and the stroke count method. In the time method, the fingers, the hands, and the arms are scrubbed for a prescribed amount of time. The total amount of time prescribed is 5 or 10 minutes. Numerous studies indicate that there is no significant difference between the 5- and 10-minute scrubs.[9]

In the stroke count method, a prescribed number of strokes are used for each surface of the fingers, the hands, and the arms. The nails receive 30 strokes and other areas of the hands and arms up to 2 inches above the elbow receive 20 strokes. To assure adequate scrubbing, the fingers are considered to have four sides. Each side, including the web spaces between them, is then scrubbed using a circular motion with firm pressure. The arm is divided into thirds; and using circular strokes, each one third is scrubbed up to 2 inches above the elbow.

The stroke count method assures that all skin surfaces are exposed to the same amount of mechanical scrubbing and germicidal solution. The time method does not provide the same assurance.

Prior to beginning the hand scrub, all personnel should check their hands and arms for the presence of any abnormal skin conditions. The skin must be free from abrasions and cuts, since microorganisms are frequently found on skin that is inflamed from minor trauma or dermatitis. Cuticles should be in good condition. Nail polish cracks and peels easily under the stress of a good mechanical scrub, thereby providing microscopic niches in which microbes can find perfect conditions for breeding.[11] The use of prosthetic fingernails should be prohibited due to reports of fungal infections in individuals wearing acrylic nails.[12] The surgical head covering is adjusted to ensure complete hair coverage, and the mask is tied securely to prevent venting at the sides. Eyeglasses should be adjusted for comfort and proper fit to avoid fogging of the lenses. Scrub dresses should be fitted or tied at the waist, and scrub shirts should be tucked into the trousers to prevent the clothing from getting wet and to avoid the scrubbed hands and arms from becoming contaminated by brushing against the loose garments.

The procedure used for the surgical hand scrub should be in writing and posted in the scrub room area. The procedure should include the following steps:

1. Remove all jewelry from hands and arms.
2. Turn on the water and adjust to comfortable temperature.
3. Check to see that the foot pedal for the soap dispenser is conveniently located and that it works.
4. Wet hands and forearms.
5. Using an antimicrobial soap or a detergent, lather the hands and arms to 2 inches above the elbows. This washing will loosen the surface debris and remove the gross contamination.
6. Rinse hands and arms so the water flows off at the elbows. Arms are flexed with the fingertips pointing upward.
7. If using a prepackaged scrub brush, the brush and the nail cleaner are removed from the package. The brush is held in one hand while the other hand cleans the nails and the subungual area of the free hand. If a disposable nail cleaner is unavailable, a sterile reusable metal or plastic cleaner may be used. The reusable cleaner must be disposed of in the appropriate location so it can be resterilized.
8. Rinse hands.
9. If the brush is impregnated with an antimicrobial soap or a detergent, wet it and begin the scrub procedure. If the brush is not impregnated, the soap or detergent is applied to the hands. See Table 9–2 for timed scrub method and Table 9–3 for stroke count method.

TABLE 9-2. PROCEDURE FOR TIMED SCRUB (10 MINUTE)

A. Left hand—1 minute
   Left arm and elbow—1½ minutes
   Rinse hand, arm, and brush

B. Right hand—1 minute
   Right arm, and elbow—1½ minutes
   Rinse hand, arm, and brush

C. Left hand—1 minute
   Left arm up to 2″ above elbow—1 minute
   Rinse hand, arm, and brush

D. Right hand—1 minute
   Right arm up to 2″ above elbow—1 minute
   Rinse hand, arm, and brush

E. Left hand—½ minute
   Rinse hand and brush

F. Right hand—½ minute
   Rinse hand and brush

10. Turn off water, discard brush, proceed to operating room holding hands and arms up and away from scrub clothes.
11. During the scrubbing procedure, if the hands or arms inadvertently touch some part of the sink, an extra 10 strokes to that area of the skin will correct the contamination.

TABLE 9-3. PROCEDURE FOR STROKE COUNT METHOD

A. Left hand	Nails—20 strokes across nails, rinsing fingertips after 10 strokes to remove dislodged soil
	Fingers—10 strokes to all sides of each digit and the web spaces
	Hand—10 strokes to palm and back of the hand
B. Left arm	Using a circular motion, scrub all the sides of the forearm to 2 inches above the elbow with 10 strokes to all surfaces
C. Rinse	Flex the arms at the elbow and rinse from fingertips to elbow, allowing water to run off elbow. Rinse the brush or sponge
D. Right hand	Repeat as in A for right hand
E. Right arm	Repeat as in B for right arm
F. Rinse as in C	
G. Left hand	Nails—10 strokes across nails
	Fingers—10 strokes to all sides of each digit and the web spaces
	Hand—10 strokes to palm and back of the hand
H. Left arm	Scrub all sides of the forearm to 2 inches above the elbow with 10 strokes to all surfaces
I. Rinse hands, arms, and brush thoroughly	
J. Right hand	Repeat as in G
K. Right arm	Repeat as in H

Drying Hands and Arms

Hands and arms must be thoroughly dried with a sterile towel to prevent contamination of the sterile gown from organisms on the skin and the scrub attire (Figs. 9–7, 9–8).

A gown package is opened on a small table for the scrub nurse. It contains one gown and one or two towels. Without dripping water on the sterile field, the scrub nurse grasps a towel and lifts it straight up and away from the sterile field. The hands and the arms are kept up and away from the scrub clothes. The nurse bends slightly forward at the waist to prevent the towel, as it is unfolded, from touching the scrub clothes.

If two towels are used, one towel is used for each hand and arm. The towel is unfolded and the hand is thoroughly dried. Then using a rotating motion, the forearm and the elbow are dried, and the towel is discarded.

In using one towel, the towel is divided mentally in half horizontally, and one half is used for each hand and arm. The towel is unfolded, and the hand is dried thoroughly. Then, using a rotating motion, the forearm and the elbow are dried. With the dried hand, grasp the dry unused end of the towel, and repeat the process on the second hand and arm. Discard the towel. In both these techniques, once the towel has been moved from the hands up to the elbow, the towel is considered contaminated and must not come in contact with the dried portion of the hand or the arm. Care must be taken not to let the edges of the towel touch the front of the scrub clothes.

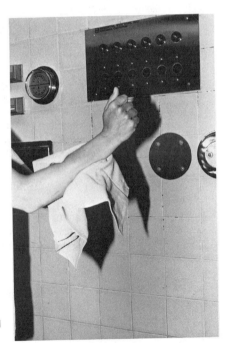

Figure 9–7. Drying with two towels. One towel is used for each hand and arm.

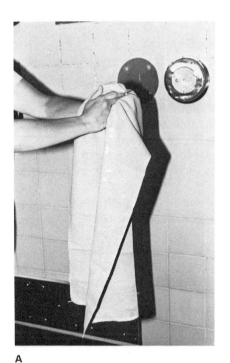

A

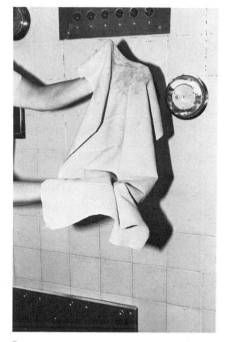

B

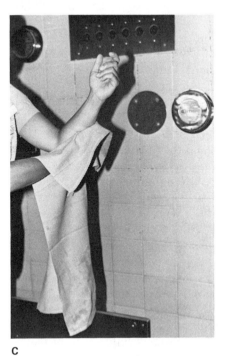

C

Figure 9-8. Drying with one towel. **A.** Dry one hand and arm using one-half of the towel. **B.** The dried hand grasps the un-used end of the towel. **C.** Dry the second hand and arm.

GOWNING AND GLOVING

Gowning

The gown is folded so the scrub nurse can put it on without touching the outer side with bare hands. The inside front neckline of the gown is visible after the towels have been removed. The following procedure is used in donning the gown:

1. Lift the folded gown upward from the sterile package, and step back from the table.
2. Grasp the gown at the neckline and allow the gown to unfold with the inside of the gown toward the wearer. The outside of the gown must not be touched with bare hands.
3. Simultaneously the hands are slipped into the armholes, holding the hands at shoulder level and away from the body.
4. The circulating nurse may assist the scrub nurse by reaching inside the gown and pulling on the inside seam. If the closed-gloving technique is used, the gown is pulled on leaving the sleeves extending over the hands approximately 1 inch. If open-gloving technique is used, then the hands are extended through the cuffs of the gown.
5. The circulating nurse ties or snaps the back of the gown, at the neck and the waist, touching only the ties or snaps. The gown is further adjusted by grasping at the bottom edge of the gown and pulling down. This will remove the blousing or ballooning effect sterile gowns frequently develop.
6. If a wraparound gown is used after the scrub nurse is gloved, the front ties are untied and the sterile gown may be wrapped in one of the following ways:
   a. The tie attached to the back (the tie on the right) is handed to another gowned and gloved team member who will remain stationary. The scrub nurse pivots to the left, which then effectively brings the flap over the back of the gown, and the gown is tied in the front.
   b. If other members of the team are not gowned and gloved, a Kocher or Allis clamp may be snapped to the end of the tie and the instrument handed to the circulating nurse. While the circulating nurse remains stationary the scrub nurse turns to the left, the circulating nurse releases the instrument, and the scrub nurse takes the tie and ties the gown. If this method is used, the instrument must be placed in an appropriate place so it will be included in the instrument count.
   c. If disposable gloves are used, the inner wrapper (provided that it is cardboard) may be used to tie the gown. The scrub nurse places the end of the tie in the center crease of the glove wrapper, folds the wrapper over, and hands the wrapper to the circulating nurse. While the circulating nurse remains stationary, the scrub nurse turns to the left and takes the tie from the glove wrapper, being careful not to touch the wrapper or the circulating nurse, and ties the gown.
   d. Some disposable gowns have the end of one tie covered with a strip of paper that can be handed to the circulating nurse. Or if it is at the back, the circulator can grasp the end without contaminating the gown. The scrub nurse turns to

the left (which closes the gown) and grasps the still sterile end of the tie from the circulating nurse. The circulating nurse then gently pulls on the strip until it is released from the sterile end and discards it. The scrub nurse then ties the gown.

Donning Sterile Gloves
Suggested procedures for closed and open gloving follow.

Procedure for Closed Gloving. For the scrub nurse, the closed method of gloving is preferred because there is no possibility of the bare hand contacting the outside of the glove (Fig. 9–9).

1. Slide the hands into the sleeves of the gown until the cuff seam is reached; the hands must not touch the cuff edges.
2. With the right hand, that is covered by the fabric of the sleeve or the cuff, pick up the left glove.
3. Place the glove on the upward turned left hand, palm side down, thumb to thumb, with fingers extending along the forearm pointing toward the elbow.
4. The glove cuff and the sleeve cuff are held together with the thumb of the left hand.
5. The sleeve-covered right hand stretches the cuff of the left glove over the open end of the sleeve.
6. The sleeve-covered right hand grasps both the cuff of the glove and the gown; as the fingers are worked into the glove, the cuff is pulled up on to the wrist.
7. The left glove is put on in the same manner with the assistance of the gloved hand.

Procedure for Open Gloving. Open-gloving technique is used when performing sterile procedures (such as a bladder catherization or insertion of an IV cutdown) and when both gloves need to be changed without assistance during a surgical procedure (Fig. 9–10).

1. Slide the hands into the gown all the way through the cuffs of the gown.
2. Pick up the cuff of the left glove using the thumb and the index finger of the right hand.
3. Pull the glove onto the left hand, leaving the cuff of the glove turned down.
4. With the gloved left hand, slide the fingers inside the cuff of the right glove, being careful to keep the gloved fingers under the folded cuff.
5. Pull the glove onto the right hand avoiding inward rolling of the cuff. Then, by rotating the arm, the cuff of the glove is pulled over the gown.
6. Place the fingers of the gloved right hand under the folded cuff of the left glove, rotate the arm, and pull the cuff of the glove over the gown.

Assisting Other Team Members with Gowning and Gloving
The scrub nurse is responsible for assisting other members of the surgical team with donning the sterile gown and gloves (Figs. 9–11, 9–12).

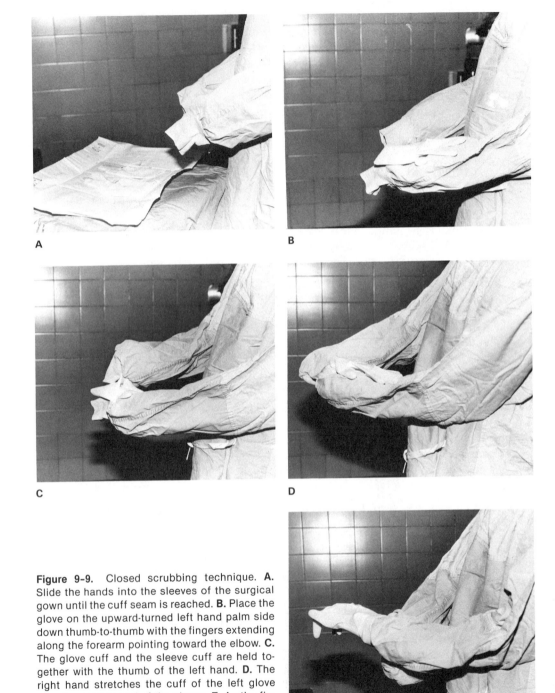

Figure 9-9. Closed scrubbing technique. **A.** Slide the hands into the sleeves of the surgical gown until the cuff seam is reached. **B.** Place the glove on the upward-turned left hand palm side down thumb-to-thumb with the fingers extending along the forearm pointing toward the elbow. **C.** The glove cuff and the sleeve cuff are held together with the thumb of the left hand. **D.** The right hand stretches the cuff of the left glove over the opened end of the sleeve. **E.** As the fingers are worked into the glove, the cuff is pulled up onto the wrist.

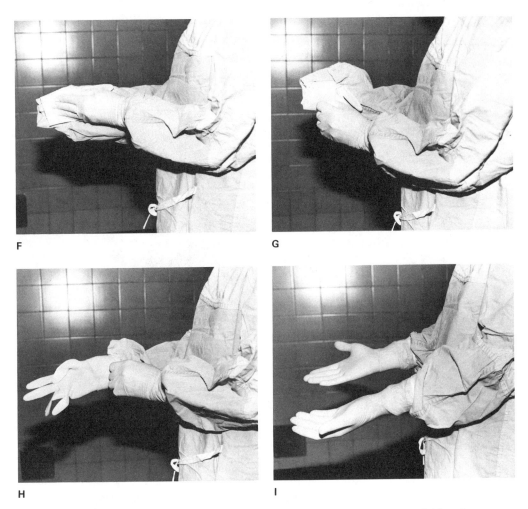

Figure 9-9. Continued. **F.** The left glove is positioned in the same manner. **G.** The glove cuff and sleeve cuff are held together with the thumb of the right hand. **H.** Fingers of the right hand are worked into the glove, and the cuff is pulled up onto the wrist. **I.** Gloves are adjusted to insure appropriate fit.

1. The scrub nurse opens the towel and places one end over the outstretched hand of the other team member.
2. The gown is picked up by the neck band and unfolded.
3. The scrub nurse makes a protective cuff of the neck and shoulder area, turns the inner side of the gown toward the person being gowned, and places the gown on the outstretched arms.
4. Once the other team member has placed his or her hands in the sleeves, the scrub nurse releases the gown. The circulating nurse assists in pulling on the gown by touching only the inside the gown.

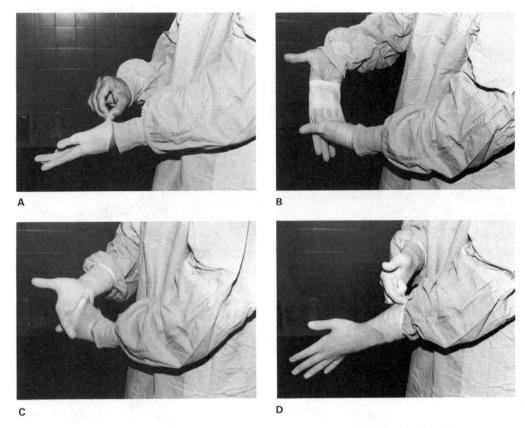

A

B

C

D

Figure 9-10. Open gloving technique. **A.** Pull the glove onto the left hand leaving the cuff of the glove turned down. **B.** With the gloved left hand, slide the fingers inside the cuff of the right glove. **C.** Place the fingers of the gloved right hand under the folded cuff of the left glove. **D.** Rotate the arm and pull the cuff of the glove over the gown.

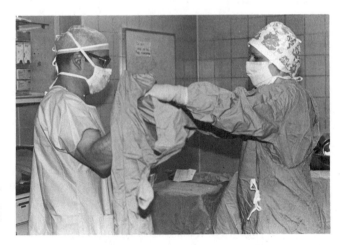

Figure 9-11. Gowning another person. The scrub nurse makes a protective cuff of the neck and shoulder area.

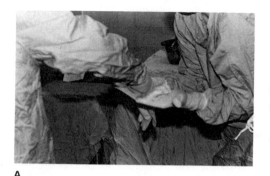
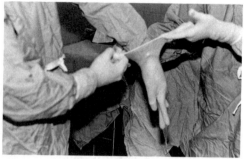

A   **B**

Figure 9-12. Gloving another person. **A.** The scrub nurse holds her thumbs out to prevent them from coming in contact with the bare hands of the other team members. **B.** Team member assists in donning second glove.

5. In gloving other team members, the right hand is always gloved first. The glove is picked up under the everted cuff.
6. The palm of the glove is held toward the other team member.
7. The glove is stretched to open the glove.
8. The scrub nurse holds her thumbs out or protects them under the cuff of the glove from coming in contact with the bare hands of the other team member.
9. As the other team member slides his or her hand into the glove, the scrub nurse exerts firm upward pressure, making certain that the gloved hand does not go below the waist.
10. The glove cuff is pulled over the cuff of the gown.
11. The procedure is repeated for the left glove.
12. If a wraparound gown is used, the scrub nurse holds the tie as the other team member turns.

Regloving

If a member of the surgical team, other than the scrub nurse, perforates or contaminates a glove during the surgical procedure, the circulator grasps the outside of the glove and pulls the glove off inside out. The scrub nurse then regloves the team member as previously indicated.

If the scrub nurse needs to change his or her gloves, the options are

1. Remove both gown and gloves
2. Have another member of the team assist in regloving
3. Use the open-glove technique

Closed gloving cannot be used to reglove, because once the hand passes through the cuff of the gown, the edge of the cuff is contaminated; therefore, the outside of the new glove would be contaminated.

Removing Soiled Gown and Gloves

At the conclusion of the surgical procedure, the gown and the gloves should be removed in a manner that avoids cross-contamination of the arms, the hands, and the scrub clothes (Fig. 9–13). The following steps should be followed:

1. The front tie is untied by the scrubbed member of the team.
2. The back neck and waist ties are released by the circulator.
3. The gown is then removed by grasping the gown at the shoulders and pulling it over the gloved hands, turning the gown inside out, and being careful not to touch the scrub clothes.
4. When the gown is removed, it is folded so the contaminated surface is on the inside. Then it is rolled before being deposited in the linen or waste hamper. Rolling the gown will ensure that any gross contamination will not soak through the laundry bag.
5. The gloves are removed by grasping the left rolled glove cuff with the right gloved hand and inverting the glove as it is pulled from the left hand (Fig. 9–14).

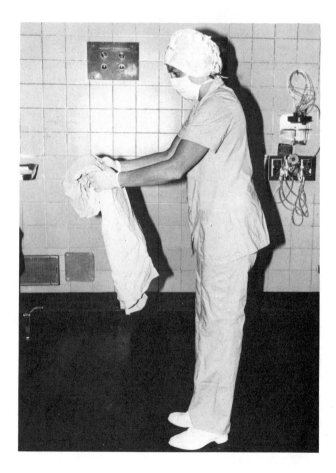

Figure 9–13. Removing soiled gown. The gown is rolled and deposited in the linen or waste hamper.

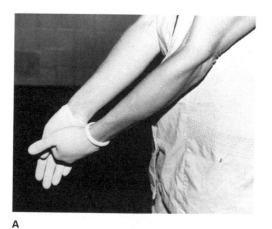

A

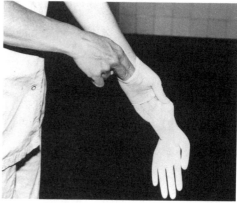

B

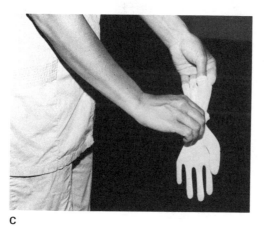

C

Figure 9–14. Removing soiled gloves. **A.** Grasp the left rolled glove cuff with the right hand and invert the glove as it is pulled from the left hand. **B.** The fingers of the left hand are then placed inside the cuff of the right glove. **C.** The glove is inverted as it is removed.

6. The fingers of the left hand are then placed inside the cuff of the right glove, along the palm of the hand; and the glove is inverted as it is removed.

If the gloves are removed prior to the gown, the contaminated gown would then be pulled off over the bare hands—causing the hands to become contaminated.

Gown and gloves are never worn outside the operating room and must be removed prior to applying the surgical dressings.

REFERENCES

1. Wilson M, Mizer H, Morello J. *Microbiology in Patient Care*, 3rd ed. New York: Macmillan; 1979:114
2. Recommended practices for preoperative skin preparation. *AORN J.* 1988; 48(5):950
3. Recommended practices for surgical scrubs. *AORN J.* 1984; 39(6):1084–1088
4. Wessel L. Freon as a solvent. *AORN J.* 1971; 14(4):88

5. Altemeier W et al. *Manual on Control of Infection in Surgical Patients*. Philadelphia: J. B. Lippincott; 1984:74

6. Seropian R, Reynolds B. Wound infections after preoperative depilatory versus razor preparation. *Am J Surg.* 1971; 121:252

7. Cruse P, Ford R. A five-year prospective study of 23,649 surgical wounds. *Arch Surg.* 1973; 107(2):208

8. Miner D. Do warmed skin cleansers affect patient heat loss? *Today's OR Nurse.* 1985; 7(3):12, 15

9. Dineen P. An evaluation of the duration of the surgical scrub. *Surg Gynecol Obs.* 1969; 129(6):1183

10. Bronside GH, Crowder VH, Cohn I. A bacteriological evaluation of surgical scrubbing with disposable iodophor soap impregnated polyurethane scrub sponges. *Surgery.* 1968; 64(4):743–51

11. Steere A, Mallison G. Handwashing practices for the prevention of nosocomial infections. *Ann Intern Med.* 1975; 83(5):687

12. Rubin D. Prosthetic fingernails in the OR. *AORN J.* 1988; 47(4):944

Chapter 10

Anesthesia

HISTORICAL INTRODUCTION TO ANESTHESIA

Historians have documented that man has consistently sought relief from pain and suffering. Mandragora wine was given by the ancient Greeks before operations, and by the Romans to relieve the sufferings of the crucified. It remained in use through the 12th century as an anesthetic agent.

In the *Annals of the Later Han Dynasty* there is reference to the performance of surgery with the assistance of a "bubbling drug medicine." The medicine, an effervescent powder added to wine, produced numbness and insensibility. The powder may well have been opium.

"Sleeping apples," sponges impregnated with potions and extracts from plants and herbs, were also used to produce sleep. The extracts included the juices of the unripe mulberry, spurge flax, mandragon, and ivy; hyposcyamus (scopolamine); lettuce seed; the shrub of hemlock; and opium. This mixture was then boiled under the sun until the mixture was soaked up by the sponge. Prior to being used, the sponge was soaked in hot water for an hour and then applied to the nostrils until the patient fell asleep. When the surgery was completed, the patient was awakened by smelling another sponge soaked in vinegar or in the juice from the hay root.[1]

The ancients, however, did not understand the strength of their potions; patients were often overdosed and killed.

Intoxication with alcohol, compression of the carotid arteries to induce unconsciousness, and hypnotism were all tried as a means of producing anesthesia and frequently failed. When appropriate anesthesia was not available, patients were strapped to the operating table or were restrained by friends or members of their family (Fig. 10–1).

Lanney, Napoleon's chief military surgeon, noticed that the half-frozen soldier had a higher pain threshold, so he used the numbing effects of cold to amputate limbs painlessly on the battlefield.

In 1772, Joseph Priestly first prepared an impure form of nitrous oxide and, in 1800, Humphrey Davy published the results of his research regarding the properties of nitrous oxide. One of his suggestions was that it appeared capable of destroying physical pain and probably could be used in surgical operations. However, no one used Davy's research for producing anesthesia. Nitrous oxide became a scientific plaything labeled "laughing gas" because of the giddy laughter induced by the agent.

Ether entered medicine as a drug that was used in the treatment of lung disease by inhalation from a saucer. The effects of an excess of ether became known and parties called "ether-frolics" were held, at which the guests made merry after inhaling ether vapor and sometimes passed out. Dr. Crawford Long of Jefferson, Georgia, witnessed the frolics and decided to substitute ether for alcohol to prevent the pain associated with

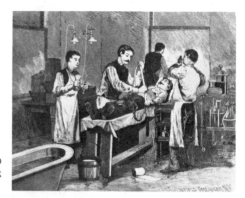

Figure 10-1. Strapping the preoperative patient to the operating table. Operating room of a New York City hospital, 1894. (*The Bettmann Archive.*)

surgery. In 1842, Dr. Long administered ether to one of his patients and successfully prevented the pain of surgery, but he did not publish his results until 1849.

Dr. William Thomas Green Morton, an American dentist, is identified as the pioneer of surgical anesthesia. The historic event took place in October 1846, at the Massachusetts General Hospital in Boston, where Dr. Morton, who had been using nitrous oxide in extracting teeth, administered ether anesthesia while Dr. John Collins Warren removed a tuberculous gland from the neck of an unconscious patient. At the completion of the procedure, Dr. Warren asked the patient to describe what he felt. The patient replied, "It felt like someone was scratching my neck."[2]

Chloroform was being used medicinally when Sir James Simpson of Edinburgh introduced it as an anesthetic agent* in 1847. For the next 60 years, chloroform became the most widely used anesthetic agent. It was more pleasant to inhale than ether and more powerful, and as a result it was easier to administer successfully. However, it was soon found that there were more deaths with chloroform, so its use as an anesthetic agent was discontinued.

Until late into the 20th century, most anesthetics were given by a mask placed over the nose and the mouth. The anesthetic was either dropped directly onto the mask or vaporized by means of a hand bellows (Fig. 10–2). Nitrous oxide was administered through a rubber mask and sometimes mixed with the vapor of ether or chloroform. These methods made operations on the head and neck difficult and dangerous, and there always was the possibility of an obstructed airway due to the relaxation of muscles and the tongue falling back into the throat. To avoid an obstructed airway, in some surgical procedures the surgeon would perform a tracheostomy through which a tube could be inserted for anesthesia.

Sir William Macewen devised the idea of passing a tube through the mouth, between the vocal cords, into the trachea. The anesthetic agent could then be administered

---

*The name for the drugs that cause complete or partial loss of feeling was proposed by Dr. Oliver Wendell Holmes. The term *anesthetic* came from the Greek term meaning "without sensation." The loss of feeling became known as anesthesia. The specialty is called anesthesiology. A physician trained in anesthesia is an anesthesiologist, and a nurse trained to administer certain types of anesthetics is an anesthetist.

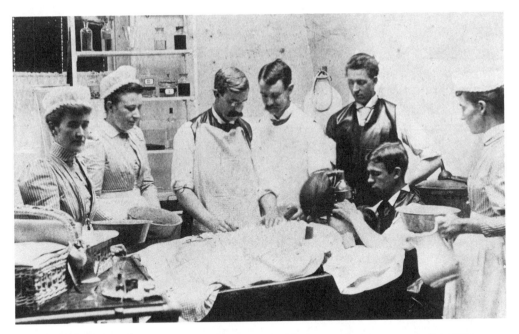

Figure 10-2. Anesthesia being administered with the surgical team ready for action, 1880. Bellevue Hospital, New York. (*The Bettmann Archive.*)

directly into the trachea without the fear of obstruction from the tongue. The tubes of silver or gum elastic could be bent to the desired angle but would retain their shape when inserted. On July 5, 1878 the first endotracheal anesthesia was administered.[2]

The continued development of anesthetic agents and techniques has not only provided patients with freedom from pain, but it has also provided prolonged operating time, allowing the surgeon to refine and to expand surgical techniques.

ANESTHESIA

Anesthesia is the partial or complete loss of sensation with or without the loss of consciousness. It may occur as a result of disease or injury or the administration of a drug or a gas. The two broad types of artificially induced anesthesia are general and regional. General anesthesia produces unconsciousness in the patient, and regional anesthesia causes a loss of feeling in some area of the body.

A third classification has recently been introduced: monitored anesthesia care (MAC). In these cases, a local anesthetic may be administered by the surgeon. However, the anesthesiologist provides the following care to the patient:

1. Preoperative evaluation
2. Preoperative medication

3. Intraoperative IV anesthetic agent/regional anesthesia
4. Monitoring of the patient during the surgical procedure
5. Transferring of the patient to the postanesthesia care unit (PACU)

The method of administering anesthesia and the agents to be used are determined after reviewing the patient. The physical status classification in Table 10–1 is one of the tools used in evaluating the patients risk for anesthesia. The following factors are also reviewed:

1. Physical and mental status of the patient
2. Age of the patient
3. Presence of coexisting disease
4. Concurrent drug therapy
5. Previous allergic reactions to drugs
6. Previous anesthesia experience
7. Site and duration of proposed surgical procedure
8. Use of electrocautery
9. Patient preference
10. Surgeon preference
11. Expertise of the anesthesiologist

The administration of anesthesia begins with the preoperative medication.

Preoperative Medication

Preoperative medications are given to allay preoperative anxiety, decrease secretions in the respiratory tract, reduce reflex irritability, relieve pain, and lower the body's metabolism so that less anesthetic is required. In general, heavy smokers, alcoholics, and hyperthyroid, toxic, and emotional patients all have a higher metabolic rate and require higher doses of medication. Conversely, debilitation and age usually reduce the need for and increase the side effects of the premedication. The side effects are confusion, restless-

TABLE 10-1. PHYSICAL STATUS CLASSIFICATION OF THE AMERICAN SOCIETY OF ANESTHESIOLOGISTS (ASA)

Class[a]	Description
1	No organic, physiological, biochemical, systemic, or psychiatric disturbances
2	Mild to moderate systemic disturbance; mild, well-controlled diabetes, asthma hypertension, or obesity
3	Severe systemic disturbance that limits activity; severe organic heart disease severe diabetes with systemic complications, poorly controlled hypertension
4	Severe systemic disorder that is life threatening; severe angina, advanced renal or hepatic diseases
5	Moribund patient not expected to survive the operation; ruptured abdominal aortic aneurysm with shock, or massive pulmonary embolus with shock

[a]Emergency operation—The letter E is appended to any of the above 5 categories to indicate that the contemplated operation is an emergency.
From A. Goldstein Jr., A. S. Keats. The risk of anesthesia. Anesthesiology. 1970; 33 (2):130.

ness, decreased respirations, hypotension, nausea, vomiting, and uncomfortably dry mouth and lips.

To ensure adequate action of the drugs, the medication should be administered 45 to 60 minutes prior to induction or as ordered by the anesthesiologist. The drugs of choice are barbiturates, narcotics, and anticholinergics. Patients medicated preoperatively must be assessed and continually observed during the preoperative period.

Barbiturates. Pentobarbital (Nembutal) and secobarbital (Seconal) are frequently used as premedications. Doses are 50 to 200 mg depending upon the route of administration. These drugs provide good sedation with minimal respiratory or circulatory depression and rarely cause postoperative nausea and vomiting.

A nonbarbiturate tranquilizer, diazepam (Valium) in a dosage of 10 mg provides sedation and tension relief without circulatory depression. Diazepam is frequently used as a premedication before local anesthesia because of its anticonvulsive properties. Convulsions are a rare but potential problem with the systemic absorption of local anesthetic drugs.

Narcotics. The narcotics primarily used are morphine in a dosage of 5 to 15 mg and meperidine hydrochloride (Demerol) in a dosage of 50 to 100 mg. They provide good preoperative sedation and are useful in the presence of pain or when painful procedures are anticipated prior to the induction of anesthesia. In short surgical procedures, narcotics decrease excitement and restlessness due to pain immediately postoperatively. However, they may prolong the emergence from anesthesia. Narcotics depress the respiratory and circulatory systems, decrease gastric motility, and may produce nausea and vomiting.

Anticholinergics. Atropine and scopolamine are given as part of the premedication to reduce secretions and to block vagal transmission. The usual dosage is 0.2 to 0.6 mg. These drugs depress the parasympathetic nervous system; therefore, the heart rate is increased. This counteracts the bradycardia that may occur as a result of (1) stimulating the carotid sinus and the vagus nerve and (2) traction on the extraocular muscles or the intraabdominal viscera. The use of these drugs may lead to a rise in the body temperature, especially in children. Scopolamine promotes amnesia; and, postoperatively, it may produce restlessness, irritability, and disorientation in the elderly patient.

Glycopyrrolate (Robinul) is a synthetic anticholinergic agent. The desired effects are the same as those for atropine and scopolamine but it decreases oral secretions more effectively. It is believed that this drug does not cross the blood–brain barrier and is less likely to cause confusion and other adverse reactions of the central nervous system (CNS). It also reduces volume and acidity of gastric secretions.

General Anesthesia

General anesthesia is a drug-induced depression of the CNS characterized by analgesia, amnesia, and unconsciousness, with a loss of reflexes and muscle tone. It is reversible upon elimination of the drug. General anesthetic agents may be administered by inhalation or IV injection.

The exact way in which general anesthetic agents produce their effect is not known. It is known, however, that the agents are carried by the blood to all the body tissue; but the chief effect is on the brain. In the brain, the anesthetic agent interrupts the activity of the nerve cells, and they temporarily cease to function. Sensory impulses are not carried to the CNS; thus, the patient feels no pain. The CNS is no longer capable of issuing motor discharges; therefore, the patient cannot move parts of the body.

The two most critical periods of general anesthesia are at the time of induction and at the time of emergence from anesthesia. It is during these crucial periods that complications such as vomiting and cardiac arrest may occur. The perioperative nurses must be alert and available to assist the anesthesiologist during these periods.

The four stages of general anesthesia and the appropriate nursing actions are identified in Table 10–2.

Anesthesia Machine. Perioperative nurses should be familiar with the anesthesia machine (Fig. 10–3) and know how to connect it and how to administer oxygen and ventilate a patient. The anesthesia machine is connected to a source of gases, either from the high pressure tanks attached to the machine or piped from a central hospital source. In

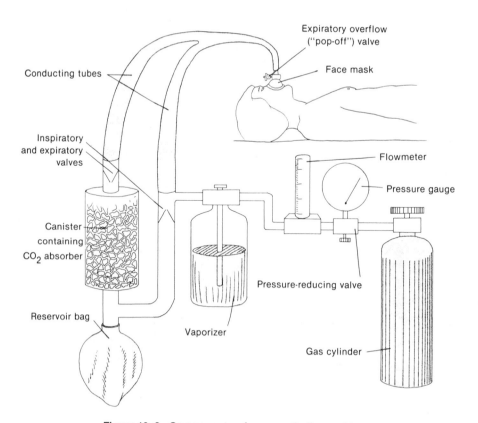

Figure 10-3. Components of an anesthetic machine.

TABLE 10-2. THE FOUR STAGES OF ANESTHESIA

Stage	Biologic Response	Patient Reaction	Nursing Action
I: Relaxation	Amnesia Analgesia	Feels drowsy and dizzy Exaggerated hearing Decreased sensation of pain May appear inebriated	Close OR doors Check for proper positioning of safety belt Have suction available and working Keep noise in room to a minimum Provide emotional support for the patient by remaining at his or her side
II: Excitement	Delirium	Irregular breathing Increased muscle tone and involuntary motor activity; may move all extremities May vomit, hold breath or struggle (patient is very susceptible to external stimuli such as a loud noise or being touched)	Avoid stimulating the patient Be available to protect extremities or to restrain the patient Be available to assist anesthesiologist with suctioning
III: Operative or surgical anesthesia	Partial to complete sensory loss Progression to complete intercostal paralysis	Quiet, regular thoraco-abdominal breathing Jaw relaxed Auditory and pain sensation lost Moderate to maximum decrease in muscle tone Eyelid reflex is absent	Be available to assist anesthesiologist with intubation Validate with anesthesiologist appropriate time for skin scrub and positioning of patient Check position of patient's feet to ascertain they are not crossed
IV: Danger	Medullary paralysis and respiratory distress	Respiratory muscles paralyzed Pupils fixed and dilated Pulse rapid and thready Respirations cease	Be available to assist in treatment of cardiac or respiratory arrest Provide emergency drug box and defibrillation Document administration of drugs

either situation, the ends of each connector must be designed so it is impossible to connect it to any source other than its own labeled source. To further guard against accidents, cylinders containing anesthetic gases and their fittings and outlets are color coded for safety. The color for oxygen is green, nitrous oxide is blue, and cyclopropane is orange.

The anesthesia machine permits the administration of inhaled gases in known and controlled mixtures of oxygen and the anesthetic agent. Using a mask or endotracheal tube, inhalation gases may be administered by an open, semiclosed, or closed system. In the open system, the patient inhales anesthetic agents and oxygen from the anesthetic machine and then exhales through a valve directly into the atmosphere. Water vapor and heat are lost, and high flows of gases are necessary for this method.

In the semiclosed system, the patient exhales gases into the atmosphere, or the gases are mixed with fresh gases and the patient rebreathes this mixture. In this system, the gases must pass through a chemical (CO_2) absorber. The chemical absorber contains granules of the hydroxides of sodium, calcium, or barium that absorb moisture and carbon dioxide from the exhaled gases. As the granules become saturated with the carbon dioxide, they change in color.

The open and the semiclosed methods of administering anesthetic gases both allow waste gases to enter the atmosphere and should not be used because of the potential health hazards of exposure to trace concentrations of waste anesthetic gases.

The closed system allows rebreathing of exhaled gases. This system is a circle arrangement consisting of an anesthetic agent, a reservoir bag, a chemical absorber, an expiratory overflow valve, and two conducting tubes (elephant hoses) connected to the face mask or the endotracheal tube. Valves in the conducting tubes allow the gases to flow in one direction only. This prevents the rebreathing of exhaled gases until the carbon dioxide has been removed by the chemical absorber.

When manually compressed, the reservoir bag forces air into the patient's lungs. This is the standard way a patient is assisted with ventilation.

Several safety features have been incorporated into anesthesia machines to avoid or reduce hazards resulting from machine malfunctions or operator errors. These features can assist the anesthetist in avoiding or rapidly correcting conditions that could lead to hypoxia, cardiac arrest, or arrhythmias. The American Society of Anesthesiologists (ASA) recommends, and the Joint Commission for Accreditation of Healthcare Organizations (JCAHO) requires the use of an oxygen monitor in the breathing system to detect hypoxic gas mixtures due to component failure, incorrect setting, or insufficient oxygen flow.

Monitors with alarms are provided to protect the patient from excessive pressure and to warn of changes in a patient's respiration or onset of unsafe operating conditions. Exhaled-volume monitors with properly adjusted alarms can be used to detect leaks and disconnections. Carbon dioxide monitors measure the level of carbon dioxide in the exhaled gas. This concentration is an indicator of the adequacy of pulmonary circulation and ventilation. This monitor can also indicate when the trachea has not been intubated. The carbon dioxide monitors are also useful for identifying leaks and disconnections because a failure to properly ventilate the lungs will result in a major change in exhaled carbon dioxide levels.

Pulse oximeters provide a widely accepted noninvasive means of monitoring the oxygen saturation of hemoglobin in the blood (SaO_2) and are emerging as part of the standard of care during anesthesia. However, an oxygen monitor is still required to provide early detection of a hypoxic gas mixture.

Inhalation Anesthetic Agents

Gaseous Agents. Cyclopropane is a colorless, sweet-smelling, flammable, explosive gas. It is a very potent anesthetic gas with rapid induction and emergence times. Cyclopropane does cause respiratory depression and can cause cardiac arrhythmias by sensitizing the myocardium to catecholamines such as epinephrine. Due to its explosive nature, cyclopropane is rarely used.

Nitrous oxide is a colorless, odorless, nonexplosive, nonirritating gas with a rapid induction and recovery period. It is a relatively weak anesthetic agent and, except for short procedures, requires the addition of other agents. Nitrous oxide can produce hypoxia as a result of administering too high a concentration of the gas.

Volatile Agents. Volatile agents are liquids that are easily vaporized and inhaled and produce anesthesia. One of the oldest anesthetic agents, ether is a colorless, volatile liquid with a pungent odor. Ether is one of the safest anesthetics, as there is a wide margin between the concentration adequate for surgical procedures and the concentration that produces respiratory and circulatory depression. The induction and the emergence are long with ether. It causes postanesthesia nausea, vomiting, and urinary retention. Ether is very irritating to the skin, mucous membranes, lungs, and kidneys. It is highly flammable and explosive; it is, therefore, rarely used as an anesthetic agent.

The most commonly used volatile agents are halothane (Fluothane), enflurane (Ethrane), methoxyflurane (Penthrane) and isoflurane (Forane)—all halogenated compounds with a sweet odor. They are nonflammable liquids that require a special vaporizor for administration.

Halothane provides a smooth induction and a rapid emergence with little excitement. It is nonirritating to the respiratory tract and produces only a minimal amount of nausea and vomiting postoperatively. Halothane depresses the cardiovascular system resulting in hypotension and bradycardia. It can sensitize the myocardium to produce cardiac arrhythmias. The use of epinephrine as a local injection for vasoconstriction may aggravate or precipitate the arrhythmias.

Due to halothane's depressant effect on the hypothalamus, shivering may be seen in the immediate postoperative period.

There is some evidence that halothane may cause liver damage in some patients and that subsequent exposures to the agent may result in severe or fatal jaundice. Therefore, most anesthesiologists avoid using halothane on patients requiring multiple surgical procedures.

Enflurane provides a rapid induction and a rapid emergence with minimal nausea and vomiting. It is nonirritating to the respiratory tract during induction. Enflurane produces adequate muscle relaxation for intraabdominal procedures. It reduces ventilation and decreases blood pressure as the depth of the anesthesia increases. The cardiac rate and rhythm remain relatively stable.

Methoxyflurane is a potent drug that provides a slow induction and a long emergence with some nausea and vomiting. It is an excellent muscle relaxant and provides good analgesia at low concentrations. Methoxyflurane causes minimal sensitization of the myocardium to catecholamines. The breakdown products of methoxyflurane are toxic to the kidney; therefore, this agent is limited to surgical procedures of short duration.

Isoflurane is the newest of the halogenated compounds and appears to be the ideal inhalation agent. It provides a rapid, smooth induction without stimulating excessive secretions. The emergence is rapid. The cardiovascular system remains stable, and the myocardium is not sensitized to catecholamines. Isoflurane provides good muscle relaxation and there is no evidence of renal or hepatic damage.

Waste Anesthetic Gases. There is a growing body of research on the occupational health hazards of long-term exposure to trace concentrations of waste anesthetic gases. These health hazards include the increased likelihood of spontaneous abortions and reproductive difficulties in females working in the operating room, and congenital defects in their children as well as in the offspring of unexposed wives of exposed men.[3,4] In Chapter 2, four methods of scavenging waste anesthetic gases were identified. In addition, the anesthesia machine should be checked daily for leaks and scheduled routinely for preventive maintenance and repairs. To ascertain the effectiveness of the gas control program, periodic air monitoring should be conducted to measure the level of waste gases present in each operating room.

IV Anesthetic Agents. IV drugs are frequently used as anesthetics and/or to supplement the inhalation agents. Unlike the inhalation agents that can be removed by ventilating the lungs, IV agents must first be metabolized and then excreted from the body. The IV drugs cannot be removed or stopped once they are injected. This technique of induction is frequently requested by patients as it is rapid and pleasant.

Barbiturates are often used for IV inductions. The barbiturates act directly on the central venous system (producing a reaction ranging from mild sedation to unconsciousness), but provide little relief of pain. The principal barbiturate used is the ultra short-acting thiopental (Sodium Pentothal). In addition to being used for inductions thiopental is used to supplement nitrous oxide during short procedures and as a hypnotic during regional anesthesia. It has a rapid onset of action, producing unconsciousness in 30 seconds. Depending on the amount and the rate of injections, thiopental is a potent depressant of respirations. It can also cause depression of the cardiovascular system, resulting in varying degrees of hypotension. An anesthesia machine and oxygen should always be available for assisting or controlling ventilations.

Narcotics may also be used to supplement the inhalation agents. The most commonly used narcotics are morphine, meperidine hydrochloride (Demerol), and fentanyl citrate (Sublimaze). The use of narcotics during surgery results in good postoperative analgesia. Morphine and meperidine hydrochloride depress the respiratory system, however, and impaired ventilation may be a major problem during the recovery phase.

Fentanyl citrate is a synthetic narcotic with a potency 80 to 100 times greater than morphine. The duration of action is shorter than with morphine or meperidine; therefore, it does not have the prolonged period of impaired ventilation associated with those drugs.

Innovar is a combination of the narcotic, fentanyl citrate, and the tranquilizer, droperidol (Inapsine). It may be used in small doses as a premedication or in larger doses during surgery to supplement nitrous oxide or a regional anesthesia. It produces a general quiescence and excellent analgesia with a lower incidence of postoperative nausea and vomiting. Innovar has a long duration of action; therefore, patients must be observed for respiratory depression, hypoventilation, apnea, and hypotension during the postoperative period.

Ketamine hydrochloride is a dissociative anesthetic drug. These drugs act by selectively interrupting associative pathways in the brain. Given intravenously or intramuscularly, ketamine results in a rapid onset of a trancelike, profound analgesic state without respiratory depression or the loss of muscle tone, thus protecting the airway. The cardiovascular system is stimulated with an increase in the heart rate and the blood pressure. Ketamine hydrochloride is excellent for diagnostic and short surgical procedures, or to supplement weaker agents such as nitrous oxide. It is useful in children because anesthesia occurs within 3 to 5 minutes after an intramuscular injection. During recovery from ketamine hydrochloride, patients may experience unpleasant dreams, hallucinations, or distorted images and they may act irrationally. These reactions are seen more often in adults than in children and can be reduced by minimizing the stimulating effects of light, noise, touch, or movement until the patient awakens naturally.

Propofol (Diprivan) is a sedative–hypnotic drug that can be used both for induction and maintenance of general anesthesia. A single IV injection produces loss of consciousness within 40 seconds and patients are awake, responsive to verbal commands, and fully oriented in less than 8 minutes after it is discontinued. Patients ambulate earlier, ingest fluids, and eat sooner than with standard anesthetic agents, therefore the drug has advantages in the outpatient setting. Adverse reactions include hypotension and apnea. The drug should be used with caution in elderly, debilitated and hypovolemic patients and in those in ASA class III or IV.

Tranquilizers and nonbarbiturate sedatives are used for induction and as adjuncts to other anesthetic agents. Their use permits the administration of lower doses of other agents. The most commonly used tranquilizers include diazepam, midazolam (Versed), and droperiodol (Inapsine). Diazepam provides sedation and amnesia and reduces anxiety and apprehension. Adverse reactions are excessive sedation, respiratory depression, preoperative or postoperative nausea, and vomiting. Droperidol is useful as an antiemetic agent. Midazolam is a potent sedative. The total dose during a procedure should not exceed 0.1 to 0.15 mg/kg for adults. If the drug is used with other narcotics, the dose of midazolam should be decreased by 25% to 30%. The safety and effectiveness of midazolam in children below the age of 18 has not been established.

Neuromuscular blocking agents are used to provide muscle relaxation during surgery or to facilitate passage of an endotracheal tube. These drugs exert their action on the striated muscles of the body by interfering with the impulses that occur at the motor end plate. The motor end plate is the point where a motor nerve fiber connects with a muscle fiber.

There are two types of muscle relaxant drugs: depolarizers and nondepolarizers.

Depolarizing agents produce a neuromuscular block by acting like acetylcholine to depolarize the membrane of the motor end plate. When these drugs are administered, the muscle fiber acts as if acetylcholine was released and the muscle contracts or twitches. The drug remains attached to the muscle fibers and prevents the repolarization necessary for another contracture from occurring; thus, the muscle remains relaxed. The most frequently used depolarizing agent is succinylcholine chloride (Quelicin, Anectine). It is a rapid-acting drug with a duration of 3 to 5 minutes and, therefore, is frequently used for intubation. It can also be administered by a continuous IV drip solution when longer periods of relaxation are required. The effects of depolarizing agents can be reversed with atropine or Robinul (glycopyrrolate).

Nondepolarizing muscle relaxants act to inhibit the effect of acetylcholine at the neuromuscular junction, but they do not cause depolarization of the motor end plate. Tubocurarine (curare), pancuronium bromide (Pavulor), gallamine triethiodide (Flaxedil), atracurium (Tracrium) and vercuronium (Norcufon) are all nondepolarizing agents. The onset time of Tubocurarine is 3 to 5 minutes and the duration of action is 20 to 60 minutes. It frequently causes hypotension and bronchospasms. Tubocurarine is potentiated by certain anesthetics such as halothane, enflurane, and methoxyflurane and by some antibiotics. Pancuronium bromide is longer acting than curare and is about five times as potent; it does cause hypertension and tachycardia. Gallamine triethiodide has a slightly shorter duration of action than curare, but it does not cause hypotension or bronchospasms. Gallamine triethiodide affects the vagus nerve and can produce tachycardia and hypertension. Atracurium and vercuronium have no significant cardiovascular effects. Atracurium results in a slight release of histamine, whereas vercuronium has no influence on histamine production.

The anesthesiologist must maintain an awareness of the amount of paralysis present. This can be accomplished by applying a nerve stimulator to the ulnar nerve at the elbow or the wrist and by observing the absence of contractions or the diminished strength of the hand muscles.

The effects of nondepolarizing agents can be reversed with the administration of neostigmine (Prostigmin) or tensiton (Edrophonium), which allows acetylcholine to accumulate at the neuromuscular junction.

Balanced Anesthesia. Balanced anesthesia is a term applied to anesthesia produced by the combination of two or more drugs (e.g., a barbiturate administered intravenously for induction, nitrous oxide and morphine for analgesia, and a muscle relaxant to provide additional relaxation of the muscle).

Malignant Hyperthermia. Malignant hyperthermia is a complication of general anesthesia that occurs in 1 out of 3,000 to 15,000 children and in 1 out of 50,000 to 100,000 adults.[3] It is characterized by a rapid elevation of temperature as high as 42.8°C to 44°C (109°F to 111°F). The complication occurs when anesthetic agents such as halothane, methoxyflurane (Penthrane), cyclopropane, or succinylcholine are administered to a susceptible patient. The patient apparently has a defect in the muscle cell membrane, allowing the anesthetic to trigger a sudden rise of calcium within the muscle cells. The increased amount of calcium then sets off a series of biochemical reactions that increase the patient's metabolic rate, eventually liberating heat. Muscle contractures also increase, liberating more heat.[4]

The most consistent, early symptom is tachycardia. Other symptoms include increased skin temperature, mottling of the skin with or without cyanosis, dark blood in the operative field, hypotension, diaphoresis, and excessive heat in the chemical (CO_2)

absorber and in the reservoir bag on the anesthesia machine. Muscle rigidity and cardiac arrhythmias usually follow.

The treatment consists of early diagnosis followed by termination of the surgical procedure, discontinuing the anesthetic agent, hyperventilating the patient with 100% oxygen and administering dantrolene sodium (Dantrium) 2.5 mg/kg either by direct IV injection or continuous rapid infusion. Dantrium interferes with the release of calcium ions within the muscle fibers and, therefore, interrupts the cycle.[5] Additional treatment may include surface cooling with bags of ice or a cooling mattress, irrigating the wound with cold saline solution, administering iced IV solutions and sodium bicarbonate, inserting a Foley catheter to monitor urinary output, inserting a CVP and an arterial line or Swan-Ganz catheter. Additional drugs to have available include procainamide, 50% glucose, and insulin.

Genetically malignant hyperthermia is an autosomal dominant gene affecting 50% of the offspring.[7] It is more common in males than females and frequently occurs in individuals with subclinical or clinical myopathy, numerous drug allergies, and a history of unexplained surgical deaths in the patient's family.

Cleaning and Processing of Anesthesia Equipment. As discussed in Chapter 6, the respiratory tract is colonized with organisms that live in harmony with the host. If these organisms are introduced into other areas of the body or are transferred to other individuals, they may multiply and cause an infectious disease. Studies[6,7] indicate that the equipment used for general anesthetics is often grossly contaminated by organisms. Therefore, the equipment should be terminally decontaminated, cleaned, and sterilized, or discarded if disposable equipment is used.[8] Disposable items are designed and manufactured for a single use; they represent a potential hazard to the patient if they are reused.

Care of Reusable Equipment. The anesthesia hoses, mask, and breathing bag must be terminally cleaned and sterilized after each use. Terminal cleaning and packaging of anesthesia equipment should be consistent with the discussion in Chapter 7. Currently, most of the rubber used in the manufacturing of these items will withstand steam sterilization. If the items are not heat stable, they should be sterilized by ethylene oxide or a solution of 2% activated glutaraldehyde. When ethylene oxide is used, the items must be aerated according to the manufacturer's recommendations.

Soda lime is not effective as a filter or bactericidal agent. Bacteria from healthy patients have been found to contaminate the valves of the anesthesia circle absorber at the average rate of 35 microorganisms per minute.[9] Since most of the absorbers are heavy, difficult to remove, and made of material that excludes heat sterilization, a sterile, single-use absorber and valve system is recommended.

The anesthesia ventilators should be disassembled and all patient-exposed parts should be steam sterilized after each use.

All ancillary equipment such as endotracheal tubes, stylettes, laryngoscopes, and airways become grossly contaminated. These items should be placed in a receptacle designated for contaminated items immediately after use. These items should not be placed on the top of the anesthesia machine.

The top of the anesthesia machine should be cleaned with a detergent germicide after each patient. All other exterior surfaces and the drawers should be cleaned once every 24 hours.

Blood pressure cuffs and tubing should be cleaned with a disinfectant solution after each use and should be washed and sterilized weekly.

As previously discussed in Chapter 6, hand washing is one of the most important controls in reducing the incidence of cross-infection. Members of the anesthesia team should wash their hands before and after each case.

Regional Anesthesia

Regional anesthesia temporarily interrupts the transmission of nerve impulses to and from a specific area or region. Motor function may or may not be involved, but the patient does not lose consciousness. The extent of the anesthetized field depends on the site of application, the total volume administered, and the concentration and the penetrating ability of the drug.

Regional anesthetics may be used on patients when a general anesthetic is contraindicated or less desirable. The advantages of regional anesthetics are

1. The technique is simple and there is a minimal amount of equipment required.
2. The drugs are nonflammable.
3. Less nausea and vomiting occur postoperatively.
4. Less bleeding occurs if a vasoconstrictor is used.
5. There is less disturbance to body function; thus, they are excellent for surgical procedures performed on outpatients.
6. They can be used when general anesthetics are contraindicated due to recent ingestion of food by the patient or when there are existing cardiac and pulmonary dysfunctions.
7. They can be used for procedures in which it is desirable to have the patient awake and cooperative.
8. They are less expensive.
9. They can be used when an anesthesiologist is not available.
10. There is no pollution to the environment.

The disadvantages of regional anesthetics are:

1. Many procedures are too complex for regional anesthetics.
2. They are difficult to administer to the very young patient and to patients who are emotionally unstable.
3. They cannot be used in the presence of skin infections or sepsis near the site of injection.
4. Patients are awake and may become apprehensive due to the sights and the sounds of the operating room.
5. There is no control over the drug once it is injected.
6. Local and general complications may occur.

If complications occur, they are usually due to overdosage, accidental intravascular injection, or the administration of a "normal dose" to a sensitive patient. The "normal dose" depends upon the area to be anesthetized, the vascularity of the tissues, the individual's tolerance, and the techniques of anesthesia. The lowest dose necessary to provide effective anesthesia should be administered. Table 10–3 outlines the general characteristics and recommended maximum dosages of the commonly used solutions for infiltration and topical anesthesia.

The local complications include edema, inflammation, abscess, necrosis, and gangrene. Inflammation and abscess are usually a result of a break in sterile technique occurring at the time of the local injection. Necrosis and gangrene may occur as a result of vasoconstriction in the area of the injection.

Vasoconstrictive drugs may be added to local anesthetic agents to constrict the blood vessels, thereby reducing the amount of bleeding. Vasoconstrictors also slow the absorption of the drug, thus minimizing toxic reactions and prolonging the operating time. The addition of a vasoconstrictor is contraindicated when injecting fingers, toes, penis, or urethra.

The signs and the symptoms of a systemic toxic reaction due to the overdose of a regional anesthetic are manifested by CNS stimulation followed by CNS and cardiovascular depression. The first signs are restlessness, excitement, incoherent speech, headache, dizziness, blurred vision, metallic taste, nausea, vomiting, tremors, convulsions, and increased blood pressure and pulse with an increased respiratory rate. Treatment is establishment of an airway, administration of oxygen, and sedation with a fast-acting barbiturate. If the toxic reaction remains untreated, unconsciousness, hypotension, apnea, and cardiac arrest will result.

When administering a local anesthetic, sterile technique is used, and resuscitation equipment must be available. This includes a patient cart with the option of Trendelenburg's position, suction, oral airways, oxygen, bag and mask for ventilation, and drugs such as vasoconstrictors and barbiturates.

Techniques of Administering Regional Anesthesia.
The techniques used to apply the drugs to the nerves include topical anesthesia, local infiltration, nerve blocks, and spinal anesthesia.

Topical Anesthesia. The local anesthetic agent is applied directly on the surface of the area to be anesthetized. This method is frequently used on the respiratory passages prior to intubation or for diagnostic procedures such as laryngoscopy, bronchoscopy, or cystoscopy. The onset of action is 1 minute and the duration is 20 to 30 minutes. Collapse of the cardiovascular system may occur following the application of the topical anesthetic to the respiratory tract.

Local Infiltration. In this technique the drug is injected into the subcutaneous tissue surrounding the incision, wound, or lesion.

Nerve Blocks. A nerve block is achieved by injecting the local anesthetic agent into or around a nerve or nerves supplying the involved area. Nerve blocks are used to prevent pain, to identify the cause of pain, to increase circulation in some vascular diseases, and to relieve chronic pain.

TABLE 10-3. DRUGS USED FOR LOCAL ANESTHETICS

	Cocaine	Novocaine (Procaine) (Hydrochloride)	Lidocaine (Xylocaine) (Hydrochloride)	Tetracaine (Pontocaine) (Hydrochloride)	Mepivacaine (Carbocaine) (Hydrochloride)	Bupivacaine (Marcaine) (Hydrochloride)	Chloroprocaine (Nesacaine) (Hydrochloride)
Topical concentration	Eye 1% Other 4%–10%	Ineffective	Eye 0.5% Other 4%	Eye 0.5% Other 1%–2%	Eye 0.5% Other 1%–2%	Not used	Not used
Onset (minutes)	Immediate		3–5	10–20	10–20		
Duration (minutes)	30–60 min		30–60	60–120	60–120		
Maximum dose	200 mg		200 mg	50 mg	500 mg		
Infiltration concentration	Not used	0.25%–1.0% 2.0, 10%	0.5%–2%	0.05%–0.1%	0.5%–2%	0.25%–0.75%	1%, 2%, 3%
Onset (minutes)		5–15	3–5	10–20	5–10	5–10	5–10
Duration of action (minutes), plain		45–60	30–60	90–120	150–240	90–120	30–60
Duration of action (minutes) with epinephrine 1:200,000		60–90	45–90	140–180	240–320	140–180	45–90
Maximum dose, plain		1000 mg or 15 mg/kg	300 mg or 6–8 mg/kg	50–100 mg or 3 mg/kg	500 mg or 6–8 mg/kg	175 mg or 4–6 mg/kg	1000 mg or 15 mg/kg

Adapted from L. Donald Bridenbaugh. Care of the surgical patient under local anesthetics. Gown and Gloves. 1979; 4 (2):13.

The nerve blocks most frequently used in operative procedures are of the brachial plexus; cervical plexus; intercostal nerves; and radial, ulnar, and digital nerves.

Field Block. This is a term used to describe regional anesthesia produced by a series of injections around the operative field.

Caudal and Epidural Blocks. When the local anesthetic solution is injected into the epidural space through the sacral hiatus and the caudal canal, the technique is termed *caudal block.* Injection of the anesthetic solution into the epidural space through the interspaces of the lumbar, thoracic, or cervical spine is termed an *epidural block.* After confirming proper placement of the catheter, the anesthetist secures it and administers a regional anesthetic. The drug is chosen on the basis of the expected length of the operation and the degree of muscle relaxation required. This catheter can be left in place postoperatively, and additional injections may be administered to assist with vasodilation or analgesia. A local anesthetic, narcotics, and steroids can be administered by continuous infusion, or the anesthetist may administer intermittent bolus doses. Blood pressure and respiratory status must be closely monitored on these patients and an apnea monitor may be ordered for the first 12 to 24 hours after surgery.

Spinal Anesthesia. Spinal anesthesia is achieved by the injection of an anesthetic agent into the cerebrospinal fluid with (1) resultant absorption by the sensory, motor, and autonomic nerve fibers and (2) blockage of nerve transmissions. The injection is performed through one of the interspaces between lumbar 2, (L_2) and the sacrum (S_1). The spinal cord usually ends at L_1 or L_2. Therefore, performing the puncture at this site or above may cause damage to the spinal cord. The site most frequently used is between L_3 and L_4.

The level of anesthesia is dependent on the following factors:

1. Dose and concentration of the drug
2. Volume injected
3. Site and rate of the injection
4. Specific gravity of the solution
5. Cerebrospinal fluid pressure
6. Length of the vertebral column
7. Position of the patient during the injection and immediately after the injection

The injection may be performed with the patient sitting on the edge of the operating room table with the arms resting on the thighs, the feet on a stool, and the chin resting on the chest, or the patient may be in the flexed lateral (fetal) position. Both of these positions straighten the natural curvature of the spine and widen the intervertebral spaces to facilitate insertion of the spinal needle.

The spread of the anesthetic agent is influenced by the specific gravity of the solution and the position of the patient immediately after the injection. The level of analgesia is usually fixed within 15 to 20 minutes and is no longer influenced by changes in the patient's position.

Spinal anesthesia can be divided into low spinal, midspinal, and high spinal anesthesia. The low spinal (saddle block) involves the sacral nerves (S_{1-5}) and provides adequate anesthesia for diagnostic and surgical interventions in the perineal and the anal regions.

The midspinal is used for surgical procedures below the level of the umbilicus (T–10) such as in appendectomies and herniorrhaphies.

The high spinal reaches the nipple line (T–4). This is achieved by lowering the patient's head immediately following injection of the drug until the desired height of anesthesia is reached. In using this method, the anesthesiologist must watch the level of anesthesia very carefully as intercostal paralysis and respiratory insufficiency may occur. The high spinal may be used on surgical procedures involving the stomach and the biliary tract. Hiccups and nausea frequently occur in the high spinal especially following vagus stimulation and manipulation of the viscera during the surgical procedure.

Spinal anesthesia produces excellent analgesia and relaxation for abdominal and pelvic procedures. The most important side effect of spinal anesthesia is hypotension caused by a preganglionic block of the sympathetic fibers, resulting in vasodilitation and a reduction in the venous return to the heart. The treatment usually consists of administering oxygen and intravenously administering vasopressors.

A spinal headache may occur 24 to 48 hours postoperatively. It occurs when the dura mater does not seal off following extraction of the needle and the cerebrospinal fluid leaks into the epidural space. This decreases the cerebrospinal pressure and puts stress on the nerves between the cranium and the brain. Treatment for the spinal headache is bed rest, hydration, and sedation and in severe cases a blood patch graft. A blood patch graft consists of an epidural injection of 10 ml of the patient's blood that plugs the leak.

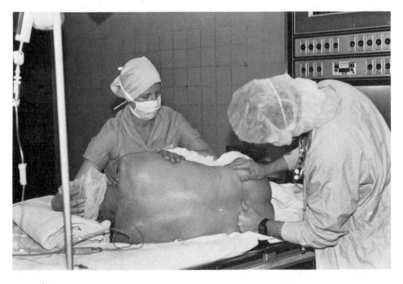

Figure 10-4. The perioperative nurse provides physical and emotional support to patients having regional anesthetics.

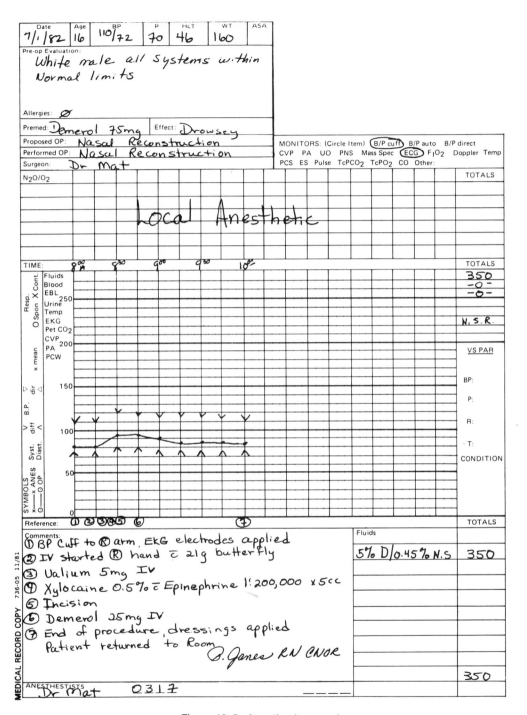

Figure 10-5. Anesthesia record.

TABLE 10-4. PATIENT CARE PLAN FOR LOCAL PROCEDURE

Nursing Diagnosis	Expected Outcome	Nursing Actions	Schedule for Assessment
1. Potential anxiety related to unfamiliar environment and/or impending surgery	1. Ability to cope with anxiety	1a. Explain preoperative and intraoperative activities	Preoperatively
		b. Encourage patient to verbalize questions and concerns	Intraoperatively
		c. Stay with patient and provide support	12–24 hours postoperatively
		d. Provide nonverbal support by touching patient	
2. Potential fear of pain	2. Pain controlled	2a. Encourage patient to verbalize discomfort	Intraoperatively
		b. Discuss with patient availability of pain medication	
3. Potential altered sensory perceptions related to preoperative medication	3. Able to respond appropriately and to follow directions	3a. Maintain quiet atmosphere	Intraoperatively
		b. Post sign on door "Patient Awake"	12–24 hours postoperatively
		c. Turn off auditory intercom	
4. Potential loss of dignity related to excessive exposure and lack of personal care	4. Dignity maintained	4a. Limit exposure of patient only to area required for surgical procedure	Intraoperatively
		b. Call patient by name	12–24 hours postoperatively
		c. Only pertinent team members permitted in room	
5. Possible discomfort related to position	5. Comfortable position	5a. Position patient anatomically	Intraoperatively
		b. Flex table slightly at knees to reduce strain on back muscles	12–24 hours postoperatively
		c. Place pillow under knees	
		d. Pad all boney prominences	
		e. Pad wrists with webril prior to restraints being applied	
		f. Ask patient about position	

Nursing Diagnosis	Goal	Interventions	Phase
6. Potential contamination of wound related to patient inadvertently touching wound	6. No wound contamination	6. Apply padded clover leaf hitch arm restraints	Intraoperatively
7. Potential alteration in body temperature related to temperature of operating room	7. Body temperature maintained within normal limits	7a. Apply warm blankets b. Use warm solutions c. Limit skin exposure to area required for surgical procedure d. Ask patient about body temperature	Intraoperatively
8. Possible adverse reaction to local anesthetic agent related to sensitivity to agent or overdose	8. Avoid or minimize cardiovascular and respiratory compromise	8a. Two nurses assigned to circulate b. Check chart for allergies c. Obtain baseline vital signs before surgery d. Monitor amount of local anesthestic administered e. Use electrocardiograph to monitor patient for cardiac arrhythmias f. Monitor and record vital signs as indicated or at least: every 15 minutes and before and after medication g. Communicate changes to surgeon	Intraoperatively
9. Potential lack in continuity of care related to patient returning to primary care nurse/ inpatient unit	9. Continuity of care maintained	9a. Inform primary care nurse what procedure was performed b. Vital signs c. All medications administered d. Amount of IV fluids infused e. Estimated blood loss f. Location of any drains or packs g. Type of dressing h. How the patient tolerated the procedure	Immediate postoperative

(continued)

TABLE 10-4. CONTINUED.

Nursing Diagnosis	Expected Outcome	Nursing Actions	Schedule for Assessment
Ambulatory Patients Only			
10. Potential latent adverse reaction or side effects to local anesthesia or surgical procedure	10. Adverse reaction and side effects treated appropriately	10. a Observe patient for minimum of 30 minutes postoperatively prior to discharge	Immediate postoperative
		b. Alert patient and significant others to signs and symptoms of adverse reaction and how to respond appropriately	
		c. Validate postoperative instructions by requesting verbal feedback	
		d. Give patient and significant others telephone number of operating room surgeon and emergency room: instruct patient to call regarding any questions or concerns	
		e. Obtain telephone number where patient can be reached for postoperative phone call in 24 hours	24 hours postoperatively

Nursing Concerns for the Patient Receiving a Regional Anesthetic. The perioperative nurse assists the anesthesiologist in assembling the equipment necessary for the regional anesthesia and in setting up for the procedure. During the procedure, the nurse observes the anesthesiologist for breaks in technique and provides physical and emotional support to the patient by staying with the patient, providing words of encouragement (Fig. 10–4), and assisting with the position required for the regional nerve block. Touch is especially important to the patient having a local anesthetic. It reassures the patient that the nurse is present and is concerned about him or her as an individual and about his or her comfort and safety.

In the absence of an anesthesiologist, such as in a local infiltration, the circulating nurse is responsible for monitoring and documenting the patient's vital signs every 15 minutes and prior to administration of a local anesthetic agent or analgesic. Intraoperative care also includes initiation of oxygen therapy and administration of IV fluids when clinical findings warrant action. All changes in the patient's condition should be reported to the surgeon. Documentation should include vital signs, a list of IV fluids and medication administered (Fig. 10–5).

At the beginning of these surgical procedures, there must be two nurses assigned to circulate, one to monitor the patient and the other one to assist the sterile members of the team. After the incision is made and the procedure is proceeding, only one circulator may be required (see Table 10–4).

The scrub nurse on a local infiltration procedure should label all drugs on the sterile field and maintain an accurate account of the amount of the drug that is injected during the course of the procedure.

Departmental policies and procedures should be formulated regarding the administration of drugs that may be given by the perioperative nurse, and the level of monitoring skills required.

REFERENCES

1. Zimmerman L. *Great Ideas in the History.* New York: Dover; 1967: 103
2. Cartwright F. *The Development of Modern Surgery.* New York: Thomas Crowell; 1968: 48, 226
3. Brodsky JA. Exposure to anesthetic gases: A controversy. *AORN J.* 1983; 38(1): 132–144
4. Mattia MA. Hazards in the hospital environment: Anesthesia gases and methylmethacrylate. *Amer J Nurs.* 1983; 38: 73–77
5. Britt BA, Kalow W. Malignant hyperthermia: A statistical review. *Can Anes Soc J.* July 1970; 293
6. Geven L. Dantrium. *Nursing.* 1980; 80: 62
7. Stallings J, Lines J. Malignant hyperpyrexia anesthesia complications. *AORN J.* 1975; 21(4): 645
8. Dryden GE. Uncleaned anesthesia equipment. *AMA.* 1975; 233 (12): 1297–1298
9. Albrecht WH, Dryden GE. Five year experience with the development of an individually clean anesthesia system. *Anesth Analg.* 1974; 51 (1): 24–28
10. Recommended practices for cleaning and processing anesthesia equipment. *AORN J.* 1987; 45 (3): 777

Chapter 11
Positioning and Draping

POSITIONING

The circulating nurse is responsible for coordinating the efforts of the team members in positioning the surgical patient. Due to preoperative medication and anesthetic drugs, the patient's normal defense mechanisms cannot guard against joint damage and muscle stretch and strain. Knowledge of anatomical structures and physiological functioning are imperative so that the circulating nurse can ensure patient safety and comfort.

The proper patient position must provide for:

1. Optimum exposure of the operative site
2. Access for the anesthesiologist to maintain the patient's circulatory and respiratory functions
3. Access for the administration of IV solutions
4. Protection of neuromuscular and skeletal structures
5. Minimal interference with circulation
6. Physiological alignment
7. Comfort and safety for the patient
8. Preservation of the patient's dignity

Nursing Considerations

During preoperative assessment, the perioperative nurse will evaluate the patient's size and identify any existing respiratory, skeletal, or neuromuscular limitations such as rheumatoid arthritis, joint replacements, or emphysema. Following the preoperative assessment, an individual patient care plan is developed. The plan may include nursing orders regarding the number of personnel required for transportation (Fig. 11–1), the appropriate mode of transportation, and the appropriate patient position during transportation.

The surgeon's preference card will determine the appropriate position. This card can be used as a guide in selecting the necessary equipment and the positioning aids and in determining the number of personnel required to achieve the position. All the equipment used to position patients should be checked for proper functioning and completeness prior to the patient's arrival in the operating room.

Factors that influence the actual time at which the patient is positioned are the site of the operation, the age and size of the patient, the anesthetic technique, and if the patient experiences pain upon moving. If the patient is going to be placed in the prone position, the anesthesiologist may want to anesthetize the patient on the transportation vehicle and then move the patient to the operating room while turning the patient to the prone position. Frequently, the anesthesiologist or the circulating nurse will hold a child during the induction phase and then place the child on the operating room table.

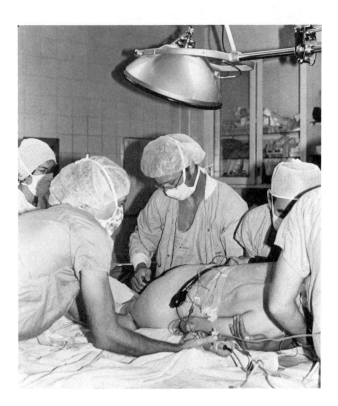

Figure 11-1. Sufficient numbers of personnel are required to safely position a patient.

If the patient experiences pain upon moving (as in the case of accident or trauma victims), the anesthesiologist may elect to anesthetize the patient on the transportation vehicle to prevent additional pain.

When transferring the patient to the operating table, it is important for the patient's safety that the transportation vehicle and the operating room table be the same height and both be locked. Two people must be in attendance when transferring the patient to the operating room table. The transportation vehicle is placed next to the operating room table with one person on each side to assist the patient in the move. The patient should be told that the table is narrow and that a safety strap is being placed across his or her legs as a reminder of this fact. The safety strap should be placed 2 inches above the knee immediately after the transfer. The strap should be applied snugly but must not restrict venous circulation or exert pressure on the nerves. The patient must never be left unattended; at least one member of the nursing staff must be present in the operating room at all times.

One of the most frequent comments from patients in regard to the operating room concerns the temperature. Every effort should be made by the perioperative nurses to provide a warm, comfortable environment. In readiness for the patient's arrival into the operating room, the operating room table may be covered with a blanket from the solution warmer; the blanket is then removed just prior to the patient being transferred to the operating room table. Additional blankets may then be placed over the patient, and a pillow offered for additional comfort.

If repositioning the patient is necessary after the induction of anesthesia, it is performed with care and the patient is lifted into position rather than rolled or pulled to avoid shearing forces and friction. Shearing occurs when two or more tissue layers slide on each other causing subcutaneous blood vessels to become kinked or stretched. This obstructs blood flow to and from the areas supplied by those vessels and contributes to pressure sores.[1] If the position of the operating table is changed while the patient is anesthetized, the weight of the torso tends to move those tissues attached to the bony structures with the patient, but due to friction between the linen and the skin, the dermal layers tend to stay in a fixed position. Skin destruction is likely to occur in the sacral area, where the blood supply to the posterior tissue exits the well-anchored deep fascia into the looser subcutaneous fascia. Angulation occurs, and thrombosis of the vessels with ischemic ulceration may result.[2,3]

Friction results in epidermal damage that significantly lowers the perpendicular pressures necessary to produce breaks in skin integrity.

Alopecia caused by prolonged immobilization of and pressure on the head has occurred following surgical intervention. It occurs early in the postoperative period as edema and a very painful seroma of the occipital scalp, followed by ulceration and transient or permanent localized hair loss. The position of the patient's head should be changed by the anesthesiologist every 30 minutes to avoid alopecia.[4-7]

Pressure may occur when a member of the surgical team inadvertently leans or rests on the patient. This additional pressure added to the patient's own weight may result in the development of pressure sores. The scrub person and the circulating nurse must monitor the position of all team members during surgery and remind them not to lean on the patient.

Disruption to the skin integrity may appear postoperatively and is identified by these stages:

1. Skin is red, unbroken, and does return to normal color 15 to 30 minutes after pressure is removed. This stage is reversible.
2. Skin is red, broken, may be excoriated, vesiculated, edematous, indurated, weeping. This stage is not reversible.
3. Presence of an open lesion with full thickness loss of skin down to subcutaneous tissue.
4. Presence of full thickness loss of skin with invasion of deeper tissues that may involve the fascia, muscle and bone.

These pressure areas are attributable to known physiological responses unique to the surgical environment; however, they are frequently erroneously described as "burns." Tissue insults precipitated by pressure occur during surgery. Perpendicular pressure (tissue compression) is an unavoidable consequence of gravity and affects capillary pressure.

Normal capillary pressure ranges between 22 to 30 mm Hg. When there is more pressure on the capillaries than in them, capillary circulation slows and blood flow in the microvasculature is obstructed. Unless the external pressure is relieved, hypoxic tissue damage will result.[8]

The tissue of any patient, whether supine, prone, or lateral is under sufficient pressure to develop pressure injuries. The following pressures are sufficient to cause tissue ischemia in a supine patient[4]:

- 20–40 mm Hg—at the occiput
- 30 mm Hg—at the spine
- 40–60 mm Hg—at the sacral area
- 30–45 mm Hg—at the heels
- 30–40 mm Hg—at the costal margins and knees (prone)

Pressure injuries can occur anywhere, but there are typical sites, as stated in the section on Common Surgical Positions and Nursing Considerations later in this chapter. Two to three hours is the longest period of time that pressure should go unrelieved, particularly during vascular procedures.[4] Without disrupting the surgery, nursing care provided by the circulator should include shifting or moving the extremities to relieve pressure and allow the cells to receive oxygen. Table 11–1 identifies factors that may predispose patients to disruption in skin integrity.

Operating Room Tables

As discussed in Chapter 2, a variety of operating room tables with accessory equipment designed to stabilize or brace the patient in a specific position are available. The perioperative nurse must be familiar with the mechanics of all the tables and the attachments available within the surgical suite. The most common table accessories are

1. Anesthesia screen
2. Armboards (these can be positioned parallel to the table to provide extra width for obese patients)
3. Head rests
4. Kidney braces

TABLE 11-1. FACTORS PREDISPOSING PATIENTS TO DISRUPTION IN SKIN INTEGRITY

1. Age extremes	12. Liver failure
2. Obesity	13. Incontinence
3. Anemia	14. Hypovolemia
4. Diabetes	15. Immobility
5. Infections	16. Vascular insufficiency
6. Fever	17. Low serum albumin
7. Cardiopulmonary disorders	18. Poor oxygenation
8. Emaciation	19. Steroid therapy
9. Poor tissue perfusion	20. Immunosuppressive drugs
10. Moisture from draining wound or diaphoresis	21. Radiation therapy
11. Dependent edema	22. Chemotherapy

5. Lateral armboards
6. Shoulder braces
7. Stirrups
8. Table extension (this can be used as an extension of the table for tall patients or placed perpendicularly to the table and padded to support the feet)

Additional items that will assist in effective positioning are

1. Blankets
2. Davis roller
3. Draw sheet (lift sheet)—A double thickness sheet is placed under the patient's trunk; the arms are placed between the flaps, and the top flap is brought down over the arm and tucked under the mattress. This positions the arm in the correct anatomical position and prevents the elbow and the fingers from resting on the edge of the table
4. Doughnut—A doughnut is used for surgical procedures on the head and face. It is made in the shape of a doughnut, using towels or foam, and then covered with webril. The head rests in the center portion, which prevents the head from rolling. If the head is turned to one side or the other, the doughnut protects the ear and the superficial nerves and blood vessels of the face
5. Elbow pads or protections
6. Laminectomy rolls (body rolls/bolsters)—These rolls consist of a solid roll of cloth or foam rubber about 6 inches in diameter and 18 inches long
7. Pillows
8. Protective padding (sheepskin, Polyurethane foam, felt, gel floatation, alternating pressure mattresses). Egg crate mattresses are flammable and should not be used in the OR
9. Sandbags
10. Surgical Positioning System (Vac-Pak) (Fig. 11–2)—This system consists of soft pads filled with tiny plastic beads; the patient is positioned on the pads, suction is attached to the pads, and as the air is evacuated the pads become firm, thus maintaining the patient's position. At the end of the procedure, the valve is released, air enters the pad, and it becomes soft
11. Tape
12. Towels

Conventional operating table pads are not capable of adequately protecting against pressure sores. The use of a full-length silicone gel pad has proven effective in preventing serious pressure injuries in surgical procedures lasting longer than 3 hours. Their effectiveness past 10 hours has not been tested. The silicone pads do not offer complete protection but extend the time that pressure can be tolerated.[3]

One disadvantage of the silicone gel pad is that warming or cooling the patient may prove difficult, since the hyperthermia blanket must be placed under the gel pad. Prewarming or precooling the gel pad prior to placing the patient on it will help alleviate this problem preoperatively but does not solve the problems during the intraoperative phase when rapid warming or cooling is required.[9]

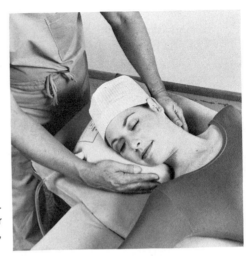

Figure 11-2. Surgical positioning system. To maintain the patient's position, this system requires air to be evacuated. (*Courtesy Olympic Medical Corp., Seattle, WA.*)

There are a number of different positions used for surgical intervention. Each of these positions has specific criteria that must be met to protect the patient from any untoward effects as a result of improper positioning. Table 11–2 delineates guidelines for nursing actions in positioning all patients.

Common Surgical Positions and Nursing Considerations

Supine or Dorsal Recumbent. In the supine position, the patient lies flat on the back, head in line with the body, arms secured at the side or one arm extended on an armboard with palms down, and legs are straight with feet slightly separated and uncrossed (Fig. 11–3A). If the arm is positioned at the side and tucked under the draw sheet, fingers and elbows should be placed close to the body. This will ensure that they do not rest on the table edge or that a team member does not inadvertently lean on the patient's arm. Small pillows or towels may be placed under the head and the lumbar curvature to assist in maintaining anatomical alignment. The safety strap is placed 2 inches above the knees. The feet are supported by a padded foot extension to prevent foot drop and to protect the feet from the weight and the pressure of the drapes.

Vulnerable pressure points that may require additional padding include: occiput, scapula, olecranon, sacrum, ischial tuberosity, and calcaneus (Fig. 11–3B). When the head is turned to one side, a doughnut or a special headrest should be used to protect the ear and superficial nerves and blood vessels of the face. The eyes should be protected from corneal abrasions or irritation by applying an eye patch or eye shield.

Trendelenburg. The Trendelenburg position is used for operations on the lower abdomen where it is desirable to tilt the abdominal viscera away from the pelvic area for better exposure. It is also used in some surgery on the extremities to assist in hemostasis. To prevent pressure on the peroneal nerves and phlebitis, the patient is positioned in the supine position with the knees over the lower break of the table. The operating room

TABLE 11-2. GUIDELINES FOR NURSING ACTIONS IN POSITIONING ALL PATIENTS

1. The anesthetized patient is never moved without checking with the anesthesiologist.
2. To prevent damage to the brachial plexus, arms are never abducted beyond 90°.
3. Legs must not be crossed as this creates pressure on blood vessels and nerves.
4. Body surfaces should not be in contact with one another.
5. Hands and feet should be protected and not allowed to hang off the table.
6. The patient should not be touching any metal part of the table. If the elbow rests on the table edge, ulnar nerve damage may result.
7. Patient exposure is limited to the area required for the surgical procedure.
8. If the patient is conscious, all activities as well as the rationale should be explained.
9. The instrument table, the mayo stand, or other equipment should not be in contact with the patient's toes or legs.
10. During the surgical procedure if the mayo stand, the instrument table, or operating table is moved, the patient must be checked for pressure points.
11. Movement of the anesthetized patient is done gently and slowly. Turning the patient too quickly may cause circulatory depression.
12. To ensure the patient's safety, adequate numbers of personnel must always be present when positioning the patient. The patient is lifted into position, never pushed or pulled.
13. When moving an anesthetized patient, the anesthesiologist guards the endotracheal tube and protects the patient's head and neck.
14. The position must not obstruct any catheters, tubes, or drains.
15. Team members should be reminded not to lean on the patient.
16. If the surgical procedure is unilateral, the consent form and the x-ray films should be checked and the proper side exposed.
17. If the surgical procedure is on an extremity, such as an amputation, both extremities should be exposed for comparison.
18. All equipment used in positioning patients is padded and terminally disinfected after use. we don't - just clean
19. The patient's position is documented as part of the intraoperative nursing notes.

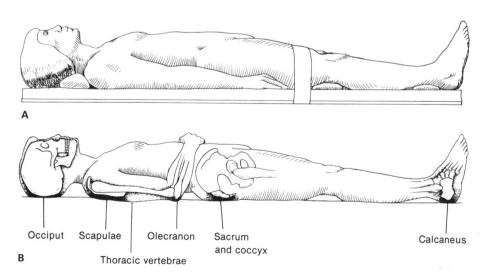

Occiput   Scapulae   Olecranon   Sacrum   Calcaneus
                                  and coccyx
B
          Thoracic vertebrae

Figure 11-3. A. Dorsal or supine position. **B.** Potential pressure points in supine position.

table is tilted downward so the patient's head is lower than the feet (Fig. 11-4). Well-padded shoulder braces assist in maintaining the patient's position. The shoulder braces are positioned away from the neck and against the acromion and the spinous process of the scapula, rather than the soft tissue, to avoid injury to the brachial plexus. The upward displacement of the abdominal viscera decreases the movement of the diaphragm and interferes with proper respiratory exchange.

When the patient is in the Trendelenburg position, blood pools in the upper torso and the blood pressure increases; when the patient is returned to the supine position, he or she may become hypotensive. Movement from this position must be slow to allow the heart time to adjust to the change in blood volume. The leg section should be raised first to reverse the venous status in the legs and then the entire table leveled. A modification of this position is used in hypovolemic shock.

Reverse Trendelenburg. In the reverse Trendelenburg position, the head is raised and the feet are lowered (Fig. 11-5). This position is used for upper abdominal surgery and for head and neck surgery. When used for abdominal surgery, it facilitates the movement of the abdominal viscera away from the diaphragm and therefore provides better visualization of the biliary tract. In head and neck surgery, it aids in hemostasis. The patient is positioned in the supine position with a well-padded footboard in place and the safety strap in position. A second safety strap may be needed for additional stability. Small pillows placed under the knees and the lumbar curvature will assist in making the patient comfortable. The head may be hyperextended by lowering the table headpiece or by placing a sandbag or a rolled towel under the patient's shoulders. If the reverse Trendelenburg is going to be used for an extended period of time, antiembolectomy hose will aid in the venous return. In this position, blood pools in the lower extremities, and caution must be exercised in returning the patient to the supine position as the cardiovascular system may become overloaded.

Sitting or Modified Fowler's. The patient is positioned over the break in the table; the footboard is placed perpendicular to the table to support the feet (Fig. 11-6A). The

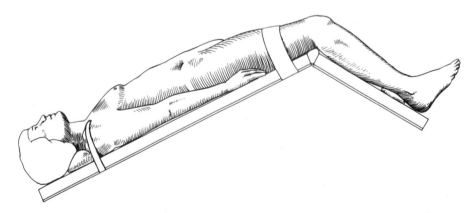

Figure 11-4. Trendelenberg position.

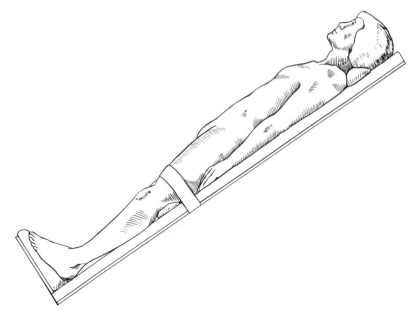

Figure 11–5. Reverse Trendelenberg position.

backrest is elevated, the knees are flexed, and the patient's arms rest on a pillow placed in the lap. The shoulders are supported with tape to prevent hyperextension, and the safety strap is positioned 2 inches above the knees. Antiembolectomy stockings will assist in venous return. Areas that may require additional padding include: sacrum, ischial tuberosity, posterior knee, calcaneus, and medial malleolus (Fig. 11–6B).

Air embolism is a threat in any surgical position where a negative gravitational pressure gradient exists between the operative site and the right atrium. The sitting position is an example. A right atrial catheter is inserted to assist in diagnosing and teating air embolisms. The following stages of the procedure are particularly critical points at which air embolisms may occur[10]:

- When muscles are being dissected free from the occiput
- When bone is being removed
- When dura is being tacked up
- When a vascular tumor bed is entered

The scrub nurse should respond with a copious amount of irrigation, wet sponges, cottonballs, cottonoid, and absorbable gelatin sponges soaked in saline. This will allow the irrigation solution to be aspirated rather than air. If bone work is being performed, bone wax will assist in closing the hole.

The circulating nurse should act quickly to assist the anesthesiologist, while making certain that the scrub nurse does not exhaust any supplies. The anesthesiologist will attempt to aspirate the embolized air via the right atrial or pulmonary artery catheter.

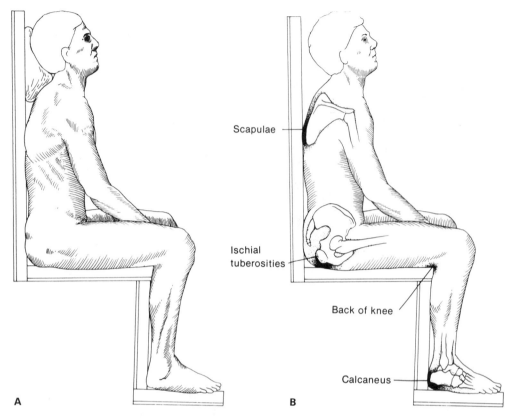

Figure 11-6. A. Sitting or modified Fowler's position. **B.** Potential pressure points in sitting position.

Lithotomy. The lithotomy position is used in surgical procedures requiring a perineal approach. The patient is positioned in a supine position with the buttocks near the lower break of the table to prevent lumbosacral strain (Fig. 11-7A). Cotton or flannel boots are placed over the feet to provide additional warmth and to contain any shedding of the epidermis from the feet. If the patient is to remain in the lithotomy position for more than 2 hours, ace bandages or antiembolectomy stockings should be applied. This will decrease the pooling of blood and thrombus formation.

Stirrups are placed on the table at the same height and at an outward angle. The height is adjusted to the length of the patient's legs. After the patient is anesthetized, two members of the surgical team simultaneously place the legs in the stirrups to avoid back strain and hip dislocation.

Nursing actions are directed toward prevention of damage to superficial veins and nerves on the medial and lateral aspects of the thigh and the knee. Unpadded or misplaced stirrups can damage the saphenous and peroneal nerves and predispose the patient to venous thrombosis. The most prevalent problem is peroneal nerve damage on the lateral aspect of the knee, which can cause footdrop. Excessive pressure on the femo-

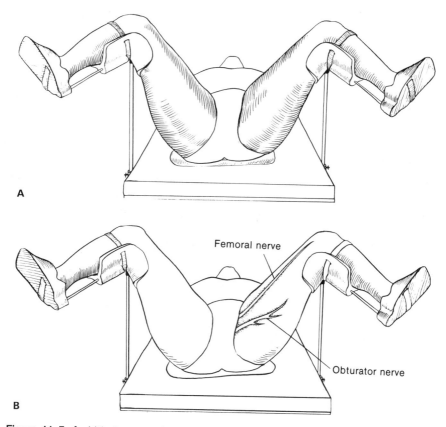

Figure 11–7. A. Lithotomy position. **B.** Nerve damage may occur to the femoral and obturator nerves in the lithotomy position.

ral and obturator nerves in the groin may cause sensory disturbances to the inner aspects of the leg (Fig. 11–7B).

If stirrups are used with popliteal knee support, they must be well padded so there is an even distribution of the thigh and leg weight. This will prevent thrombosis of the superficial vessels from occurring.

In the lithotomy position, most of the weight rests on the sacrum; to avoid pressure, additional padding may be required for lengthy procedures. A small lumbar pad will help reduce strain.

To prevent damage to the digits when raising or lowering the bottom portion of the table and to prevent peripheral nerve damage, the arms are placed on armboards positioned parallel to the table or are positioned loosely over the patient's abdomen and supported with a sheet or the patient's gown.

In this position, circulatory pooling occurs in the lumbar region. Venous flow may be reduced because of interference with lung expansion due to the pressure of the thighs on the abdomen and the pressure of the abdominal viscera against the diaphragm. Blood loss during surgery may not immediately produce clinical symptoms due to the pooling in the lumbar area. However, when the legs are lowered, 500 to 800 mL of blood may drain from the lumbar area into the legs, causing severe hypotension. When surgery is completed, the patient's legs must be lowered simultaneously and slowly returned to the normal supine position.

Prone. The prone position is used for surgical procedures on the posterior surface of the body (Fig. 11–8A). Induction of general anesthesia and intubation of the patient frequently occurs in the supine position on the transportation vehicle. After the anesthesiologist indicates that the patient may be moved, the patient is turned carefully onto the abdomen with the lumbar spine over the center break of the table. Four team members are used in turning the patient prone and in the return to supine, as it must be done gradually and slowly to allow the patient's cardiovascular system to adjust to the change in position. Rapid turning of the patient can result in hypotension.

The patient is positioned on two large body rolls placed longitudinally from the acromioclavicular joint to the iliac crest. This allows the diaphragm to move freely and the lungs to expand and decreases pressure on female breasts. Male genitalia should be positioned between the legs and free from pressure.

All head rests must be well padded and special care must be taken to prevent damage to the ears, the eyes, and the superficial nerves and blood vessels of the face.

The arms are placed at the patient's side or are placed on padded armboards with

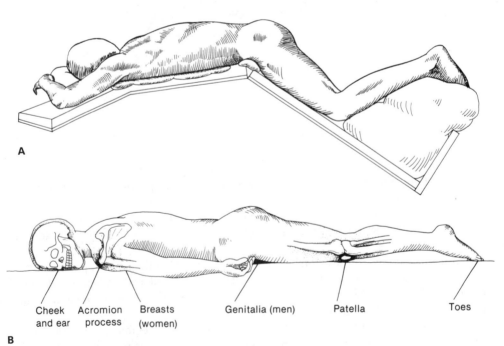

A

B

Cheek and ear   Acromion process   Breasts (women)   Genitalia (men)   Patella   Toes

Figure 11–8. A. Prone position. **B.** Potential pressure points in prone position.

the arms extended outward and upward, palms down, with elbows slightly flexed to prevent overextension of the shoulder. The feet are elevated off the table with a pillow to prevent plantar flexion and pressure on the toes. Additional padding may be required on the shoulder girdle, olecranon, anterior–superior iliac spine, patella, and dorsum of the foot (Fig. 11–8B). The safety strap is positioned 2 inches above the knees.

Jackknife or Kraske's Position.   The patient is placed in the prone position with the hips over the table break and the table is flexed at a 90° angle, raising the hips and lowering the upper portion of the body (Fig. 11–9). The arms are placed on padded armboards with the arms extended outward and upward, palms down, and elbows slightly flexed. A small towel roll placed under each shoulder will protect the brachial plexus. A pillow is placed under the lower legs and the ankles to prevent pressure on the toes. The safety strap is positioned across the thighs.

When this position is used for rectal procedures, hemorrhoid straps assist in optimum exposure and visualization. Hemorrhoid straps are wide strips of adhesive tape applied to both sides of the buttocks, at the level of the anus a few inches from the midline; they are pulled tight and fastened to the underside of the table.

The same principles in regard to turning the patient in the prone position apply to the jackknife position.

Lateral.   The lateral position is used for surgical procedures on the kidney, the chest, or the upper ureter. The patient is anesthetized in the supine position and then positioned by four team members on the unaffected side, with the back close to the edge of the mattress.

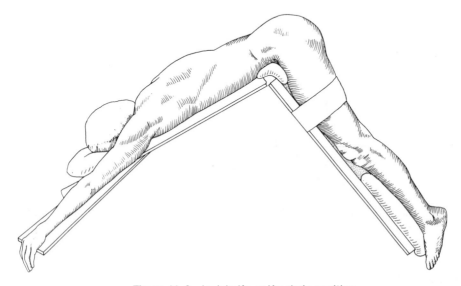

Figure 11-9. Jack-knife or Kraske's position.

Positions for Kidney Procedures. When used for kidney procedures, the flank region is positioned over the kidney elevator so the area between the twelfth rib and the iliac crest will be elevated when the table is flexed and the kidney elevator raised (Fig. 11–10A). The lower leg is flexed and the upper leg is straight, with pillows positioned between the legs to minimize the pressure and the weight from the upper leg to the lower leg. To prevent peroneal nerve damage to the lower knee, additional padding may be required. The ankles and the feet should be protected from pressure and foot drop (Fig. 11–10B).

The position is maintained by using sandbags or two well-padded kidney braces; the short kidney brace is positioned at the back, and the long brace is attached in front of the patient. Adhesive tape is placed across the hip and the shoulder and secured to the underside of the table for additional support. As in the prone position, female breasts and male genitalia should be free from pressure.

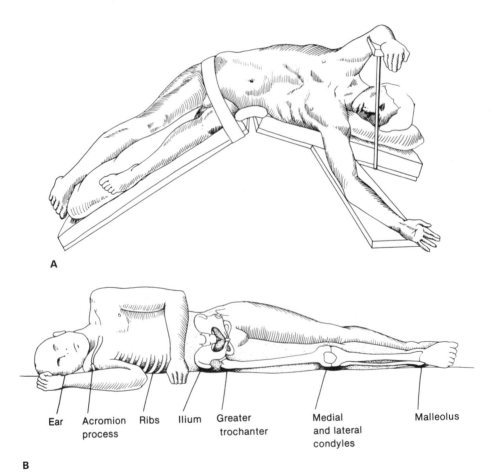

A

B

Ear   Acromion   Ribs   Ilium   Greater   Medial   Malleolus
       process   trochanter   and lateral
                                                  condyles

Figure 11–10. A. Lateral or kidney position. **B.** Potential pressure points in lateral position.

The upper arm is placed on a raised armboard, and the lower arm is flexed near the face on the mattress (or a double armboard may be used). Padding should be placed under the lower axilla to assist in chest expansion. The safety strap is positioned across the hip for stabilization.

The entire table is tilted downward so the operative area is horizontal; the upper shoulder, the hip, and the ankle are in a straight line.

Positions for Chest Procedures. In chest procedures the legs may be positioned in three ways: the lower leg may be flexed and the upper leg straight, or both legs may be flexed, or the upper leg may be flexed and the lower leg straight. In all three of these positions, pillows are placed between the legs, and the ankles and the feet are protected from pressure (Fig. 11–11).

The lower arm is slightly flexed and positioned in front of the patient on an armboard and the upper arm is positioned over the head to elevate the scapula from the operative site and to separate the intercostal spaces. A rolled sheet or towel placed between the patient and the mattress, below the level of the axilla, will relieve pressure on the dependent arm and allow chest movements. The patient's head is supported on a pillow.

The body is stabilized with the use of braces, sandbags, and body rolls. If braces are used, they should be well padded; the front brace should be positioned between the xyphoid and the umbilicus, the back brace in the lumbar area. Adhesive tape placed across the upper hip and fastened to the table on both sides assists in stabilization.

Circulation in the lateral position is compromised due to blood pooling in the lower limbs and the additional pressure placed on the abdominal vessels when the kidney elevator is raised.

Respiratory function is compromised as the vital capacity is decreased due to the weight of the body on the lower chest.

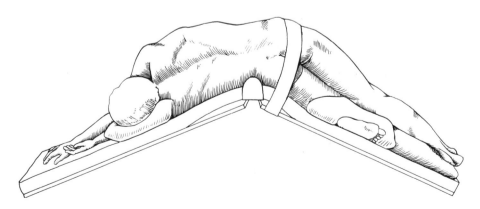

Figure 11–11. Lateral or chest position.

DRAPING

The purpose of draping is to provide a sterile operative field by placing drapes over the patient, leaving only a minimum area of skin exposed around the site of the incision.

Criteria for Surgical Drapes

Surgical drapes should establish an effective barrier eliminating the passage of microorganisms between nonsterile and sterile areas. Draping material should be resistant to blood and aqueous fluid, abrasion resistant, lint free, sufficiently porous to eliminate heat buildup, and should meet the requirements of the National Fire Protection Association.[11] In addition, the drapes should be memory free, possess a high degree of drapability, and be penetrable by gas or steam for sterilization.

The types of drapes available are reusable woven or disposable nonwoven materials and plastic adhesive skin drapes. The woven materials are made of muslin (140 to 160 thread count) and cotton (280 + thread count) with special waterproofing treatment. Nonwoven materials are made of processed cellulose fibers either alone or in combination with reinforcements of various types including polymeric films.

The components of a draping system are towels, sheets in various sizes, fenestrated drapes, specialty drapes (eye, perineal, thyroid, chest sheets), and mayo stand covers. The drapes must be of adequate size to drape the patient without proximity to the floor. Nonperforating towel clips should be used on all surgical drapes.

Reusable Drapes

The basic requirements for reusable surgical drapes are the same as those described in Chapter 8 ("Packaging Materials") for wrappers. Woven drapes must be checked for defects, lint, and stains. Inspection must be done over an illuminated table. Defects are patched with a vulcanized heat seal patch.

Muslin with a thread count of 140 to 160 per square inch is available as surgical drapes. Muslin drapes do not retard the passage of fluids, and this results in migration of bacteria to the operative site. If the drapes become wet during the surgical procedure, they must be covered with another layer of draping material. The perioperative nurse must exercise caution in the number of layers of linen placed over the patient as excessive layers will interfere with heat dissipation from the patient's skin through the drapes.

Cotton with a thread count of 280 + per square inch can receive a special waterproofing treatment that provides a barrier to liquids and abrasions up to 75 washing–sterilizing cycles and uses.[12] Due to this limitation, a system of accounting for the number of uses of each drape must be implemented.

Disposable Drapes

Disposable or "paper" drapes refer to those made of nonwoven material designed for onetime use. They can be manufactured with either absorbent or nonabsorbent properties. The nonwoven drapes are adaptable to lamination and bonding, which results in moisture repellency. Disposable drapes are compact, lightweight, permeable to air, and lint free and are available in presterile form in packs or single-wrapped items.

Some disposable drapes tend not to conform as well as linen on areas around the

TABLE 11-3. PROPERTIES OF WOVEN VERSUS NONWOVEN SURGICAL DRAPES

Properties	Woven (140–160)	Woven (280+)	Nonwoven
Bacterial filtration	Low	High (up to 75 washings)	High
Fluid strikethrough	Immediate	Resistant	None
Wicking	Immediate	Resistant	None
Air permeable	Yes	Yes	Yes
Linting	Sheds lint	Sheds lint	Lint-free
Size of pack	Bulky	Bulky	Compact
Weight of pack	10–12 lbs	10–12 lbs	3–5 lbs
Fenestration	Fixed	Fixed	May be enlarged
Drapability	Excellent	Excellent	Some limitations
Shelf life	28 days	28 days	Indefinite—provided conditions of sterility are maintained
Quality control inspection required	Yes	Yes	Random checking prior to use
Penetrated by gas or steam for sterilization	Yes	Yes (check manufacture guidelines for time–temperature heat profile)	Presterile
Meets NFPA Requirements	Yes	Yes	Yes

face, the head, and the extremities. In addition, solvents and volatile liquids tend to penetrate the drapes. Table 11–3 contrasts the properties of woven and nonwoven materials.

Documented studies are available to support both nonwoven and woven materials as surgical drapes.[13] The nurse manager will incorporate these studies into an analysis of the departmental needs in determining whether woven or nonwoven drapes will be used. Areas to be included in the analysis are the total cost of repair and replacements, the cost of inspection and delinting, the type and condition of laundry equipment, the amount of storage space available, pilferage of woven items, the adequacy of the laundry service including the length of time that elapses before soiled linen is washed. To assure that the blood protein is removed, a period of 11 hours is suggested as the maximum amount of time that should elapse.[13] Additional areas to be explored are the acceptability of the items to the users, an analysis of the impact nonwovens would have on the waste system, and the concerns of the ecologist in using nonwovens.

Custom Packs

Custom procedure packs have gained wide acceptance for cases performed in high volume or when quick turnover time is essential. A custom pack is a vendor-supplied collection of disposable surgical supplies, assembled in predetermined sequence, aseptically wrapped, sterilized, and delivered as requested by the institution. The principal reason for these packs is to assist in reducing the nonrevenue set-up time and, therefore, increase the time available for revenue-producing surgical procedures. Analysis by the OR manager regarding "cost reductions" and set-up time is essential prior to implementation of a custom pack program.

Plastic Adhesive Drapes

Plastic adhesive drapes are available in various sizes and configurations for surgical draping. The plastic drapes may be applied directly to the dry skin prior to draping or over the sterile drapes (Fig. 11–12). When applied over the sterile drapes, plastic drapes assist in holding them in place, thus eliminating the need for skin towels and towel clips. The incision is made through the plastic drape; the cut edges remain adherent to the skin and keep the surgical incision sealed off from the migration of bacteria. The drapes are clear, allowing visibility of the patient's skin; they conform to irregular body surfaces; and they may be used to wall off contaminated areas such as a colostomy, the anus, and infected wounds.

Three sterile team members can effectively apply a large plastic drape. Two members stand on opposite sides of the operating room table holding the drape about 12 inches above the patient. The third member removes and discards the backing, holding the drape taut; and the first two members lower the drape until it touches the patient's skin surface. The third member uses a towel to smooth the drape out, starting in the center and moving to the periphery (Table 11–4).

Plastic adhesive drapes should be removed carefully from patients, particularly those with fragile skin, to prevent denuding of the skin.

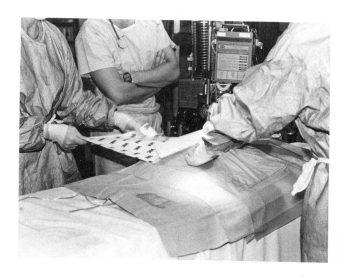

Figure 11-12. Plastic drapes may be applied directly to the dry skin prior to draping or over sterile towels.

TABLE 11-4. GUIDELINES FOR NURSING ACTIONS IN SURGICAL DRAPING

1. The skin around the incision must be dry before drapes are applied.
2. Sufficient time should be allowed to observe proper technique and application of the drapes.
3. Sterile drapes should be handled as little as possible; shaking linen should be avoided.
4. The drapes are carried folded to the operating room table. To avoid contamination of the front of the gown, care must be taken to maintain an appropriate distance from nonsterile areas (Fig. 11-13).
5. Drapes should be held high enough to avoid touching the nonsterile areas of the table.
6. To protect the sterile gloved hands, form a cuff from the drapes or towels (Fig. 11-14).
7. When placing drapes, never reach across the nonsterile area of the operating table to drape the other side; go around the table.
8. If a drape is incorrectly placed, it should be discarded. The circulating nurse will remove the drape without contaminating other drapes or the operative site.
9. If the drape falls below waist level, it should be discarded because the area below the waist is considered unsterile.
10. A towel clip that has been placed through a drape or to the patient's skin is considered contaminated. It must not be repositioned during the procedure.
11. Draping is always done from a sterile area to an unsterile area, draping the nearest area first.
12. The area around the incision is draped first and then the periphery.
13. Whenever sterility is in doubt, consider the drape to be contaminated.

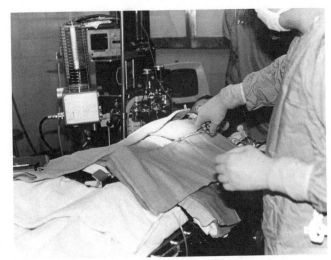

Figure 11-13. To avoid contamination of the front of gown, care must be taken to maintain an appropriate distance from nonsterile areas.

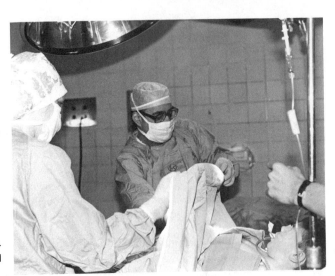

Figure 11-14. To protect the sterile gloved hands, a cuff is formed from the drape.

REFERENCES

1. Gruis M, Innes B. Assessment: Essential to prevent pressure sores. *Am J Nurs*. 1976; 76 (11):1762
2. Reichel SM. Shearing force as a factor in decubitus ulcers in paraplegics. *JAMA*. 1958; 166 (7):762
3. Gendron F. Burns occurring during lengthy surgical procedures. *J Clini Engin*. 1980; 5 (1):22, 24

4. Gendron F. *Unexplained Patient Burns: Investigating Iatrogenic Injuries.* Brea, Cal: Quest; 1988: 170, 173, 238
5. Lawson NW, Mills NL, Ochsner JL. Occipital alopecia following cardiopulmonary bypass. *J Thor Cardiovasc Surg.* 1976; 71 (3):347
6. Elden WJ. Occipital alopecia. *J Thorac Cardiovasc Surg.* 1977; 73 (2): 322
7. Poma PA. Pressure induced alopecia: Report of a case after gynecologic surgery. *J Reprod Med.* 1979; 22 (4):220
8. Chagares R, Jackson B. Sitting easy: How six pressure-relieving devices stack up. *Am J Nurs.* 1987; 87 (2):191
9. Skin injury in the OR and elsewhere. *Health Dev.* October 1980; 313
10. Temple A, Katz J. Air embolism, a potentially lethal surgical complication. *AORN J.* 1987; 45 (2):399
11. Recommended practices: Aseptic barrier materials for surgical gowns and drapes. *AORN J.* 1988; 47 (2):572
12. Laufman H, Siegal J, Edberg S. Moist bacterial strikethrough of surgical materials: Confirmatory tests. *Ann Surg.* 1979; 289 (1):74
13. Ryan P. Reusables vs. disposables? Defending your position. *AORN J.* 1979; 30 (3):419, 423

Chapter 12
Surgical Instruments

Skulls found by archaeologists dating back to 350,000 BC showed evidence that one of the first operations to be performed was trephining—used as a surgical intervention "for the release of demons"—in which an opening was chiseled through the skull of the patient. An ancient tool or instrument maker sharpened flints and made the crude hammers necessary for these procedures. Sharpened animal teeth were later used for bloodletting and drainage of abscesses.

The surgical instruments used in the United States during the period of 1776 to 1826 were imported or made by skilled American artisans under the direction of the surgeon. The surgeon used the services of steelworkers; coppersmiths; silversmiths; needle-grinders; turners of wood, bone, and ivory; sewers of leather; glass-blowers; and silk and hemp spinners in designing and manufacturing instruments that were crude and expensive.

> The cutlers who made and sold knives kept small assortments of surgical instruments and changed their signs from "Cutler and Scissor Grinder" to "Cutler and Surgical Instrument Maker." Thus, began the physicians' supply houses and surgical instrument making in America.[1]

During the early 1800s, the physicians' principal tools were his eyes, ears, and keen observation. Surgeons were scarce and surgical instruments almost nonexistent. Kitchen and penknives doubled as scalpels, and table forks were used as retractors. Federal records disclose that three of four operations during the Civil War were amputations and the carpenter's saw worked as well as a forged instrument.

The use of ether and chloroform as anesthetic agents in 1846 brought with it new surgical procedures never before considered possible. As a result, there were new ideas and demands for surgical instruments.

During the late 19th and early 20th centuries, general surgery divided into specialties, and there was an increased demand for smaller and more delicate instruments (Fig. 12–1). German silver, brass, and steel that could withstand repeated sterilization replaced the wood, ivory, and rubber formerly used on instrument handles (Fig. 12–2).

The development of stainless steel in Germany during World War I provided a superior material for manufacturing surgical instruments. This paved the way in 1924 for instrument craftsmen to be brought to the United States from Germany, Sweden, and England to teach their craft to apprentices.

Currently, most surgical instruments are made of stainless steel and are from the United States, Germany, France, and Pakistan. However, since there are no standards for instrument manufacturing, the quality of instruments may vary among manufac-

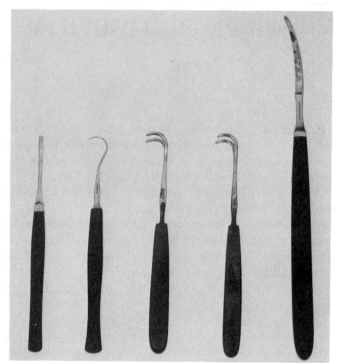

Figure 12-1. Minor operating instruments with ebony handles, 1880. Left to right: $5\frac{1}{2}''$ knife, aneurysm needle, 2 tenaculum, 7″ knife. (*Courtesy Codman & Shurtleff, Randolph, Massachusetts.*)

turers. Instruments should be examined prior to purchase to ascertain their quality. A well-made instrument when properly cared for will last at least 10 years.

Steels capable of stainless qualities are compounds of iron, carbon, and chromium. Some also contain small amounts of nickel, magnesium, and silicone. The classification and the type of steel such as 410, 416, 420, are dependent on the amounts of carbon and chromium used.[2] The subsequent processing will determine the degree to which the steel is "stainless."

The metal is first forged or cast into tubes or sheets and then machined or milled, ground, or lathed into instrument blanks. These blanks are then die-forged into specific pieces, the excess metal is trimmed away, and the two halves are assembled. The instrument is then heat treated to temper and harden the metal. The finishing operation consists of grinding, buffing, polishing, and inspecting.

There are three kinds of joints used in manufacturing instruments. In the screw joint, the two halves of the instrument are connected with a screw or a pin. These instruments must be checked routinely as the screw or pin may work loose due to repeated use. Instruments with semibox joints have two separate halves that are disassembled for cleaning purposes. In the box lock, one arm passes through a slot in the other arm. This method of manufacturing is most frequently used on instruments that require accurate approximation of the tips.

Instruments may be finished in one of three ways. The bright polished finish reflects

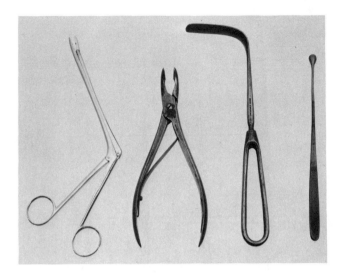

Figure 12-2. Cushing hypophyseal instruments, 1911. Left to right: pituitary rongeur, bone rongeur, hypophyseal speculum, and pituitary curette. (*Courtesy Codman and Shurtleff, Randolph, Massachusetts.*)

light and may cause eye fatigue. The satin or dull finish is used more frequently, as it eliminates glare and decreases eye fatigue. Instruments with this finish should always be used when taking photographs or filming surgical procedures. The third finish is black or ebonized and is most frequently used with lasers.

Surgical instruments are very expensive. New instruments and replacements constitute a sizable portion of the operating room's annual budget. Perioperative nurses can assist in controlling the amount required to be expended on replacement items by being knowledgeable about the proper care and handling of instruments.

Instruments are manufactured in a wide variety of sizes and shapes in four main categories: sharps, clamps, graspers, and retractors.

Sharp instruments include scalpels, scissors, bone cutters, rongeurs, chisels, osteotomes, saws, curettes, and dermatomes. These instruments are designed to incise and dissect tissue and bone. Scalpel handles have one end for attaching a disposable blade. This allows the blade to be changed at intervals during the procedure. To prevent lacerations, blades should be applied and removed with a needle holder, touching only the dull side of the blade.

Scissors are manufactured in various sizes, the blades are curved or straight, and the tips may be blunt or sharp (Fig. 12–3). Heavy scissors (such as the curved mayo) are used on heavy tough tissue, and the lighter metzenbaum scissors are used for the dissection of delicate tissue. Straight mayo scissors, frequently called suture scissors, are used to cut sutures. When the procedure is being performed in a cavity, 9-inch scissors and scalpels are used to allow visualization and better control of the dissecting site.

Clamping instruments are most frequently used to control bleeding and maintain hemostasis; however, in some instances they may be used as graspers or retractors. The grasping end of these instruments have serrations that are meshed to prevent the clamp from slipping off a blood vessel. The jaws of vascular clamps are designed with finely

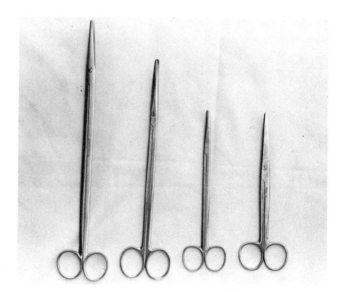

Figure 12-3. Scissors are manufactured in various sizes.

meshed multiple rows of longitudinal teeth to prevent leakage and to minimize trauma to the vessel walls (Fig. 12–4).

Grasping or holding instruments are used to grasp and hold tissue or bone for dissection or retraction or to assist in suturing. This group includes tissue forceps (Fig. 12–5), tenacula, rib approximators, stone forceps, bone holders, sponge forceps, towel clips, and other special holding instruments.

Tissue forceps are designed to get a grip on tissue with a minimum amount of trauma. These instruments vary in length and are available with or without teeth. Forceps with teeth are used on thick or slippery tissue. Forceps without teeth can be used on delicate thin tissue.

Tenacula are designed with a sharp point and are used to pierce an organ, such as the uterus, to facilitate retraction or dissection.

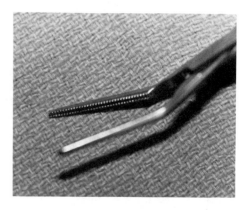

Figure 12-4. The jaws of vascular clamps have multiple rows of longitudinal teeth.

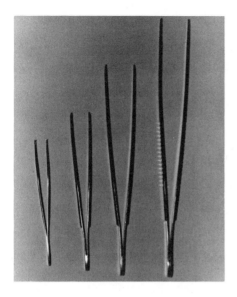

Figure 12-5. Tissue forceps are available with or without teeth.

Towel clips are available as nonpiercing or piercing clamps. The most frequent use of towel clips is to hold the drapes in place or to clip towels or sponges to the edges of the wound. Piercing clamps damage both the linen and the tissue, and their use should be discouraged.

Sponge forceps can be used to hold tissue; however, they are most frequently used to hold gauze sponges. A 4 × 4 sponge can be folded in thirds and placed on the sponge stick and then be used for "prepping," retracting tissue, and absorbing fluids.

Needle holders are designed to retain a firm grip on needles (Fig. 12–6). Diamond

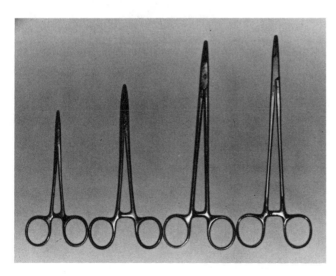

Figure 12-6. Needle holders are designed to prevent the rotation of the needle.

jaw needle holders have a tungsten carbide insert designed to prevent rotation of the needle. The longitudinal groove in the jaw releases tension and prevents flattening of the needle. Needle holders need to be repaired or replaced on a frequent basis, as grasping and holding the needles shortens the life of the instrument. One of the advantages of the diamond jaw needle holder is that the inserts can be replaced as often as required, thus decreasing the expense of replacing the entire instrument.

There are several special holding forceps designed with special tips or jaws for use on specific tissue. Allis and allis-adair forceps have multiple sharp teeth that do not crush or damage tissue. These instruments are frequently used in perineal surgery. A Kocher or Ochsner clamp has one sharp tooth and is used on tough heavy tissue. The Babcock forceps has a curved fenestrated jaw without teeth and is used on delicate tissue such as the intestine or the ureter.

Retractors are used to assist in visualization of the operative field (Figs. 12–7, 12–8). This caterogy of instruments is designed to provide the best exposure with a minimum of trauma to the surrounding tissue. Retractors come in various sizes with the blade usually at a right angle to the handle. The width and the length of the blade and the use of sharp or dull blades depends on where the retractor is used (Fig. 12–9). A malleable retractor is made of a special stainless steel that permits repeated bending and shaping by the surgeon without hardening the metal. Self-retaining retractors have a frame to which blades may be attached, or they may consist of two blades held apart with a ratchet.

When handing instruments to the surgeon, the following guidelines will be useful to remember:

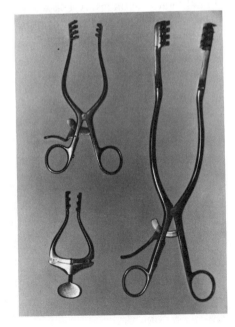

Figure 12-7. Self-retaining retractors. Mastoid, Wheatlander and laminectomy.

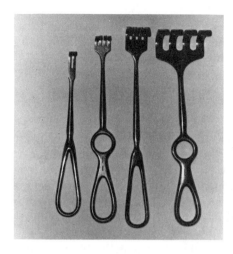

Figure 12–8. Hand-held rake retractors.

1. Scalpels are always handed to the surgeon so he or she has control of the handle.
2. All instruments with curves are handed so the curve of the instrument is in the same direction as the curve of the surgeon's palm. The scrub assistant holds the instrument by the hinged area so the surgeon can view the tips.
3. When mounting needles on a needle holder, the needle must point in the direction it will be used. This will depend on whether the surgeon is right- or left-handed.
4. Retractors are handed so the surgeon can grasp the handle of the retractor.

A card file with pictures of instruments, vendor's name, order number, principal use of the instrument, method of sterilization, and cost will assist new personnel in learning instruments. Grouping the instruments within the card file by surgical specialty and by instrument set or special trays will add clarity to the learning process.

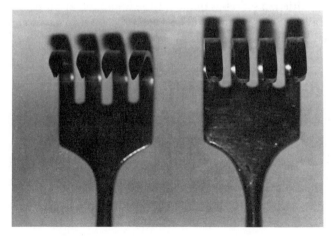

Figure   12–9. Retractors   have sharp or dull blades.

Access to the instrument room or instrument cupboards should be controlled to prevent pilferage and indiscriminate use. An instrument inventory should be conducted at least annually to assess the effectiveness of inventory control.

INSTRUMENT SELECTION

Standard basic instrument sets containing the minimum number and types of instruments will facilitate instrument counts. A basic instrument set includes instruments required to open and close the incision and provides the majority of instruments needed to complete the surgical procedure. Table 12–1 identifies a basic major instrument set appropriate for use in the following surgical specialties: gynecology, genitourinary, vascular, and general. Basic sets should be assessed at regular intervals to identify instruments that need to be added or deleted.

Proper selection of additional instruments is based on information obtained during the preoperative assessment and includes the age and the size of the patient, the selected surgical approach, the anatomy, the possible pathologic condition, and the surgeon's preference.

INSTRUMENT COUNTS

Instruments should be counted on all surgical procedures to ensure patient safety and to prevent loss of the instruments. To assist in accomplishing this, instruments are assembled in a predetermined manner with all instruments accounted for. The count is verified in the operating room prior to the beginning of the surgical procedure by the scrub assistant and the circulating nurse. Instruments added during the case are added to the instrument count sheet by the circulating nurse. The instrument count should not be finalized until the wound is closed and the surgical drapes are removed. Instruments broken or disassembled during the procedure are accounted for in their entirety. If a count is incorrect, the surgeon is notified, a search is made for the item, and appropriate measures are taken (i.e., an x-ray of the patient is taken before he or she leaves the operating room) and documented by the circulating nurse according to hospital policy.[3]

GUIDELINES FOR THE CARE OF INSTRUMENTS

The following are guidelines that should be observed in the care of instruments.

1. Instruments are used only for the purpose for which they were designed.
2. Instruments are handled gently. Sharp and delicate instruments should be placed in a separate tray for terminal cleaning.
3. Instruments are sterilized open so the steam can penetrate the box lock.
4. During a surgical procedure, instruments are soaked, rinsed, or wiped off at frequent intervals.

TABLE 12–1. BASIC MAJOR INSTRUMENT SET

Sharps		Forceps		Clamps		Retractors	
#4 Knife handle	2	6" Thumb forceps	2	Large towel clip	6	Loop	2
#7 Knife handle	1	6" Tissue forceps	2	Small towel clip	12	USA	2
Straight mayo scissors	1	8" Thumb forceps	2	Short needle holder	2	Vein	2
Curved mayo scissors	1	8" Tissue forceps	2	Long needle holder	3	Small Richardson	2
7" Metzenbaum scissors	2	10" Thumb forceps	1	Providence	6	Medium Richardson	2
9" Metzenbaum scissors	1	Adson forceps	2	Straight Kelly	6	Large Richardson	2
				Curved Kelly	6	Narrow Deaver	2
				Mayo	8	Wide Deaver	2
				Kocher	6	Harrington	1
				Allis	4	Balfour with blade	1
				Short Babcock	2	Narrow Crile	1
				Long Babcock	2	Wide Crile	1
				Long straight Kelly	6		
				Long curved Kelly	6		
				Mixter	6		
				Pean	6		
				Sponge forceps	4		

5. Instruments must not be soaked in saline as the sodium chloride will increase rusting and discoloration.
6. All instruments with removable parts are disassembled after use to expose all surfaces for terminal sterilization.
7. Following a surgical procedure, instruments are processed through a washer–sterilizer and then a sonic cleaner to ensure adequate cleaning. Detergents should be noncorrosive and low sudsing with a pH close to neutral (see Chapter 7).
8. Abrasives such as steel wool and scouring powders are not to be used, as they will scratch and remove the finish on the metal, thus increasing the possibility of corrosion.
9. Instruments are checked after each use. Damaged or stiff instruments are repaired or replaced.
    a. Forceps and hinged instruments are inspected for alignment of the jaws and the teeth.
    b. The tips of clamps must be even, and when the instrument is held up to the light, fully closed: no light should be visible between the jaws.
    c. Clamps should be closed on the first rachet, held by the box lock, and tapped lightly against a counter top; if the clamp springs open, it is faulty.
    d. Heavy scissors such as mayos should cut through four layers of gauze at the tips; delicate scissors should cut through two layers of gauze.
    e. Needle holders are checked with a needle in place; if the needle can be moved easily by hand, the needle holder needs repair.
    f. Chrome-plated instruments are checked for chips, sharp edges, and worn areas.
10. Stiff instruments should be treated with a water-soluble lubricant. Oils form a bacterial-protecting film and prevent sterilization.
11. Instrument milk should be used routinely as a preventive maintenance measure.
12. Instruments are marked with an electroetching device rather than a vibrating marker to avoid hairline cracks. All markings are on the shank of the instrument to avoid fracturing the box lock. The date of purchase should be indicated on the instrument so the life of the instrument can be properly assessed. This will also assist in identifying defects that may be associated with the manufacturing process.

INSTRUMENTS FOR SPECIAL USES

Microsurgery Instruments

Lightweight metals such as titanium and tungsten carbide are now being used in the manufacturing of microsurgery instruments. These lightweight and high-strength materials provide sharper cutting edges and are easier for the surgeon to manipulate. These metals are more corrosion resistant than stainless steel. Titanium and tungsten carbide, however, will corrode if not properly cared for.

Microsurgical instrument trays are designed to safely position and secure instru-

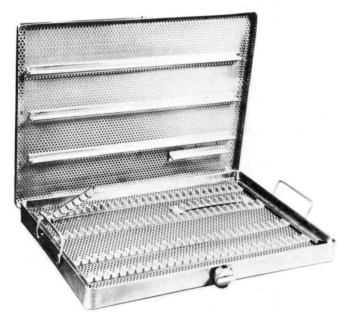

Figure 12-10. Microsurgical instrument trays are designed to safely position and secure instruments. (*Courtesy Edward Weck Co., Princeton, New Jersey*)

ments (Fig. 12–10). These trays are usually lined with posts constructed of polyfoam, silicone, or Teflon to prevent direct contact between instruments. Contact between instruments during storage, use, or processing can cause sufficient damage to require repair or replacement.

When the instruments are on the mayo stand, the tips should be elevated in the air by placing a rolled towel under the handles. Protective guards should be left on until the surgeon is ready to use the instruments.

At the end of the procedure, the gross soil should be removed with a soft toothbrush and the instrument placed back into the instrument tray and terminally processed in the washer–sterilizer and the ultrasonic cleaner. Prior to storage, the instruments must be thoroughly dried, especially the tips and the box locks, to prevent corrosion. If hand drying is required, a chamois is preferable, as it will not leave lint on the instrument. Following the cleaning process, the tips should be checked with a magnifying glass to detect any defects.

Air-powered Tools

During the past 20 years, air-powered instruments have been used successfully in neurosurgery, orthopedic, dental, plastic, and reconstructive surgery. These instruments are powered by compressed nitrogen and are controlled with a foot pedal or a hand switch.

The instruments are used for cutting, shaping, and beveling bone; taking skin grafts; and for dermabrading.

The bone instruments have a rotary, reciprocating, or oscillating action. The rotary action is used to drill holes and to insert screws, wires, or pins. The reciprocating cutting action is from front to back, and the oscillating action is from side to side; both are used to cut or remove bone.

All blades and attachments must be seated properly before activating the instrument. The instruments should always be tested for proper working condition prior to being given to the surgeon. When air-powered instruments are used on bone, saline solution is dripped from a plastic bulb syringe by the scrub assistant or the first assistant to cool the bone and wash away the particles.

The use of high-speed burrs in conjunction with metal suction tips generates a dispersion of very fine metallic particles due to the abrasion of the metal into the soft tissue adjacent to the operative area. Although this by itself does not have immediate clinical effects, it may have a deleterious effect if the patient requires further magnetic resonance imaging (MRI) studies of the area, as it causes a distortion defect in the image analogous to a starburst configuration. Therefore, plastic suction tips should be substituted for high-speed burrs or drills.[4]

It is important that all personnel associated with using these instruments understand all aspects of proper surgical use including cleaning, maintenance, repairing, and sterilization. Critical to all these procedures are the manufacturer's directions for the use, care, cleaning, and lubrication of the instruments.

There is some air leakage from all air-powered instruments. The amount varies from instrument to instrument and from manufacturer to manufacturer. This exhausting of propellant gas is an important consideration in recommending cleaning procedures and sterilization exposure times. If the air-powered instrument is bacteriologically contaminated internally, there is a possibility of direct wound infection caused by forward exhaust of this gas during the operation.[5]

Drills should be disassembled before cleaning and are not to be immersed in water or any other solution. It is preferable that they be disassembled before sterilizing. With proper care and maintenance, air-powered tools have an indefinite lifespan.

Electrically Powered Tools

Dermatomes, drills, and saws may also be powered electrically. The motors must be designed to be explosionproof and have sparkproof connectors. The anesthesiologist should be alerted to the use of equipment requiring an electrical motor, as these units should not be used in the presence of a flammable anesthestic agent. With the switch in the off position, equipment with a motor must be plugged into the electrical outlet before anesthesia begins and must not be removed until after the anesthestic agent is discontinued.

As with air-powered tools, it is important that the hospital staff adhere to manufacturer's directions for the use, care, cleaning, and lubrication. The motor must not be immersed in any liquid; however, the power cord and the foot pedals must be cleaned following each use. Cords must be removed from the outlet by grasping firmly on the plug, not by pulling on the cord. All power cords and plugs should be checked prior to each use for any cracks or breaks.

Nonlensed Endoscopic Instruments

Laryngoscopes, bronchoscopes, and esophagoscopes consist of a tubular instrument with removable light carrier. They are powered by using a battery cord or fiberoptic cable and power or light source. These instruments are very delicate. The accidental dropping of an instrument, handling the instrument with forceps, or placing a heavier instrument on a lighter one may result in dents or scratches, requiring repair or replacement.

These instruments should be cleaned immediately following the procedure to prevent the formation of encrustations. The instruments should be washed in a mild soap solution with a soft brush. A water pistol with interchangeable nozzles that can be attached to any water faucet or air outlet will assist in cleaning and drying the interior of the instrument. These instruments do not contain any optics; therefore, autoclaving is the preferred method of sterilization.

Lensed Endoscopic Instruments

Endoscopic instruments that contain lenses require special care and handling to ensure their safe and efficient operation. To prevent scratching and potential injury to the patient, the instruments are never handled with another instrument. They are handled one at a time and are picked up by the proximal end, the eyepiece. On a sterile setup, these instruments should be placed in the center of the table to prevent the instrument from rolling over the edge of the table. Excessive bending, loosening, or removal of the eyepiece should be avoided. For cleaning, instruments are disassembled and washed with a mild detergent in warm or tepid water with an appropriately sized soft brush and a water pistol. The water pistol assists in the cleaning of small channels, holes, and hinges. Plastic pans should be used for the disinfecting process to avoid the reaction of metals with the disinfectant and to prevent scratching the instrument's surface.

The proximal and distal lenses are cleaned with 70% isopropyl alcohol on a cotton applicator or sponge. After the instrument is cleaned and dried, the lenses are checked for visual clarity. A "half moon" but otherwise clear view could indicate that the instrument has a dent on the outside sheath. Fogging and loss of image are a result of condensation within the optical system.

The instruments should be placed in perforated metal containers with towels folded loosely around each to prevent direct contact between them during processing and storage.

For efficient and effective operation of these instruments, it is important that the manufacturer's guidelines be followed regarding the proper sterilization procedure. Some of the lensed instruments are autoclavable; however, even under ideal conditions, heat and pressure during a steam autoclave cycle will reduce the life of any optical system.[6] Ethylene oxide gas sterilization may be used on all lensed instruments provided they are thoroughly dried before packaging. Aeration should be in accordance with the sterilizer manufacturer's instructions. An alternative to ETO sterilization is high-level disinfection in 2% glutaraldehyde for 45 minutes. The 45-minute soak time is to assure 100% mycobactericidal activity. The instrument should then be rinsed and dried.

Fiberoptic Cables

Fiberoptic cables are made of high-refractory optical glass and contain many hundreds of tiny fibers. These fibers transmit light from the light source to an instrument. To avoid unnecessary damage to the cables, they must not be pulled or stretched. This requires that the cables be long enough so that there is adequate slack when in the operating position. Only nonperforating or plastic towel clips should be used to secure the fiberoptic cables to the drapes.

The light source should be turned on with the rheostat at the lowest setting and then turned up slowly to avoid blowing out the bulb. If the cable and the optics are in good condition, a medium position should provide the required brightness for the examination. Bulbs will deteriorate and give less light before they burn out. The consistent need to turn the light source above the normal setting may be an indication that the bulb needs replacement. If the illuminator does not have a built-in second standby lamp, an extra bulb should be available in the operating room.

After the procedure is completed, the circulating nurse should turn the rheostat to zero and let the fan run 2 to 3 minutes to cool the bulb. If the light cable is left on for an extended period of time, it may burn a hole in the drapes and result in a burn to the patient.

The cable should be removed from the illuminator by grasping the stainless steel ferrule and pulling firmly. If the cable is yanked from the illuminator, the fibers will break.

Fiberoptic cables should be washed by hand in a mild detergent with warm water, rinsed, air-dried, and checked for light transmission and breakage of fibers. The cable can be checked for broken fibers by directing one end of the cable to a light and observing the opposite end. Any black spots indicate broken fibers. If 25% or more of the fibers appear black, the cable needs to be repaired or replaced.

For sterilization, the cable should be coiled loosely, placed in a sterilizing case, or wrapped according to departmental procedure. Some fiberoptic cables may be steam sterilized; however, this may reduce the life of the cable. All fiberoptic cables can be sterilized with ethylene oxide. Cables should withstand 12 months of normal usage without noticeable deterioration.[7]

REFERENCES

1. Crawford M. Surgical instruments in America. *AORN J.* 1976;24(1):152
2. Ginsberg F. Stainless steel instruments. *AORN J.* 1964;2(6):66
3. Recommended practices for sponge, sharp, and instrument counts. *AORN J.* 1984;39(4):699–706
4. Groah L, Skinner H. Practical innovations. *AORN J.* 1989; 49(3):882
5. Kereluk K, et al. Sterilization of air-powered instruments by steam: Recommended exposure times. *Hosp Top.* 1973, 51(3):56
6. *Gynecological Laparoscopy Instruments.* Rosemount, Ill.: Richard Wolf Instrument Co.: 1980:10
7. *Pilling Endoscopic Instruments.* Fort Washington, Pa.: Pilling Co.: 1976: D

Hemostasis and
Wound Closure

INCISION SITES

The most important factors determining where the incision occurs are the patient's diagnosis and the pathology the surgeon expects to encounter. Additional factors that are important are maximum exposure, ease of extending the incision, ease of closure, minimum postoperative discomfort, maximum postoperative wound strength, and cosmetic effect, and, in emergencies, the ease and speed of entering the affected area. Figure 13–1 indicates frequently used incision sites and the types of surgical procedures for which each is used.

HEMOSTASIS

Hemostasis is the arrest or control of bleeding. It can occur either by the natural clotting of blood, by artificial means, or by a combination of the two. Hemostasis during surgical intervention is essential to prevent hemorrhage, to allow visualization of the surgical field, and to promote wound healing.

Natural Method of Hemostasis

Blood clotting is a normal defense mechanism whereby the soluble blood protein, fibrinogen, is changed into the insoluble protein, fibrin. The exact way this occurs is not known, but there are five known blood components that take part in the reaction: prothrombin, factor V, thromboplastin, calcium, and fibrinogen. The data below demonstrate the basic chemical reactions in blood clotting.

$$\text{Prothrombin} + \text{``Factor V''} \xrightarrow{\text{(Thromboplastin, Ca}^{++}\text{)}}$$

$$\text{Fibrinogen} \xrightarrow{\text{(Thrombin)}} \text{Fibrin}$$

Basic chemical reactions in blood clotting. Vitamin K catalyzes liver synthesis of prothrombin; factor V and fibrinogen come from the liver; and both injured platelets and tissue cells release thromboplastin into the blood to form thrombin.

Thromboplastin is released from the disintegrating platelets and the injured tissue cells. "Roughening" of the endothelial lining of a blood vessel by cutting or bruising

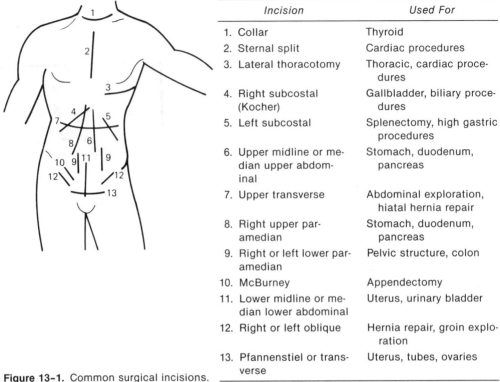

Incision	Used For
1. Collar	Thyroid
2. Sternal split	Cardiac procedures
3. Lateral thoracotomy	Thoracic, cardiac procedures
4. Right subcostal (Kocher)	Gallbladder, biliary procedures
5. Left subcostal	Splenectomy, high gastric procedures
6. Upper midline or median upper abdominal	Stomach, duodenum, pancreas
7. Upper transverse	Abdominal exploration, hiatal hernia repair
8. Right upper paramedian	Stomach, duodenum, pancreas
9. Right or left lower paramedian	Pelvic structure, colon
10. McBurney	Appendectomy
11. Lower midline or median lower abdominal	Uterus, urinary bladder
12. Right or left oblique	Hernia repair, groin exploration
13. Pfannenstiel or transverse	Uterus, tubes, ovaries

Figure 13-1. Common surgical incisions.

causes platelets to adhere to the rough area, start to disintegrate, and release sufficient thromboplastin to enter the blood and form thrombin.[1]

Prothrombin and factor V, both globulins, are formed by the liver. Vitamin K catalyzes the synthesis of prothrombin. Since vitamin K is fat-soluble, its absorption depends upon the presence of adequate amounts of bile in the intestinal tract. Therefore, patients with bile duct obstructions and those with liver diseases may not synthesize enough prothrombin, and a bleeding tendency results. These patients may receive an injection of vitamin K preoperatively.

Fibrinogen, also a globulin, is formed by the liver. Only in rare instances of extreme liver damage is fibrinogen so deficient that clotting is hindered.

Calcium ions come from ingested foods, and the blood always contains enough calcium to catalyze the clotting reaction.[1]

Artificial Methods of Hemostasis

Instruments. Clamping the end of a bleeding vessel with a hemostat is the most common method of achieving hemostasis. This stops the flow of blood until the vessel is ligated (tied) or pressure applied. The vessel may be ligated with a free tie or a suture ligature (transfixion suture). A suture ligature is accomplished by pushing a needle holder with a needle and suture material through a piece of tissue and then tying the suture around the vessel's end.

Pressure. Manual pressure may be used directly on small vessels, as it delays bleeding until the blood begins to form a clot. When sponging an area with a gauze sponge or sponge stick, light pressure applied and released assists in identifying the source of bleeding.

Heat. Heat is used to speed up the clotting mechanism by dilating the vessels and allowing more blood to get to the area. This stimulates the platelets and tissues to liberate more thromboplastin.

Bonewax. Bonewax is refined beeswax that is used to control bone marrow oozing. It is frequently used in neurosurgery and orthopedic surgery. Pieces of bonewax are rolled into balls and handed to the surgeon for application to the bone.

Ligating Clips. Ligating clips, small clips made of tantalum or stainless steel, are used to ligate arteries, veins, or nerves. Serrations across the wire prevent them from slipping off the vessel. The clips are in various sizes with applicators and are also used to mark biopsy sites and tumor margins. This allows visualization on the x-ray film to detect postoperative complications and to observe the size of the tumor.

Tourniquets. Tourniquets are used on the extremities to prevent the flow of blood to a designated area and thereby conserve the patient's blood volume and create a bloodless field. Following the release of the tourniquet, the bleeding must be controlled.

Prior to the application of the tourniquet, the patient's skin is protected by applying a towel or cotton padding around the extremity. The tourniquet is then applied directly over the padding.

Selection of the proper tourniquet cuff should be determined by the patient's age, anatomy and medical condition.[2] The potential for nerve damage is affected by the width of the cuff in relation to the size of the limb, the amount of soft tissue between the cuff and nerve, and the degree and duration of cuff pressure.[3] Tourniquets applied to the lower extremities should be applied to the proximal third of the thigh to avoid vulnerable neurovascular structures.[4] To drain the venous blood from the limb, the extremity is elevated and wrapped with an Esmark or Martin rubber bandage; the tourniquet is then inflated in adults to 250 to 300 mm Hg for arms or 400 to 500 mm Hg for legs. Children and thin patients will require less pressure.

There is no rule as to how long the tourniquet may be safely inflated. The duration of tourniquet time is determined by the patient's age and the presence of vascular disease in the limb.[5] In the average healthy adult under 50 years of age, it is preferable not to leave the tourniquet inflated on an arm more than 1 hour or on a thigh more than $1\frac{1}{2}$ hours.[6] If the operation requires more time, the tourniquet is deflated for 10 minutes. Safe limits after reinflation are unknown. The circulating nurse informs the surgeon of the tourniquet time every 30 minutes. Information regarding the cuff location, cuff pressure, time of inflation and deflation, and identification number of the specific tourniquet should be recorded on the patient's record.[7]

When prepping patients with tourniquets, care must be exercised to prevent the pooling of solutions under the tourniquet, as a burn may result.

Tourniquet gauges should be checked for accuracy prior to each use, and monitored during use to prevent tourniquet paralysis. The use of tourniquets is contraindicated in patients with vascular disease or poor peripheral circulation.

Thrombostat. Thrombostat (thrombin, USP) is an enzyme extracted from dried beef blood. It unites with fibrinogen to accelerate the coagulation of blood and to contain capillary bleeding. It is supplied as a powder and may be applied on the surface of bleeding tissue as a solution or a powder. Solutions of Thrombostat are prepared in sterile distilled water or isotonic saline and should be made just prior to use and the solution appropriately labeled.

Thrombostat may be used in conjunction with an absorbable gelatin sponge. The sponge is immersed in the Thrombostat solution, and the scrub assistant kneads the sponge to remove trapped air and to facilitate saturation of the sponge. The saturated sponge is then applied to the bleeding area.

Thrombostat must never be injected or allowed to enter large vessels, as extensive intravascular clotting may occur.

Gelatin Sponge. Gelatin sponge (Gelfoam) is made from a specially cured gelatin solution beaten to a foamy consistency, dried, and sterilized. The sponge is dipped in saline or a solution containing epinephrine or Thrombostat and then placed on the bleeding area. Fibrin is deposited in the interstices of the sponge, and the sponge swells as it absorbs 45 times its own weight in blood. The gelatin sponge may be left in the body as it will be absorbed in 20 to 40 days.

Gelatin sponge is available as a pad, powder, or film. The pads may be cut to the appropriate size without crumbling.

Oxidized Cellulose. Oxidized cellulose (Oxycel, Surgicel) is a specially treated gauze or cotton that is placed directly over the bleeding area. It absorbs an amount of blood seven to eight times its own weight and forms coagulum. The hemostatic activity results from the coagulum and the pressure of the swelling cellulose.

The hemostatic effect of oxidized cellulose is greater when it is applied dry; therefore, it should not be moistened with water or saline.

Oxidized cellulose may be left in situ, as it is absorbed in 7 to 14 days with minimal tissue reaction. When it is used to help achieve hemostasis around the spinal cord or the optic nerve and its chiasm, it must always be removed after hemostasis is achieved, as the swelling of the cellulose could exert unwanted pressure on these structures. When it is used on bone, it must also be removed, as it may interfere with bone regeneration.

Open, unused oxidized cellulose must be discarded because resterilization results in the physical breakdown of the product.

Microfibrillar Collagen Hemostat. Microfibrillar collagen hemostat or MCH is an absorbable topical hemostatic agent prepared from purified bovine dermis collagen. It achieves hemostasis by the adhesion of platelets and the formation of thrombi in the interstices of the collagen. MCH adheres to wet gloves and instruments; therefore, dry, smooth forceps should be used to apply the powder or sponge directly to the source of bleeding. It is then necessary to apply pressure over the site with a dry sponge. The period of time required for the pressure will vary with the force and severity of the bleeding. After several minutes, the excess MCH should be teased away. If breakthrough bleeding occurs, additional MCH may be applied.

Unused portions of MCH should be discarded as MCH may not be resterilized.

Styptic. One category of styptics includes chemicals that cause a blood vessel to constrict. Two examples are epinephrine and tannic acid. Epinephrine may be added to a local anesthetic agent to prolong the drug's action and to decrease the amount of bleeding when the incision is made. Epinephrine 1:1000 may also be used to soak gelatin sponges prior to applying them to bleeding surfaces. Tannic acid is a powder used on the mucous membranes of the nose and the throat to control capillary bleeding.

Sponges. Sponges of various sizes are used to control capillary oozing, to wall off the viscera, and to keep tissues moist. When sponges are used to control capillary oozing, the sponges are moistened with hot saline, placed on the tissue, and pressure applied. When used for walling off the viscera, it is essential that the scrub assistant maintain an accurate account of the number used to assure that all sponges are removed prior to the closure. This may be accomplished by setting aside an equal number of empty suture packages or instruments. Gauze 4 × 4 sponges may be opened and used for finger dissection in the perineal area, or they may be folded into 2 × 2 squares and used on a sponge forceps. Since these sponges could easily be lost in the wound, they should not be used as free sponges in large wounds.

Compressed rayon or cottom "patties" are commercially available in assorted sizes with strings (Fig. 13–2). They are used for sponging delicate tissues such as the spinal cord and brain. Before the patties are used, they are moistened in saline and the excess moisture is pressed out between the fingers. If the patties are cut, they must be accounted for in their entirety during the sponge count.

Cotton-filled gauze balls or heavy cotton tape is available for dissection or for the absorption of fluids. These sponges are always used on a sponge stick or a pean clamp.

All sponges and patties used on the operative field must be labeled x-ray detectable or radiopaque. These sponges are manufactured with either a small radiopaque insert sewn into the material, or they are impregnated with a radiopaque substance such as barium sulfate. Radiography can then be used to locate sponges or patties suspected of being in the patient.

Each size and type of sponge should be kept separate from the other sponges and from the linen. This will prevent sponges from inadvertently being carried into the wound. X-ray detectable sponges are never used for dressings.

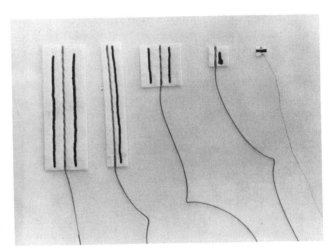

Figure 13-2. Compressed rayon or cotton patties are available in assorted sizes with strings.

Sponge Count. The scrub personnel and circulating nurse count all sponges prior to the beginning of the operation. The scrub person separates each sponge and counts audibly with the circulator. The circulator records the number and the type of sponges on the count sheet or the count board. Sponges placed on the sterile field during the surgical procedure are counted and recorded following this procedure. If the package does not contain the appropriate number of sponges, the sponges should be handed off the sterile field, placed in a bag, and marked with the number. Some institutions may require that the sponges be removed immediately from the room.

As the surgical procedure progresses, soiled sponges are discarded into a polyethylene-lined kick bucket. A sponge forcep or disposable gloves are used to handle the soiled sponges. The discarded sponges are then secured in a clear polyethylene bag according to the type and the number contained in the original package. The bags are then placed in an area of the room where the anesthesiologist can observe the contents to ascertain the patient's blood loss. As the sponges are bagged, they are subtracted from the count sheet or the board. When sponges are used for packing the wound, the scrub person should inform the circulator of the number used so this number can be recorded with the sponge count.

The first count of closure occurs when the surgeon begins to close the incision. All soiled sponges are discarded for the circulating nurse to count and bag; the sponges remaining on the field are then counted audibly by the scrub person and the circulator. The number of sponges bagged or in the kick bucket and the number remaining on the sterile field should equal the initial count plus any sponges added during the surgical procedure. If the count does balance, the circulating nurse informs the surgeon, "The first count is correct." The second count begins with the skin closure and uses this same procedure. If the count is correct, the surgeon is informed, and the count is documented on the intraoperative nurse's note.

A third count is performed when a body organ (such as the bladder or the uterus) is opened but not removed. This count is taken prior to the closure of the organ.

Linen and waste containers are never removed from the operating room until all counts are completed. If the count is inaccurate, a recount of all sponges not bagged is performed. If the count remains incorrect, the circulating nurse opens all the bags and recounts the discarded sponges. If necessary, the laundry and the trash are then checked. If the missing sponge is not found, an x-ray is required to determine whether or not the missing sponge is in the patient. If the sponge is not found, an incident report must be completed. The report should document all the steps taken to find the missing sponge and should be signed by the surgeon and the circulating nurse.

Weighing Sponges. Weighing sponges is one way to assess blood loss and to accurately identify the amount of blood that needs to be replaced. Sponges should be weighed routinely on pediatric, elderly, and critically ill patients, and on extensive surgical procedures. A scale calculated in grams is used to weigh sponges; 1 g is equal to 1 cc. The scale platform is covered with wax paper or plastic sheeting to protect it from contamination.

Each type of sponge is weighed dry, and this weight is posted in each operating room or attached to the scale. If the sponges are used dry, the weight of the blood-soaked sponge is subtracted from the dry weight. This calculates the amount of blood loss.

If the sponges are used wet, the weight of the wet sponges should be calcuated for each case because varying amounts of solution will be removed by each individual when wringing out the sponges. One of each type of sponge should be wrung out by the scrub person and handed off the field for the circulating nurse to use as a baseline weight. The weight of the wet sponge is then subtracted from the blood-soaked sponge to give the amount of blood present in the sponge. Sponges should be weighed frequently, as they will dry out and thus not accurately reflect the blood loss.

To assess the amount of blood lost in suction, the amount of irrigating solution used is subtracted from the total amount of liquid in the suction bottle. In addition, the amount of blood on the drapes is estimated and added to the total. The total blood loss is kept accurately and recorded in the full view of the anesthesiologist and the surgeon.

Electrosurgery. Heat or fire applied to a wound to stop bleeding was used as far back as 3000 BC. The discovery of electricity in the middle 1800s led to the development of electrocautery around 1875. Electrocautery is achieved by passing an electric current through a wire hoop until it is red hot. The heat is then transferred to the tissues by touching the red-hot wire to the tissue.

During this period, Nicholai Tesla and d'Arsonval in France were both working on the production of high-frequency electric currents for possible application in medicine. In 1893, Oudin developed a special resonator for use with spark gaps to produce the first high-power, high-frequency source. In 1900, Riviere used this current to treat skin cancer.

In 1907, Lee DeForest built the first vacuum tube generator for medical use and called it the "cold cautery." It was rejected in this country but adapted for use in Vienna and Paris.

In the 1920s, surgical technique began to expand, and the need to control bleeding became important to the success of these procedures. Dr. Harvey Cushing attempted to use the cold cautery in neurosurgery, but found it unacceptable because it was not effective in controlling capillary oozing. Ed Flarsheim and Henry Liebel, working with Dr. Cushing and Dr. W. T. Bovie, a physicist at the Massachusetts Institute of Technology, developed the first spark gap electrosurgical unit in this country. This unit remains the unit of choice.

In the 1970s, solid-state electrosurgical units became available. These units use transistors, diodes, and rectifiers to generate the current.

Electrosurgery is used for controlled cutting, dehydration, or destruction of tissue. If the active electrode is held a short distance away and the spark "jumps" to the tissue, fulguration occurs. This is used when superficial drying or dessication of tissue is desired. If the electrode is in direct contact with the tissue and more power is used, coagulation occurs. When used for cutting, the current forms an arc between the tissues. The active electrode cuts through the tissue and at the same time coagulates capillaries. Although the electrosurgical units are effective in cutting and coagulating blood vessels, they do significant tissue damage. If they are used extensively and a large amount of coagulated tissue is present, sloughing may occur and interfere with wound healing.

The appropriate functioning of the electrosurgical unit depends on two electrodes: the active and the inactive or ground electrode. The tip of the active electrode is small, and the current density is high; as the surface temperature increases, the tissue is burned. The inactive electrode is large, the current density is small, and little heat is generated.

The tip of the active electrode may be a blade, ball, loop, or needle that fits into a a pencil-shaped handle; or it may be a suction tip. The active electrode is activated by a hand control or foot switch and introduces the electrical current into the patient's body. The inactive or ground electrode provides the electrical current with a return path to the electrosurgical unit.

Newer electrosurgical units have isolated outputs. They are designed so that the unit will not work unless the active and inactive electrodes are connected and functioning properly. Many units have a built-in alarm that warns personnel when a malfunction exists; these do not, however, ensure that the plate is in proper contact with the patient. Safety precautions must be observed and instituted to assure the safe use of all electrosurgical units.

The active electrode may be disposable or reusable. If it is reusable, the cable must be examined for cracked or frayed insulation and the handpiece inspected for damage after each use. The active electrode and the cable are checked for electrical continuity. During use, the tip must be clean and free from dried blood and tissue.

There are several forms of inactive or ground electrodes available: reusable metal plates, disposable foil plates, and self-adhesive plates. If a reusable metal plate is used, the ground cable must be inspected for broken, frayed, or damaged insulation and for maintenance of the electrical continuity. Cables that are spliced or taped or have cracked insulation must not be used. If the cable is designed for permanent attachment to a ground plate, this connection must be firm. The use of alligator clips for ground plate attachments is unacceptable. The surface of the metal plate must be flat, free from cracks or creases, clean, and free from corrosion.

The reusable metal plate and the disposable foil plate require that a conductive gel be applied to reduce tissue heating at the point of the electrode contact with the patient. Only gels designed for use with electrosurgery should be used. The electrolyte gel should be spread completely and evenly over the conductive surface. Missed spots may cause burns, and too thin a coat may dry out during lengthy surgical procedures.

Another type of disposable inactive ground plate is foil covered with a foam pad impregnated with an electrolyte gel. The inactive electrode is usually referred to as a ground pad or plate. Generally, this type of inactive ground plate is flexible and self-adhering. It provides more uniform contact with the patient and presents fewer pressure point problems. Pressure points due to boney protuberances can be grounding hazards as the pressure exerted at these areas can cause increased current density and result in "hot spots." Electrosurgical current tends to heat at the small, low-resistance area created by the pressure point, and a burn may result.

The greatest hazard in using the electrosurgical unit is a radiofrequency electrical burn. The damaged tissue of an electrosurgical burn is hard and has a translucent tan color. Blanching of the skin may show immediately postoperatively; however, the injury may not develop fully for about 24 hours after the incident. The lesion usually has a red rim and is very painful to the touch. The necrosed area eventually blackens to form a typical eschar. Unlike burns associated with noxious liquids, electrosurgical burns do not heal well and may require debridement and skin grafting.[10]

Improper placement of the inactive or ground electrode accounts for most burns associated with electrosurgical units. If the patient is not in adequate contact with this electrode, the current will find other paths to ground through ECG electrodes, stirrups, the operating room table, towel clips, or any other conductive material in contact with the patient. In such an instance, too much current flows through too small an area, there is an excessive temperature rise, and a burn results. ECG electrodes should be placed as far as practical from the active site.

Contact with the ground electrode is not the only hazard in using the electrosurgical unit. Since the circulating nurse is responsible for applying the inactive electrode to the patient, it is important that this nurse be knowledgeable about electrosurgery to prevent injury to the patient.

Guidelines Prior to Use

1. The use of explosive anesthetic gases is contraindicated for procedures using electrosurgery.
2. Flammable skin preparations must dry thoroughly and the fumes dissipate prior to activating the electrosurgical unit. Flammable agents, such as alcohol and tinctures, may ignite when the electrosurgical unit is used.
3. Be familiar with the unit and how to connect all the cables.
4. Place the electrosurgical unit in a location that will avoid stress on the cables and the hazard of personnel tripping over the cables.
5. Whenever possible, eliminate patient contact with any device that offers a potential alternate return path for the electrical current (i.e., OR table, towel clips).
6. Inspect the electrical plug, cord, foot switch cord, and all electrical connections for damage.
7. Test all the safety features (lights, activation, sound).

Guidelines For Ungelled Pads

1. Apply a smooth, even film of electrolyte gel over the entire plate.
2. Select a site for the ground plate that is muscular, clean, and dry and as close as possible to the operative site. Avoid boney protuberances, sites where fluids might pool, skin folds, scar tissue, areas of excessive adipose tissue or hair, and sites to be x-rayed. The electrode must make contact with the patient's bare skin in an area of good blood supply.
3. Lift or turn the patient to position the plate. Do not slide the plate under the patient.
4. Avoid any insulator, such as the drapes, to come between the plate and the patient.
5. In surgical procedures with excessive fluid runoff, the foot pedal should be placed in a plastic bag.

Guidelines During Use

1. Operate the generator at the lowest effective power setting. If the surgeon repeatedly requests higher than normal power settings, check the ground plate and the connections of the active and inactive electrodes; during urologic procedures, make certain that a nonconductive irrigation solution is being used.
2. If the patient is repositioned or moved during surgery, recheck the position of the ground plate and the connection of the cable.
3. The unused active electrode should be positioned in such a way that accidental activation of the unit will not harm the patient or the surgical team members or burn the drapes.
4. If the surgical procedure is long and a reusable metal or a disposable foil plate is used, check to ensure that the gel has not dried out; if necessary, regel the electrode.
5. Do not use the top of the generator as a storage area. Solutions may leak inside and damage the unit.
6. The unit is activated only when touching the active electrode to tissue.

Guidelines Following Use

1. Turn all dials to the off position.
2. Disconnect the power supply cord first and then the active and the inactive electrode cables.
3. Remove the ground plate and inspect the site for skin damage. If a self-adhering pad was used, it must be removed carefully by peeling it back slowly to avoid denuding the skin.
4. The generator and all reusable parts are wiped off with a disinfectant; do not immerse or pour fluid over the electrosurgical unit.
5. Remove all gel and foreign material from the reusable metal ground plate and wipe dry.
6. The foot switch should be stored appropriately, with the electrical cord coiled.

Routine preventive maintenance should be performed and documented. The generator is checked to confirm power output versus control settings. All connections for active and ground electrodes are tested for secure fit. Foot switches and electrical cords are checked for fraying or breaks, internal connections are tightened, and spark gaps are changed if needed. If alarms on isolation circuits are present, they are checked for appropriate function, and the unit receives a routine electrical safety check.

In using electrosurgical units designed for a specific purpose, such as laparoscopy or other endoscopy procedures, the manufacturer's guidelines must be followed.

Pacemakers and Electrosurgery. Electrosurgery can disrupt the operation of pacemakers, particularly external-demand pacemakers. These tend to be more susceptible to electrical interference since, unlike implanted pacers, they are not shielded by body fluids.

In addition to the previously discussed precautions taken for electrosurgery, the following steps should be implemented for the patient with a pacemaker:

1. The distance between the active electrode and the ground plate should be as short as possible and both should be as far as possible from the pacemaker.
2. All electrosurgical cords and cables must be as far as possible from the pacemaker and the leads.
3. Monitor the patient's ECG continuously during the procedure.
4. The surgeon should use short activation periods so the heart can be paced normally between activations.
5. A defibrillator should be available in the operating room.[11]
6. Postoperatively evaluate the pacemaker for proper function.

Bipolar Electrosurgical Units. The bipolar unit uses forceps for coagulation. One side of the forceps is the active electrode, and the other side is the inactive electrode or ground. Therefore, this unit does not require a ground plate. The current flows only between the tips of the forceps rather than through the patient. The bipolar unit is controlled with a foot switch and provides precise hemostasis without stimulation or current spread to adjacent structures.

Heated Scalpel. This unit uses a steel scalpel that is heated and used to seal small vessels as it cuts, resulting in less tissue damage than when the spark-gap or solid-state electro-surgical units are used. The heated scalpel thermally transfers heat to the tissue and is electrically insulated from the patient. There is no electric current that passes through the patient's body; therefore, a ground pad is not required, and the risk of electrical burns is eliminated.

The unit does require that the surgeon develop a different technique than is used with electrosurgical units or with a conventional scalpel. To eliminate the need to "go back" over the area to coagulate bleeding vessels, the incisions must be made at a low speed and through thin layers of tissue.

Documentation Regarding the Electrosurgical Unit. The brand name of the electrosurgical unit, the serial number, the settings used, and the location of the ground plate are documented on the intraoperative nurse's notes.

During the preoperative assessment, all abnormal skin lesions are identified and documented on the preoperative assessment form. This will ensure that these lesions will not be confused with lesions acquired during the intraoperative period.

Postoperatively, if a skin lesion is observed, a full investigation of the injury with a report of the findings is appropriate. Dependent upon hospital policy, an incident report may be required.

Hypotension

Hypotension may be induced and controlled by the anesthesiologist to reduce the amount of blood loss and to provide a bloodless field. It is frequently used in total hip replacement and vascular surgery to control oozing and in neurosurgery on vascular tumors and cerebral aneurysms. It is also used when compatible blood is not available or when receiving blood transfusions are against the patient's religious beliefs.

During induced hypotension, adequate oxygenation of the heart, the liver, the kidneys, and the lungs is essential to prevent damage to these vital organs. Complications of induced hypotension are coronary thrombosis, anuria, and reactionary hemorrhage.

Hypothermia

Hypothermia may be used to lengthen the period of circulatory interruption, ischemia, or hypoperfusion. Decreasing the body's temperature decreases cellular metabolism; therefore, the need for oxygen is reduced, and bleeding is decreased. Hypothermia may be light, 37° to 32° C (98.6 to 89.6° F); moderate, 32° to 26° C (89.6° to 78.8° F); deep, 26° to 20° C (78.8° to 68° F); or profound, 20° C or below (68° F or below).

Hypothermia may be achieved by surface cooling, internal cooling, or extracorporeal circulation. Surface cooling can be accomplished with thermal blankets (temperature control unit), packing the patient in ice, or immersing the patient in an ice bath. Thermal blankets warm or cool patients by circulating fluids through blankets that are placed under or over the patient. Internal cooling is achieved by irrigating with cold fluids or placing ice packs around the internal organs. Moderate and profound hypothermia are accomplished through the heat exchange device of the heart–lung machine.

When a thermal blanket is used, a sheet is placed between the blanket and the patient. After moving the patient onto the blanket, the blanket is checked to assure that there are no creases or folds present that would concentrate heat in one area. The temperature of the heating fluid must be monitored constantly and never allowed to exceed 42° C.

When surface cooling is used, nursing care measures should be directed at preventing frostbite by wrapping the extremities in cotton sheeting or towels. Other complications include cardiac arrhythmias, metabolic acidosis due to shivering, impaired renal and hepatic functions, disturbance of blood coagulation, downward drift of the temperature, and pressure areas from the thermal blankets.

Urinary output, the electrocardiogram, and the temperature are carefully monitored during hypothermia. A nasopharyngeal temperature probe reflects the brain temperature, an esophageal probe monitors the heart temperature, and a rectal probe monitors the core temperature. The location of all temperature probes must be checked when the patient is repositioned.

The patient is rewarmed slowly to prevent vasoconstriction and shivering. Shivering increases the need for oxygen requirements by 400% to 500%; without an appropriate increase in cardiac output, metabolic acidosis will occur. This is called "rewarming shock." Rewarming is accomplished with the heat exchange device of the heart-lung machine, warm blankets, thermal blankets and convective warming therapy in the immediate postoperative phase. Convective warming is a system that directs a gentle flow of warm air across the patient using a warming cover.

Thermal burns or pressure necrosis may occur in patients when thermal blankets are used. Most of these injuries occur during lengthy surgical procedures in which extracorporeal circulation or cross-clamping of the aorta is part of the procedure. In some cases, excessive temperature may be the cause, and the patterns of the burns match the pattern of the tubing in the thermal blanket. These injuries tend to be concentrated in sites where pressure is the greatest, such as over the sacrum.[12]

There also have been incidents when the unit was not used in the heating mode, but injuries occurred as a result of prolonged immobility. In these cases, the prolonged pressure on subcutaneous blood vessels obstructs the blood flow to the tissues, and tissue necrosis occurs.[12]

The use of hypothermia is documented on the intraoperative nurse's notes and includes all nursing care measures instituted. If a temperature control unit is used, the brand name, the serial number, and the temperature at which the unit was set, as well as the patient's temperature, are charted.

Routine inspection, preventive maintenance, and user education and observation during use are essential to ensure safe operation of temperature control units.

Investigating a Skin Lesion

When a skin lesion occurs, it is important to avoid the tendency to assume that a particular device such as the electrosurgical or temperature control unit was at fault. It is, therefore, important to refer to the injury as a "skin lesion" rather than a burn and to investigate all possible causes for the injury.

When a skin lesion occurs, the location, size, and shape of the lesion are evaluated. If the lesion is relatively large and is either an irregular shape or symmetrical around the skin folds or the body crevices, the possibility of a liquid or chemical burn should be considered. If it is located on a surface where there may have been pressure, a pressure sore should be considered. A thorough investigation should occur as soon as possible.

If an electrosurgical burn is considered, all the members of the staff involved in the placement and the checking of the ground pad should be interviewed. The electrosurgical unit should be removed from service and checked by the biomedical engineer or the manufacturer's representative. If the area is noted immediately following surgery, the active electrode and the ground plate should be saved and sent with the generator for investigation.

If the lesion appears to be associated with a temperature control unit, the unit and the thermal blanket are removed from service and examined for appropriate function by the biomedical engineer.

Color photographs of the lesion as soon as it is discovered and periodically as it heals will assist in identifying any characteristic patterns of skin destruction and may assist in identifying the causative mechanism.[12]

The written report should contain all of the facts discovered during the investigation and recommendations for preventing similar occurrences in the future.

AUTOLOGOUS BLOOD TRANSFUSION

Concern about the transmission of the AIDS virus has heightened awareness of the complications of blood transfusion and caused an increased interest in autologous transfusion. Autotransfusion or autologous transfusion is the process of reinfusing a patient's own blood rather than relying on banked stores of homologous blood. Presently, four autologous techniques are available:

1. Predonation of blood
2. Recycling of blood during surgery
3. Hemoconcentration (blood dilution)
4. Postoperative collection for retransfusion

In the predonation program, blood is collected from the patient and banked several weeks before elective surgery. If the donor is acceptable as a homologous donor, unused products may be transfused to other patients.

If the blood lost intraoperatively is not contaminated by bacteria or tumor cells, it can be salvaged and used for transfusion. To transfuse this blood, it must be collected sterilely, not allowed to clot, and placed in a suitable container for administration. Intraoperative salvage systems are of two types—those that transfuse the salvaged product without further treatment and those that "wash" the collected blood by saline suspension and centrifugation. If washing is not used, care must be taken to avoid excessive dilution of the product with surgical irrigants and to prevent hemolysis caused by vigorous suction.[8]

Hemoconcentration is used for patients undergoing open heart surgery. The patient's blood is usually diluted preoperatively with crystalloid or colloid solutions to extend its volume to accommodate the added volume of the heart–lung bypass circuit. After this is done, the patient's blood may be centrifuged to remove the added liquid volume while preserving the cellular components.[9]

Postoperatively, blood can be collected sterilely from mediastinal or chest drainage and transfused. Anticoagulation is not required since the blood is defibrinogenated and does not clot.[8]

Autotransfusion also offers a safeguard against serious transfusion reactions and offers the patients whose religious beliefs will not allow them to receive transfusions of banked blood a viable alternative.

Cyroprecipitated Fibrinogen Concentrate

Autologous and donor-directed blood can also be used to procure fibrinogen that aides in hemostasis.

Cyroprecipitated fibrinogen concentrate is prepared by thawing fresh-frozen plasma and recovering the cold precipitate: this is then warmed and transferred under sterile conditions to a sterile bottle. The fibrinogen is then refrozen for storage. Prior to use, the component is warmed to 37°C and applied topically with thrombin to the surgical site via a syringe or aerosol dispenser. Cyroprecipitated fibrinogen assists in the control of hemostasis, tissue sealing, and wound healing.

Sutures

A Historical Perspective

The use of linen strips and animal sinews for wound closures and for ligatures is described in the literature as far back as 3000 BC in the Edwin Smith Papyrus. Since then, many materials have been used for these purposes: dried gut, dried tendon, strips of hide, horsehair, human hair, bark fibers, and textile fibers of various kinds.

Among the more exotic methods of suturing was the use of the Sauba ant to accomplish skin closure. In the historical publication, "Surgery Through the Ages," the technique is described as follows[13]:

> An ant is set on the margin of the open wound and promptly sinks its claws into the wound. The edges are then drawn together and the rear claws of the ant grip the other side of the wound. The insect is then beheaded and the shriveling of its body draws together the edges of the cut. The ant, even in death, will not release its grip.

Another unusual method of skin closure was practiced by the Masai and Zulu Africans.[13]

> The witch doctors, in addition to their incantations and voodoo, sutured open wounds by inserting tiny sharp slivers of wood on each side of the edges of a cut. They then used a bast, which is the phloem or inner bark tissue of plants, to draw the slivers together and tied the bast forming a suture line. The suture closed the wound and allowed healing to take place. The wound was bandaged with leaves purported to have medicinal properties, following suturing.

In the first century AD, a Roman physician, Celsus, described the excision of the thyroid gland for treatment of goiter, the removal of tonsils, and the repair of penetrating wounds of the abdomen. He advocated ligation of blood vessels and referred to the use of gold and iron threads to close wounds.

The use of silk suture was reported as early as 150 AD by Hua Tu. This early Oriental surgeon used silk on intestinal cases. When the great caravans returned with products and knowledge of the East, silk was adopted for surgical use in Europe.[14]

The first recorded use of surgical gut is found in the writings of Galen, about 200

AD. The Arabian surgeon, Rhazes, in 600 AD contributed to the misnomer of the term kitgut. Derived from the intestines of sheep, this material was first used as a string on a small instrument called a kit; thus, the term kitgut evolved. Since a small cat is called a kit, the word catgut replaced kitgut.

The Japanese of the 10th century did not use ligatures. They preferred to control hemorrhage by compression or application of various plasters of powdered oyster shells. They did, however, suture large wounds with threads from the bark of the mulberry tree.[14]

During the Middle Ages, surgical techniques regressed, and sutures fell into disuse. During this period, the accepted treatment for bleeding and infection was boiling oil and hot irons. It was a French surgeon, Ambroise Paré, who revived the use of ligatures in the 16th century.

As a surgeon with the French army, Paré had been taught that the treatment of traumatic wound injuries was the cauterization of tissue by holding the edges of the wound wide apart and pouring into it a mixture of treacle and scalding hot oil from elders. On one occasion, he ran out of the oil and substituted a mixture of egg yolk and oil of roses in turpentine. To his amazement these patients recovered equally as well and with much less discomfort than the ones treated with the boiling oil. This led Paré to challenge many of the accepted surgical techniques and to restore the use of ligatures to bleeding blood vessels during amputation. In 1552, Paré explained to other surgeons the advantages of using ligatures.[14]

In 1825, Phillip Syng Physick of Philadelphia discovered that leather disintegrated when it was exposed to tissue fluids; thus, he saw the possibility of eliminating wound complications caused by the prolonged presence of nonabsorbable ligatures. Buckskin, parchment, and kid were tried; but gut fabricated from tanned intestines of sheep and beef was the most satisfactory.[14]

During this period, when a surgeon used sutures, he would leave the ends long and dangling from the wound. These sutures were thought to be the cause of the pus and the infection that occurred postoperatively. Secondary hemorrhages from abscess and sutures sloughing out prematurely were also a common complication. It was not until 1867 that Lister supplied an answer to the problem of contamination by spraying sutures with carbolic acid.

The development of asepsis and general anesthesia (1842) provided the necessary information for surgeons to perform new surgical procedures. Thus, the need developed for better suture material and advanced suturing techniques.

An important step came with Lister's promotion of chrome treatment of catgut to delay its absorption in tissues and thus contribute to the longer lasting strength of sutures.

Following the use of carbolic acid, heat was used to sterilize sutures; and in 1902, Claudius introduced sterilization by chemical treatment with potassium iodide. By 1901, sterile surgical gut was available in boilable glass tubes (Fig. 13–3A). These tubes were wrapped in muslin and placed in the instrument sterilizer to be boiled with the instruments for each case. In the 1920s, a different method of packaging sutures was developed, and the tubes were changed to nonboilable (Fig. 13–3B). These tubes were washed by the operating room nurse in green soap and then placed in a glass jar containing a formaldehyde solution, which sterilized the exterior of the tubes (Fig. 13–3C). The fumes of

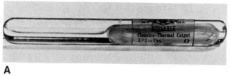

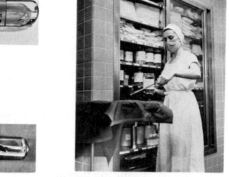

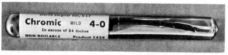

Figure 13-3. A. Suture packaging, 1909—Boilable gut in glass tubes had to be boiled or autoclaved to sterilize exterior surface. **B.** Suture packaging, 1949—Nonboilable gut in glass tubes immersed in germicidal solution became available to hospitals. **C.** In the 1940s and 50s nurses were assigned the uncomfortable routine of restocking suture jars. (*From* Perspective on Sutures, *Copyright 1978, American Cyanamid Company, Wayne, New Jersey, with permission.*)

the solution were irritating, and many individuals developed allergic reactions to the formaldehyde solution; more importantly, the solution was not effective against the hepatitis virus.

Efforts to improve upon the package and the sterilization process continued and, in 1956, the precursor of today's package was introduced in the form of a double plastic envelope. The outer envelope could be opened so the inner package containing the suture could be delivered safely to the sterile field. This system eliminated the use of formaldehyde, saved time, was safer, and reduced shipping costs. In a few years all manufacturers adopted the sterile dry-pack system. This basic system is still in use.

Regulating Standards and Sutures

In 1820, a group of physicians created a nonprofit organization to establish a United States Pharmacopeia (USP) that would include all substances and preparations they believed to be of substantial worth in medical practice. Until 1906, the standards included in the USP were followed on a voluntary basis; then on June 30, 1906, the United States federal government passed the Pure Food and Drug Act. The standards in this act were those of the USP and the *National Formulary (NF)*, a publication of the American Pharmaceutical Association. Federal law now required that drug preparations conform to these standards if the label carried the USP or NF reference.

In 1937, sutures were included in the USP. The USP indicates standards and tests for suture size, diameter limits, and tensile strength. The diameter of each suture strand must fall within the minimum and maximum limits for the gauge. The tensile strength is measured on the basis of the knot-pull strength. The minimum knot-pull strength is specified for each size and type of suture. The knot-pull strength is the force that can be applied to the free ends of a suture, tied with a surgical knot around a $\frac{1}{4}$"-diameter rubber tubing, before it breaks. For example, for size 3/0 surgical gut, the diameter limits are 0.30 to 0.339 mm, with a minimum tensile strength of 1.25 kg. Size 0 surgical gut (which is larger) has diameter limits of 0.40 to 0.499 mm, with a minimum tensile strength of 2.77 kg. In addition, the standards cover suture packaging, labeling, needle attachment, dyes, and sterility.

In 1976, the Medical Device Amendment gave the Federal Food and Drug Administration (FDA) regulatory control over all medical devices. For purposes of this amendment, the term "device" means an instrument, apparatus, implement, machine, contrivance, implant, in vitro reagent, or other similar or related article, including any component, part, or accessory, that is[15]:

1. Recognized in the USP
2. Intended for use in the diagnosis, cure, mitigation, treatment, or prevention of disease
3. Intended to affect the structure or any function of the human body

The legislation classified all devices into one of three categories based on the extent of control necessary to ensure the safety and effectiveness of each device. The three categories established are[15]:

- Class I, General Controls: This includes simple medical devices and requires that the company follow good manufacturing practices and report information to the FDA regarding the safety, efficacy, and proper labeling of these devices.
- Class II, Performance Standards: These devices require performance standards to assure that the items are safe, effective and labeled correctly. Sutures, which previously did not require a New Drug Application prior to being marketed, are included in this category.
- Class III, Premarket Approval: These devices are represented to be either life sustaining, life supporting or implanted in the body, or present a potential unreasonable risk of illness or injury. Devices classified into this category will be required to have approved applications for premarket approval. All new materials manufactured for use as a suture will be a Class III.

Although the FDA had been involved with the efficacy of synthetic absorbable sutures, it was not until 1976 that the Medical Device Amendment required manufacturers to submit proof of suture safety and efficacy prior to the marketing of the sutures. The USP minimal standards remain voluntary; however, the USP standard must be met if the product label indicates that the sutures conform to these standards.

Classification of Suture Material

Sutures are used for two primary purposes: (1) to occlude the lumen of blood vessels and (2) to approximate wound edges until healing is complete.

There are two classifications of suture material: absorbable and nonabsorbable.

Absorbable sutures are digested by body enzymes or hydrolysis. These sutures first lose strength, then gradually disappear from the tissue. The minimal standard for absorbable surgical suture as defined in the United States Pharmacopeia, Twentieth Revision (USP XX) are[16]:

Absorbable Surgical Suture is a sterile strand prepared from collagen derived from healthy mammals, or from a synthetic polymer. Its length is not less than 95.0 percent of that stated on the label. Its diameter and tensile strength correspond to the size designation indicated on the label, within the limits prescribed herein. It is capable of being absorbed by living mammalian tissue, but may be treated to modify its resistance to absorption. It may be impregnated or coated with a suitable antimicrobial agent. It may be colored by a color additive approved by the Federal Food and Drug Administration.

The USP requirements for diameter and tensile strength are different for surgical gut and synthetic absorbable sutures. For example, on 2/0 surgical gut, the limits are 0.35 to 0.399 mm, with a minimum tensile strength of 2.00 kg.; size 2/0 synthetic absorbable suture has diameter limits of 0.30 to 0.339, with a minimum tensile strengh of 2.68 kg.

Materials that are not affected by enzyme activity or absorption in living tissue are classified as nonabsorbable materials. Nonabsorbable sutures become encapsulated in fibrous tissue during the healing process and remain embedded in body tissues unless they are surgically removed. The USP XX provides this description of nonabsorbable surgical sutures[16]:

Non-absorbable Surgical Suture is classed and typed as follows: Class I Suture is composed of silk or synthetic fibers of monofilament, twisted, or braided construction. Class II Suture is composed of cotton or linen fibers or coated natural or synthetic fibers where the coating forms a casting of significant thickness but does not contribute appreciably to strength. Class III suture is composed of monofilament or multifilament metal wire.

Non-absorbable Surgical Suture is a strand of material that is suitably resistant to the action of mammalian tissue. Its length is not less than 95.0 percent of that stated on the label. Its diameter and tensile strength correspond to the size designation indicated on the label, within the limits prescribed herein. It may be nonsterile or sterile. It may be impregnated or coated with a suitable antimicrobial agent.

Nonabsorbable Surgical Suture may be modified with respect to body or texture, or to reduce capillarity, and may be suitably bleached. It may be colored by a color additive approved by the Federal Food and Drug Administration.

Monofilament suture consists of a single strand of suture material that is noncapillary and is designated by USP as type B. Multifilament suture consists of more than one strand of suture held together by spinning, twisting or braiding. All multifilament sutures have a certain capillarity, which means that fluid is soaked into and along the thread. The USP identifies this as type A suture. The capillarity can be reduced by coating the thread with silicone or paraffin. Type A sutures elicit a higher degree of tissue reaction.

The diameter (size or gauge) of suture is designated in descending sequence from No. 5, 4, 3, 2, 1, 0, then 2/0, 3/0, and so on, down to 11/0. Size 5 is the heaviest material and 11/0 the smallest diameter suture. There is less tissue reaction with smaller diameter sutures.

TABLE 13-1. USP SPECIFICATIONS FOR SYNTHETIC ABSORBABLE SUTURE

USP Size	Metric Size (Gauge No.)	Limits on Diameter (mm)		Limits on Knot-Pull Tensile Strength (kg)
		Minimum	*Maximum*	
12-0	0.01	0.001	0.009	
11-0	0.1	0.010	0.019	
10-0	0.2	0.020	0.029	
9-0	0.3	0.030	0.039	0.045
8-0	0.4	0.040	0.049	0.07
7-0	0.5	0.050	0.069	0.14
6-0	0.7	0.070	0.099	0.25
5-0	1.0	0.10	0.149	0.68
4-0	1.5	0.15	0.199	0.95
3-0	2.0	0.20	0.249	1.77
2-0	3.0	0.30	0.339	2.68
1-0	3.5	0.35	0.399	3.90
1	4.0	0.40	0.499	5.08
2	5.0	0.50	0.599	6.35
3 and 4	6.0	0.60	0.699	
5	7.0	0.70	0.799	

United States Pharmacopeia Twentieth Revision, United States Pharmacopeial Convention—1980 (Rockville, Md), 759.

For the USP specifications for absorbable and nonabsorbable sutures, see Tables 13–1, 13–2, and 13–3.

Absorbable Suture Material

Natural Absorbable Sutures (Surgical Gut). Except for specialized uses, surgical gut has been abandoned. Surgical gut, formerly called catgut, comes from the submucosa of sheep intestine or the serosa of beef intestine and is about 98% collagen. The intestines are first washed and stripped of all impurities; next the collagen is stretched and slit into long ribbons; then it is inspected for color and condition and identified for either plain or chromic gut. Chromic surgical gut resists digestion by tissue enzymes for a longer period than plain gut because it is subjected to a "tanning" process called chromicizing. This tanning process can occur either to the ribbons before they have been twisted or spun into strands, or to the finished strand. The diameter of the strand is dependent upon the number and the width of ribbons it contains. The plain gut strand is made in the same manner but is not chromicized.

After the strands are dried, they are polished and ready for needles to be attached or for packaging. Surgical gut is packaged in an inner packet in a small amount of conditioning fluid to maintain pliability.

Surgical gut should be handled only when it is moist; therefore, it should remain in the package until it is needed. Gut should be straightened when it is removed from the packet with a steady gentle pull. Needle–suture combinations should be straightened

TABLE 13-2. USP SPECIFICATIONS FOR COLLAGEN SUTURE (SURGICAL GUT)

USP Size	Metric Size (Gauge No.)	Limits on Diameter (mm)		Limits on Knot-Pull Tensile Strength (kg)
		Minimum	Maximum	
	0.01	0.001	0.009	
	0.1	0.010	0.019	
	0.2	0.020	0.029	
9-0	0.3	0.030	0.039	0.023
	0.4	0.040	0.049	0.034
8-0	0.5	0.050	0.069	0.045
7-0	0.7	0.070	0.099	0.07
6-0	1.0	0.10	0.149	0.18
5-0	1.5	0.15	0.199	0.38
4-0	2.0	0.20	0.249	0.77
3-0	3.0	0.30	0.339	1.25
2-0	3.5	0.35	0.399	2.00
1-0	4.0	0.40	0.499	2.77
1	5.0	0.50	0.599	3.80
2	6.0	0.60	0.699	4.51
3	7.0	0.70	0.799	5.90
4	8.0	0.80	0.899	7.00

United States Pharmacopeia Twentieth Revision, United States Pharmacopeial Convention—1980 (Rockville, Md), 759.

in the same manner except that the strand should be grasped about 2 inches from the needle attachment to avoid stress on the needle–suture junction. If surgical gut is opened and prepared in advance, such as for individual ties, it should be stored in the folds of a dry towel and moistened in cool saline solution or water for 4 to 6 seconds before handing it to the surgeon. If gut is soaked for a longer period, it will absorb moisture, swell, and lose tensile strength. Surgical gut should be handled as little as possible; excessive handling or running gloved fingers up and down the strand can cause fraying.

Surgical gut is absorbed by phagocytosis and this results in varying degrees of inflammatory reaction. The rate of absorption is influenced by the following factors:

1. Plain gut absorbs more rapidly than chromic gut.
2. Absorption of gut takes place more rapidly in the presence of infection and proteolytic enzymes in the gastrointestinal tract.
3. Surgical gut is absorbed much more rapidly in serous or mucous membrane than in muscle tissue.
4. In undernourished, debilitated, anemic, or elderly patients, surgical gut may be absorbed faster than desired.

Additional disadvantages of surgical gut are

1. Surgical gut is inconsistent in absorption and has poor tensile strength in comparison to synthetic absorbable sutures.

TABLE 13-3. USP SPECIFICATIONS FOR NONABSORBABLE SUTURES

USP Size	Metric Size (Gauge No.)	Limits on Diameter (mm)		Limits on Knot-Pull Tensile Strength (kg)		
		Minimum	*Maximum*	*Class I*	*Class II*	*Class III*[b]
12-0	0.01	0.001	0.009	0.001	—	0.002
11-0	0.1	0.020	0.029	0.005	0.004	0.017
10-0	0.2	0.020	0.029	0.016	0.012	0.05
9-0	0.3	0.030	0.039	0.036	0.024	0.06
8-0	0.4	0.040	0.049	0.06	0.04	0.11
7-0	0.5	0.050	0.069	0.11	0.06	0.16
6-0	0.7	0.070	0.099	0.20	0.11	0.27
5-0	1.0	0.10	0.149	0.40	0.23	0.54
4-0	1.5	0.15	0.199	0.60	0.46	0.82
3-0	2.0	0.20	0.249	0.96	0.66	1.36
2-0	3.0	0.30	0.339	1.44	1.02	1.80
1-0	3.5	0.35	0.399	2.16	1.45	3.40
1	4.0	0.40	0.499	2.72	1.81	4.76
2	5.0	0.50	0.599	3.52	2.54	5.90
3 and 4	6.0	0.60	0.699	4.88	3.68	9.11
5	7.0	0.70	0.799	6.16	—	11.4
6	8.0	0.80	0.899	7.28	—	13.6
7	—	0.90	0.999	9.04	—	15.9
8	10.0	1.00	1.099	—	—	18.2
9	11.0	1.100	1.199	—	—	20.5
10	12.0	1.200	1.299	—	—	22.8

United States Pharmacopeia Twentieth Revision, United States Pharmacopeial Convention—1980 (Rockville, Md), 760.
[a]The limits on knot-pull tensile strength apply to nonabsorbable surgical suture that has been sterilized. For nonsterile sutures of class I and class II, the limits are 25% higher.
[b]The tensile strength of sizes larger than metric size 3 or monofilament class III (metallic) nonabsorbable surgical suture is measured by straight pull.

2. The knot security is poor.
3. Surgical gut must be packaged moist for pliability.
4. It is difficult to handle because is has memory.

The only advantage to surgical gut is that it is absorbable. Due to the many disadvantages of surgical gut, researchers began to experiment with a more acceptable absorbable suture. In the early 1960s, reconstituted extruded collagen was developed but, except for specialized uses, was abandoned due to problems with absorbtion. It was not until 1971 that a superior absorbable suture was available. This suture, Dexon, is made from a polymer of polyglycolic acid and creates minimal tissue response.

Synthetic Absorbable Sutures. Synthetic polymers are extruded to form monofilament and braided absorbable sutures. These sutures are absorbed through hydrolysis, a process whereby the polymer reacts with water to cause a breakdown of the molecular structure. The byproducts of this metabolism are excreted by the urinary, digestive, and respiratory systems; therefore, tissue response is very mild.

The absorption time and the loss of tensile strength are not affected by infection, the inflammatory process, or the proteolytic enzymes in the gastrointestinal tract. The tensile strength of synthetic absorbable sutures exceeds that of surgical gut of a comparable diameter and compares favorably with most of the nonabsorbable sutures.

Polyglycolic acid suture (Dexon) is a synthetic polymer of glycolic acid that was first marketed in 1971. The second generation of Dexon "S" is constructed of filaments finer than in the original Dexon to provide optimal handling properties and increased tensile strength. Dexon "S" is also available as Dexon Plus. This synthetic absorbable is coated with poloxamer 188, an inert surfactant, which is subsequently excreted in the urine.

Polyglactin 910 (Vicryl) is a copolymer of lactide and glycolide. Vicryl is coated with polyglactin 370 and calcium stearate.

Monofilament absorbable sutures have also been developed. One is a copolymer of glycolic acid and trimethylene carbonate (Maxon) and the other is extruded from the polyester poly (p-dioxanone) PDS. These monofilament sutures are becoming widely accepted, as they are easier to tie, and the material goes through tissue with less resistance than does braided suture. This allows the surgeon to use a running closure, thus saving time at the close of the procedure. In addition, there has always been concern that in the case of infection bacteria could migrate through the interstices of braided suture.

All absorbable suture, including synthetic absorbable suture, is contraindicated where extended or prolonged approximation is required.

Metallic Sutures (Nonabsorbable)

Stainless Steel. Stainless steel sutures are made of a ferrous alloy wire. It is available as a monofilament and as a twisted multifilament stainless steel suture.

Stainless steel wire has the greatest tensile strength of any suture material. It is inert, nonmagnetic, and electropassive in tissue fluids. It is useful in the presence of infection, when minimal tissue reaction is desired, and where slow healing is anticipated. It is often used in secondary repairs of wound disruption, eviscerations, and tendon repairs and as retention sutures.

Stainless steel wire requires special handling techniques as it kinks easily, rendering it useless. Care must be exercised in handling the ends to avoid tearing gloves. Only wire scissors should be used in cutting stainless steel sutures.

In addition to the diameter-size range defined by the USP XX (Table 13–3), stainless steel wire is frequently identifed by the Brown and Sharp (B & S) scale for diameter (i.e., No. 40, No. 35). Table 13–4 identifies wire diameter equivalents in USP and B & S gauges.

When a prosthesis is implanted, it is important to know the composition of the metal. If it is made of Vitallium, titanium, or tantalum, stainless steel sutures must not be used to close the wound, for two different kinds of metals create an unfavorable electrolytic reaction.

Silver Wire Sutures. Silver wire is available as a monofilament. It is soft and pliable and easier to handle than stainless steel. It has antibacterial characteristics and a high

TABLE 13-4. WIRE DIAMETER EQUIVALENTS

Steel Size	Equivalent B & S Gauge
7	18
5	20
4	22
3	23
2	24
1	25
0	26
00	28
000	30
4–0	32/34
5–0	35
6–0	38/40

tensile strength. It is available only in size 7 swaged to a large needle for closure after dehiscence.

Natural Fiber Nonabsorbable Surgical Sutures

Silk Sutures. Surgical silk sutures are made from the thread spun by silkworm larvae in making cocoons. The raw silk is degummed and bleached before being braided or twisted together to form a multifilament suture strand.

Surgical silk loses up to 20% of its tensile strength when it is wet. Therefore, it is treated with silicone or paraffin, thus reducing capillarity and improving the handling characteristics. The substances used for treatment can cause tissue reaction. Silicone is physiologically inert and therefore provokes less tissue reaction than does paraffin.

The tensile strength of silk is stronger than cotton; however, it is not as strong as comparable sizes of synthetic materials. Silk loses substantial tensile strength 90 to 120 days after implantation and is not used if long-term support is vital, for example, in suturing a vascular prosthesis or a heart valve.

Silk is frequently used in the eye, the gastrointestinal tract, the brain, the cardiovascular system, and as a skin closure.

Silk is contraindicated in the presence of infection or contamination, and in the biliary or urinary tract.

Virgin Silk Sutures. Virgin silk suture is bleached but not degummed or treated for capillarity. Available in 8/0 or 9/0 and in white or dyed black, it is primarily used in ophthalmic surgery.

Cotton Sutures. Cotton sutures are made by twisting long, staple cotton fibers into a smooth multifilament strand. The strands are smoother, more uniform in diameter, and stronger than ordinary cotton thread. Cotton sutures are weaker than silk, but moistening cotton before use increases the tensile strength by 10%. Moistening also reduces the tendency of surgical cotton to cling to gloves.

Cotton sutures are used in repairing the fascia, the brain, and the thyroid gland, and in the serosal layer of gastrointestinal anastomosis.

Like silk, cotton sutures are contraindicated in wounds known or suspected to be contaminated.

Synthetic Nonabsorbable Sutures. Advances in synthetic technology have resulted in a decrease in the use of the natural fibers of cotton and silk and an increase in the use of synthetic nonabsorbable suture. The materials in the latter group are polyesters and polyamides. These materials were originally developed for use in the textile industry. Synthetic fibers cause less tissue irritation than natural fibers, have a higher tensile strength, and retain their strength in tissue. Braided synthetic fibers are capillary as are natural fibers. To reduce capillarity, they may be coated. The coating can be applied to the twisted or braided thread or to the individual fibers before twisting or braiding.

Nylon Sutures. Nylon is made of a polyamide derived from coal, air, and water. Nylon is available as a monofilament or a multifilament. Monofilament nylon is available in clear, blue, black, and green colors.

Like silk, multifilament nylon is tightly braided and treated to prevent capillary action. When treated, it handles like silk; but it is 40% stronger, passes more smoothly through tissue, and produces less tissue reaction than silk. It may be used in all tissue where cotton and silk are used. Like silk, nylon should not be used if long-term support is vital.

Monofilament nylon is very smooth and inert; therefore, it is used in general skin closure and for plastic surgery procedures. It can be extruded in gauges as fine as 11/0 and is used in ophthalmic microvascular and peripheral nerve repairs.

Polyester Sutures. Surgical polyester fiber, Dacron, is made from a polymer of polyethylene terephthalate. The raw material is first produced as pellets that are melted and extruded into filaments and then stretched and braided into a multifilament suture strand. It is available in two forms, treated and untreated.

Untreated polyester is rough and stiffer than treated polyester and has a tendency to drag through the tissue.

Treating polyester suture aids in handling and smooth passage through tissue. Polyester sutures are considered to have the highest tensile strength of all the synthetic nonabsorbable sutures. They retain high tensile strength even after prolonged implantation and produce minimal tissue reaction. This suture material is used when extended approximation is required, such as implanting heart valves, vascular grafts, and revascularization procedures.

Polyester sutures are treated with three types of material:

1. Silicone is physiologically inert and becomes liquid at a low temperature, allowing it to vulcanize to the Dacron strand without a bonding agent.
2. Polytetrafluoroethylene (Teflon) requires a high temperature to become liquid. Therefore, it is applied to the Dacron suture in a solid dispersion that requires a bonding agent.
3. Polybutilate coating is now used on some polyester sutures instead of Teflon.

Polybutester Suture (Novafil). A recent addition to nonabsorbables is a polybutester suture. This is a monofilament synthetic material available in either clear or blue. It is indicated for approximation in all types of soft tissue except those involving microsurgery and neural tissue.

Polypropylene Sutures Polypropylene is made from a linear hydrocarbon polymer extruded into smooth monofilament strands. It is available clear or pigmented with cyan blue. Since it is smooth, it passes through tissue or vascular prosthesis with minimal drag. Polypropylene has a high tensile strength that is retained during extended periods of implantation and causes minimal tissue reaction.

Polypropylene suture can be used when delayed or retarded healing is anticipated, in the presence of infection, and when extended support is required, such as in cardiovascular surgery.

The method of packaging polypropylene is vital because it has "memory." When removed from some types of packages, it has a tendency to kink and is therefore difficult to handle.

Surgical Needles

Surgical needles are made of a special steel alloy with a high carbon content. A properly balanced heat treatment and tempering of the material is important for the wire to acquire the necessary firmness but still retain its elasticity to avoid breakage under heavy strain. The steel wire is then formed into various sizes and shapes of needles. The thickness of the needle depends on the diameter of the wire.

Reusable eyed needles were formerly the most popular; however, during the last two decades they have been replaced with disposable eyed needles and needle–suture combinations.

All suture needles have three basic components: the point, the body or shaft, and the eye. The body or shaft of the needle is straight or curved (Fig. 13–4). The various curvatures are $\frac{3}{8}$, $\frac{1}{2}$, and $\frac{5}{8}$ circle. Variations include $\frac{1}{4}$ and 160° for ophthalmic surgery. Needle points are tapered (noncutting), cutting, and blunt (Fig. 13–5).

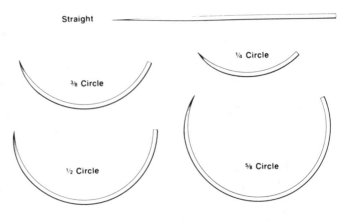

Straight

¼ Circle

⅜ Circle

Figure 13–4. Surgical needles vary in shape, size, type of point, and body, and how suture is attached (swaged or threaded). (*From* Perspective on Sutures, *Copyright 1978, American Cyanamid Company, Wayne, New Jersey, with permission.*)

½ Circle

⅝ Circle

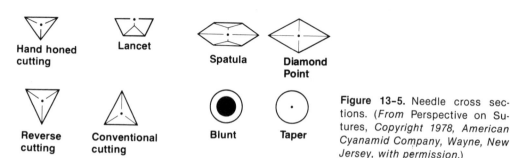

Figure 13-5. Needle cross sections. (*From* Perspective on Sutures, *Copyright 1978, American Cyanamid Company, Wayne, New Jersey, with permission.*)

Points of the Needle. Tapered needles do not have a cutting edge and are used for tissue offering little resistance, for example, the intestines and the peritoneum. These needles tend to push the tissue aside as they go through rather than cutting it.

Conventional cutting needles have a triangular point with two edges in the horizontal plane and one edge in the vertical plane following the inner curvature of the needle. In a reverse cutting needle, the sharp edge follows the outer curvature of the needle and on cross section appears as an upended triangle. Cutting needles are used in tough tissue, such as skin and tendons.

Another variation of a cutting needle is a spatula. Spatulas have a somewhat flattened needle shaft ending in a spatulate point, with the cutting edge in the horizontal plane. These needles are primarily used in ophthalmic surgery.

A trocar needle has a highly sharpened point combined with a tapered body. It provides cutting action with the smallest hole as it penetrates tissue. These needles are useful in tough tissue such as cartilage.

A straight needle with a sharpened triangular blade used for skin closure without a needle holder is called a Keith needle.

Blunt needles terminate in a rounded end. This type of needle is used for suturing the liver and the kidney where neither cutting nor piercing properties are required.

Eye of the Needle. The eye of the needle is where the suture attaches. The eye may be round, oblong, or square. These needles are threaded from the inside curvature with 2 to 3 inches of the suture pulled through the eye. A single twist of the double strand near the needle will lock the suture and help prevent the suture from pulling out of the needle.

French eyes or spring-eye needles have a split from the inside of the eye to the end of the needle through which the suture is drawn. To thread a french eye, place the needle in the needle holder, hold the needle holder in the left hand with 3 inches of the suture secured by fingers of the left hand, and use the right hand to bring the suture strand over the top of the spring and down into the eye of the needle (Fig. 13-6). French eyes are used with fine sizes of suture material.

Selection of the appropriately eyed needle depends upon the area being sutured, the type of tissue, the diameter of the suture material, and the surgeon's preference. The diameter of the needle should be about the same size as the suture.

Eyed needles may be reused or disposable. If they are reused, the needles must be

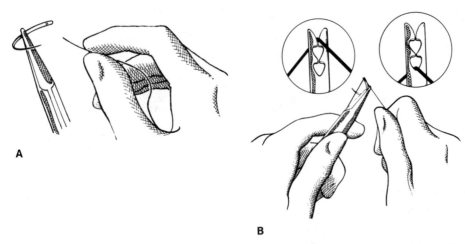

Figure 13-6. A. If eyed needle is threaded from inside curvature, take care to avoid pricking glove on sharp needle point. **B.** Holding suture strand taut with left hand, bring strand down over top and string into eye. Pull through about three inches. (*From* Perspective on Sutures, *Copyright 1978, American Cyanamid Company, Wayne, New Jersey, with permission.*)

cleaned and checked for burred points and eye damage after each use. Dull or burred points can cause tissue damage and defects in the eye will cut the suture material during threading. Prepackaged disposable needles are now available, thus eliminating this time-consuming task.

Eyed needles cause trauma to the tissue due to the excessive bulk created by the needle and the two suture strands passing through the tissue. For this reason many surgeons prefer atraumatic sutures.

Atraumatic Needles. When the needle and suture are one continuous unit, it is referred to as a swaged or atraumatic suture. In atraumatic suture, the diameter of the needle matches the size of the suture as closely as possible.

Atraumatic suture is available with single- and double-armed needle attachments. The needles on double-armed suture may be dissimilar and are designed for a specific surgical procedure such as a tendon repair. Double-armed suture is frequently used in cardiovascular surgery when the surgeon wants to approximate tissue on both sides from a midpoint in the suture.

A recent modification of atraumatic sutures is the development of needles that can be released from the suture by means of a light tug. These sutures are used for bowel anastomosis and general closure when rapid placement of interrupted sutures is desired.

Needles such as those used in ophthalmic and plastic surgery require extra manufacturing techniques. These needles are polished and hand honed under magnification using special equipment. The needle ends are drilled and carefully matched to the diameter of the suture, and the surface of the needle undergoes a special process to provide for easier penetration through tissue.

Preparing Sutures

The surgeon's preference card will designate the type of suture used for each surgical procedure. A minimum amount of suture should be prepared prior to the procedure to eliminate waste and to control costs.

Sutures should be prepared in the order of use. Sutures will first be used to ligate or tie off bleeding vessels. These sutures may be handed as a free tie, placed in the end of an instrument for a deep tie or on a needle for a suture ligature. Nonneedled suture material is placed in a "suture book," a fan-folded towel, with the ends of the suture extending for visualization and rapid extraction (Fig. 13–7). The largest size is placed in the bottom fold and the smallest in the top fold. The suture is pulled from the book toward the operative field to prevent possible contamination.

The scrub assistant should exercise care to avoid damage when handling the suture. Crushing or crimping with surgical instruments such as needle holders or forceps should be avoided except when grasping the free end of the suture for an instrument tie.

Suture for ligating is available in precut lengths, continuous ties on radiopaque ligating reels, or standard lengths that can be cut to meet the requirements of the surgical procedure.

For large blood vessels, the surgeon may request a suture ligature or a stick tie. This may be a swaged suture or a taper-point eyed needle threaded with suture.

The size of the needle holder depends upon the size of the needle and the location of the area to be sutured. A small needle requires a needle holder with fine jaws. When the area to be sutured is deep inside a cavity, a longer needle holder will be needed than in superficial areas.

The needle is placed at approximately one-third the distance from the swaged or eyed end of the curved needle to its point (Fig. 13–8). The needle holder is never clamped

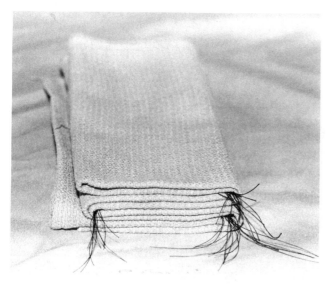

Figure 13-7. A "suture book."

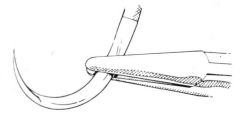

Figure 13-8. Clamp the needle holder approximately one third the distance from swage or eye to point of needle. (*From* Perspective on Sutures, *Copyright 1978, American Cyanamid Company, Wayne, New Jersey, with permission.*)

over the swaged area as this is the weakest area of the needle. The needle holder is closed to the first or second ratchet.

The needle holder is handed to the surgeon with the point of the needle down and directed toward the surgeon's thumb, ready for immediate use. The free end of the suture is held in one hand while passing the needle holder with the other hand. The free end of the suture is handed to the first assistant; it must be allowed to drag across the sterile field.

To assist in identification, atraumatic suture may be armed, placed on a needle holder, and left in the package until it is needed (Fig. 13-9).

Needle Counts

Needles are counted in the operating room by the scrub assistant and the circulating nurse prior to the beginning of the operation, before closure begins, and when skin closure is started.[17] The scrub assistant should maintain an accurate account of all needles by handing them to the surgeon on an exchange basis. Needles must never be left free on the sterile field as they may be inadvertently dragged into the incision. Any needle broken during the procedure must be accounted for in its entirety. If the final needle count is incorrect, the floor and surgical drapes are searched. If the needle is not found,

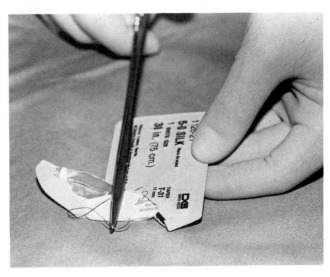

Figure 13-9. Atraumatic suture may be armed and left in the package until it is needed.

an x-ray is required to determine whether or not the missing needle is in the patient. If the needle is not found, an incident report must be completed and signed by the circulating nurse and the surgeon.

Disposable needle count pads are available commercially to assist in performing needle counts. Due to the cost of these items, guidelines should be established for use. For example, when fewer than 20 needles are used on a surgical procedure, a needle pad is not required; with more than 20 but less than 50 needles, a small size pad is used; and when more than 50 needles are used, a large needle pad is appropriate.

Suture Packaging

Suture packages are made to protect the sterile suture from contamination and to allow extraction of the suture from the package ready for immediate sterile use.

Sutures are supplied packaged in a double envelope. The suture is sealed inside the primary envelope, which is then placed in an outer peel-package cover. The unit is then sterilized by ethylene-oxide gas or by cobalt 60 irradiation. Sutures are packaged in boxes, each containing one to three dozen envelopes. To simplify identification of different types of material, a color code appears on the envelopes and the boxes of the suture material.

Each envelope and box contains all the information required by the USP (Fig. 13–10). This will include the trade name, the generic name, size, color, length, number of sutures in the package, needle description, suture construction (braided, twisted, monofilament), any coating material used, the catalogue number, date of manufacturing and/or date of expiration, and an indication if the suture meets the USP standards.

To transfer the sterile primary suture packet to the field, the circulating nurse peels apart the outer wrapper exposing the sterile inner package for the scrub assistant to retrieve (Fig. 13–11). Flipping of sutures onto the sterile field should occur only in an emergency situation, as the field may inadvertently become contaminated by the circulating nurse's hands extending over the sterile surface.

Suture Techniques

The primary suture line refers to the line of sutures used to approximate the edges of the incision during healing by first intention. An interrupted or a continuous suture technique can be used.

Interrupted sutures are placed and tied separately. If one of these sutures breaks, the entire suture line is not disrupted; therefore, there is less opportunity for infection to spread to other interrupted sutures.

A continuous or running stitch is one suture that approximates the edges from one end of the incision to the other end, and is tied only at the ends of the suture line. If a break occurs at any point in the suture, the entire suture line is in danger of disruption.

Both interrupted and continuous sutures can be placed in several different ways. Some of the most common types of suture techniques are illustrated in Figure 13–12.

Buried sutures are those placed under the skin.

A pursestring suture is one suture stitched around a lumen, drawn tight, and tied to close the lumen. This stitch is used when inverting the stump of the appendix.

Subcuticular stitches are short lateral stitches taken beneath the epithelial layer of

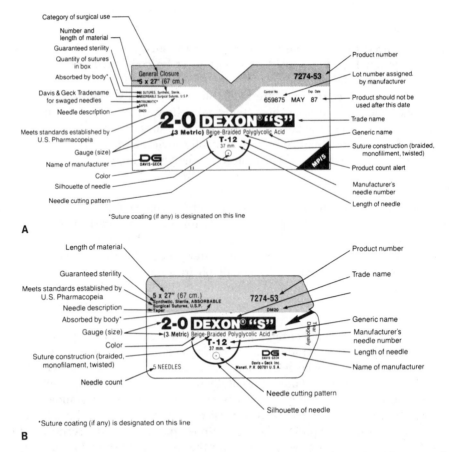

Category of surgical use
Number and length of material
Guaranteed sterility
Quantity of sutures in box
Absorbed by body*
Davis & Geck Tradename for swaged needles
Needle description
Meets standards established by U.S. Pharmacopeia
Gauge (size)
Name of manufacturer
Color
Silhouette of needle
Needle cutting pattern

General Closure
5 x 27" (67 cm.)
SUTURES, Synthetic, Sterile.
ABSORBABLE Surgical Sutures, U.S.P.
ATRAUMATIC*
TAPER
DM20
2-0 DEXON® "S"
(3 Metric) Beige-Braided Polyglycolic Acid
T-12
37 mm
DG
DAVIS-GECK
MPI5

7274-53
Control No   Exp. Date
659875   MAY 87

Product number
Lot number assigned by manufacturer
Product should not be used after this date
Trade name
Generic name
Suture construction (braided, monofilament, twisted)
Product count alert
Manufacturer's needle number
Length of needle

*Suture coating (if any) is designated on this line

A

Length of material
Guaranteed sterility
Meets standards established by U.S. Pharmacopeia
Needle description
Absorbed by body*
Gauge (size)
Color
Suture construction (braided, monofilament, twisted)
Needle count

5 x 27" (67 cm.)
Synthetic, Sterile, ABSORBABLE
Surgical Sutures, U.S.P.
Taper
2-0 DEXON® "S"
(3 Metric) Beige-Braided Polyglycolic Acid
T-12
37 mm.
DG
DAVIS-GECK
Davis + Geck Inc.
Manati, P.R. 00701 U.S.A.
5 NEEDLES

7274-53
DM20
Tear Diagonally

Product number
Trade name
Generic name
Manufacturer's needle number
Length of needle
Name of manufacturer
Needle cutting pattern
Silhouette of needle

*Suture coating (if any) is designated on this line

B

Figure 13-10. A. Suture box label information. **B.** packet label information. (*Courtesy of American Cyanamid Company, Wayne, New Jersey*)

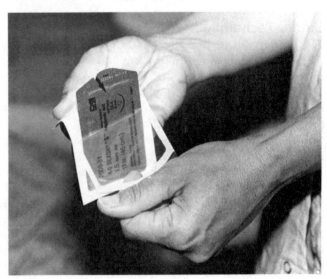

Figure 13-11. Opening suture package. The circulating nurse peals apart the outer wrapper exposing the sterile inner package for the scrub assistant to retrieve.

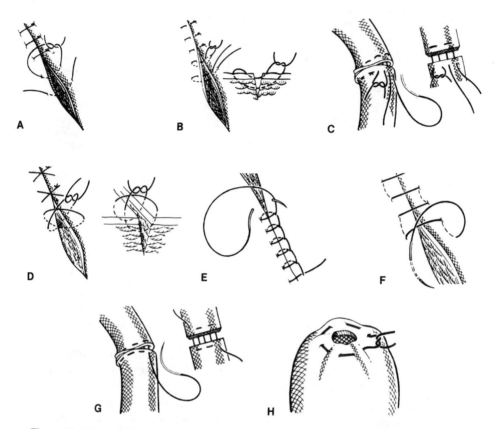

Figure 13-12. A. Interrupted skin closure. **B.** Interrupted vertical mattress. **C.** Horizontal mattress. **D.** Figure-of-8 mattress. **E.** Continuous skin closure (lock stitch). **F.** Continuous inverting mattress. **G.** Continuous everting mattress. **H.** Purse String. (*From Perspective on Sutures, Copyright 1978, American Cyanamid Company, Wayne, New Jersey, with permission.*)

the skin. The suture comes through the upper layer of the skin at each end of the incision. The suture is drawn tightly enough to hold the skin edges in approximation and leaves a minimal scar. If a nonabsorbable suture is used, it is removed by cutting off the knot and pulling the strand through the length of the incision. If an absorbable suture is used, the risk of trauma and breakage during removal is eliminated.

Traction sutures are used to hold tissue out of the way during the surgical procedure. A heavy-nonabsorbable suture may be placed through the tissue, such as the tongue, and then retracted to the side. Dacron or cotton umbilical tape may be put around large vessels or tendons to retract them out of the way.

A mattress suture is placed through the tissue from one side of the wound to the other, then back through the tissue again. Most of the suture is buried. Only a small loop on one side of the incision and the knot on the other side are visible on the skin.

When there is an indication that the wound requires additional support beyond

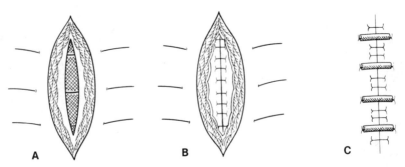

Figure 13-13. A. Retention sutures may be placed from inside the abdominal cavity through all layers to the skin, or **B.** the peritoneum may be closed first and retention sutures passed from fascia through skin. **C.** Bolsters often are used to protect skin from pressure of heavy retention sutures. (*From* Perspective on Sutures, *Copyright 1978, American Cyanamid Company, Wayne, New Jersey, with permission.*)

that provided by the primary suture line, a secondary suture line can be used. Sutures used for this purpose are referred to as retention, stay, or tension sutures (Fig. 13–13).

Heavy, nonabsorbable sutures on large cutting needles are placed from the fascia to the skin on each side of the primary line. Closure of the primary suture line is completed, and the stay sutures are then tied.

Each retention suture may be threaded through a short length of rubber or plastic tubing (bolster, bumper, boot) to protect the skin and the suture line. This prevents the heavy sutures from cutting into the skin and the suture line.

Retention sutures are frequently used when slow healing is anticipated due to obesity, malnourishment, carcinoma, or infection. They may also be used to prevent wound disruptions when postoperative stress on the primary suture line is anticipated due to coughing, vomiting, and straining and for secondary closure following a wound dehiscence or evisceration.

Suturing Drains in Place
Drains may be placed in the wound to prevent the accumulation of blood and serum. These drains are frequently sutured to the skin with a nonabsorbable material so they will not slip in or out of the wound.

Tubes placed in an organ or duct are sutured in place with an absorbable suture.

Stapling Instruments
Stapling instruments mechanically close tissue. The instruments are used for ligation and division, resection, anastomosis, and skin and fascia closure.

Tissue manipulation and handling are reduced by the mechanical application of the instrument. The instruments fire from presterile, preloaded, disposable cartridges, either a single staple or simultaneously one or two straight lines of multiple staples. Different instruments are used for various surgical procedures.

The staples are shaped like a capital "B" and are noncrushing; thus, nutrition is permitted to pass through the staple line to the cut edge of the tissue. This promotes healing and reduces the possibility of necrosis. The staples are essentially nonreactive; therefore, the occurrence of tissue reaction or infection is reduced. Anastomosis performed with staples appears to function sooner than those with manual technique.

The reusable instruments are expensive and are not always reliable in their operation. The surgeon is responsible for choosing the appropriate instrument and must receive instructions outside of the operating room regarding the proper use and function. Inappropriately placed staples are much more difficult to correct than manually placed sutures.

The nursing personnel must know how to assemble the instrument, as inappropriately assembled instruments may misfire. The instruments are cared for in a routine manner. They are disassembled after use, terminally sterilized in the washer–sterilizer, placed in the ultrasonic cleaner, and then sterilized for use by steam or ethylene oxide gas.

Second-generation stapling instruments have been developed that are preassembled and disposable. This eliminates the need for assembling, cleaning, and repairing the instruments (Fig. 13–14).

A variety of disposable skin staples are commercially available for the approximation of the skin edges. All the staplers implant stainless steel staples in varying size cartridges and widths. The wide staples are easier to use as they span a wider area before closing and thus assist in everting the skin edges. Regular width staples require more

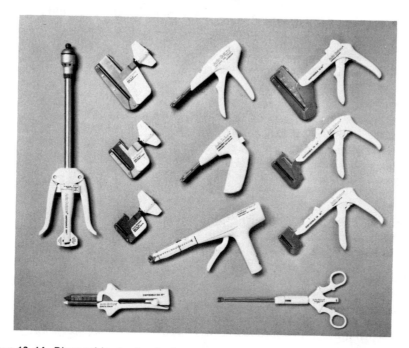

Figure 13–14. Disposable stapling instruments. (*Courtesy, United States Surgical Corporation, Stamford, Connecticut.*)

careful approximation and eversion of the skin edges. The length of the incision will determine which size cartridge to use.

Skin staples represent the fastest method of skin closure and have a low level of tissue reactivity. They are removed 5 to 7 days postoperatively.

Skin Clips

Skin clips are made of noncorroding metal and may be used for skin closure or for securing towels to the skin. They can be steam-sterilized, used in the presence of infection or drainage, and applied quickly. Skin clips create more discomfort postoperatively than do suture material or skin staples, and they leave more of a scar than other skin closures.

Skin Strips

A reinforced micropore surgical tape with an adhesive for immediate adherence to the skin has been developed for skin closures. The tape can be used to close superficial lacerations in conjunction with subcuticular sutures or with interrupted skin sutures. When used with interrupted skin sutures, the sutures may be removed in 32 to 48 hours postoperatively; the skin strips will continue to provide the necessary wound support.

The ease with which wounds can be closed by skin strips varies according to the anatomic site and the biomechanical properties of the wound site. Areas over a joint require additional support from sutures, whereas linear wounds are easily approximated by this method. Areas of the body with excessive secretions (for example, the axilla, the palms, and the soles) discourage tape adherence. The use of an adhesive adjunct such as compound benzoin tincture will enhance the adhesion of the tape to the skin.

Adhesive skin strips are available in widths of $\frac{1}{8}$, $\frac{1}{4}$, and $\frac{1}{2}$ inch, and lengths from $1\frac{1}{2}$ to 4 inches, which can be cut to meet the needs of the patient.

REFERENCES

1. Anthony C. *Textbook of Anatomy and Physiology*, 5th ed. St. Louis, Mo: C. V. Mosby; 1959: 279
2. Recommended practices for preparation, utilization, and maintenance of the pneumatic tourniquet. *AORN J.* 1984;39
3. Bolton CF, McFarlane RM. Human pneumatic tourniquet paralysis. *Neurology.* 1978;28: 787–793.
4. Arenson DJ, Weil LS. The uses and abuses of tourniquets in bloodless field foot surgery. *J Am Pod Assoc.* 1976;66:854–861.
5. Flatt AE. Tourniquet time in hand surgery. *Arch Surg* 1972;104:190–192
6. Edmonson A, Crenshaw A. *Campbell's Operative Orthopaedics*, 6th ed. St Louis, Mo: C. V. Mosby; 1980:vol 1, 2
7. Recommended practices for documentation of perioperative nursing care. *AORN J.* 1987; 45(3):777
8. Thurer R. Autologous blood transfusion. *Surgic Rounds.* 1987;53–57
9. Automated intraoperative processing autotransfusion machines. *Health Dev.* 1988;17(8): 219–243

10. *Biomedical Engineering Guideline Reports.* Los Angeles: Hospital Council of Southern California, 1978:2

11. *Safer Electrosurgery.* Cayton, Ohio: NDM Corp; 1979:21

12. Skin injury in the OR and elsewhere. *Health Dev.* 1980;9:313, 316

13. Riall CT. Surgical and medical devices and their origins. *J OR Res.* 1981;(2):35

14. Riall CT. Surgical and medical devices and their origins, chapter 11. *J OR Res Inst.* 1981; (3):68, 70

15. *Everything you always wanted to know about the medical device amendments—and weren't afraid to ask.* Silver Spring, Maryland: U.S. Department of Health, Education and Welfare, Food and Drug Administration; 1977:6

16. *Pharmacopeia Twentieth Revision.*Rockville, Md: United States Pharmacopeial Convention; 1980:759

17. Recommended practices for sponge, sharp and instrument counts. *AORN J.* 1984;39 (4):699–706

Chapter 14

Wound Healing
and Dressings

WOUND HEALING

The healing of a wound means restoring the continuity in the tissue after injury or surgical intervention by replacing dead tissue with viable tissue. Wounds are considered open if the skin has been divided, and closed if the continuity of the skin is uninterrupted (Table 14–1).

Open Wounds

In an *abrasion*, the injury is confined to the epidermis or the mucous membrane. An abrasion is usually caused by a glancing blow in which varying amounts of the epidermis or the mucous membrane are scraped off, leaving defects in the surface. Frequently, these defects are filled with small particles of dirt or other foreign material. If not removed, these particles retard healing and may result in a "tattoo" that remains following healing.

Treatment consists of irrigating with copious amounts of saline to remove any foreign particles; washing the area with an antiseptic solution; applying a mild antiseptic or antibiotic ointment; and if appropriate (depending upon the location and the extent of the injury), applying a dressing.

Incised and *lacerated* wounds consist of division of the skin with exposure or possible injury to the underlying structures. Incised wounds are caused by sharp cutting objects, and the edges are smooth and even. These wounds may be either aseptic or infected depending upon the circumstances that caused them. A surgical incision is an aseptic wound; healing will occur without incidence if the patient's condition is not compromised and if there is no contamination due to pathogenic organisms or foreign material entering the wound.

A laceration results from the application of force that tears or splits the skin, leaving the edges ragged. This wound is not clean, as it is usually caused by an implement that may be contaminated with pathogenic bacteria. This wound is cleaned with an antiseptic solution and the ragged edges trimmed; the wound is frequently left open to heal by secondary intention.

A *puncture* wound is made by piercing the skin with a sharp object such as a needle, a nail, an ice pick, or a bullet. These wounds are characterized by a small surface opening that gives no clue to the depth or the extent of the internal damage. The treatment frequently involves surgical exploration of the wound to assess the internal damages.

In a *compound fracture*, the bone is broken and there is an external wound leading

TABLE 14-1. TYPES OF WOUNDS

Open	Closed
Abrasion	Blister
Incision	Contusion
Laceration	Sprain
Puncture	Dislocation
Compound fracture	Simple fracture

down to the site of the fracture. Before treating the fracture, hemostasis is achieved, the wound is cleaned with an antiseptic solution, the fracture is then treated, the soft tissue sutured, and a cast applied.

Closed Wounds

A *blister* is a superficial closed wound that occurs following chemical, thermal, or frictional irritation of the skin. The damaged epidermis is raised and separated from the dermis by an excessive collection of serum. If blisters become extremely painful due to pressure of the fluid, they can be aseptically punctured and then treated as an open wound.

A blow of adequate force on the skin produces a *contusion*. The blood vessels beneath the skin rupture and cause discoloration and edema. If the extravasated blood becomes encapsulated, it is termed a *hematoma;* if it is diffused, an *ecchymosis.* Treatment consists of cold compresses, rest, and elevation of the affected area.

A *sprain* is the forcible wrenching of a joint, with partial rupture or other injury to the tendons or ligaments at the joint. It occurs without dislocating the bones. The signs of a sprain are rapid swelling, heat, discoloration, and limitation of function. The treatment consists of cold compresses, bandaging, and elevation of the joint.

The temporary displacement of a bone out of the normal position in a joint is termed a *dislocation.*

A *simple fracture* is a broken bone without an external wound. Treatment consists of reducing the fracture and then immobilizing the bone until union has taken place.

Forms of Healing

Open wounds heal in three different ways: primary or first intention, secondary or second intention, and tertiary or third intention.

First intention healing occurs when the tissue is clearly incised and accurately approximated and contamination is held to a minimum. In these wounds, functional and cosmetic results are optimal.

Healing by second intention differs from first intention in that the wound edges are not approximated and healing occurs through the formation of granulation tissue (the red, granular, moist tissue that appears during the healing of open wounds), which is finally covered by epithelial cells. Most infected wounds, traumatic wounds with excessive loss of tissue, and burns heal by secondary intention.

Initially, these types of wounds may seep serosanguineous drainage. If infection does occur, the drainage is purulent with a color characteristic of the dominant organism. In burns, the open area becomes covered with dried plasma proteins and dead cells called the *eschar*. To maintain cleanliness and promote epithelialization, these wounds may require debridement at frequent intervals. As the healing progresses, the appearance changes to that of granulation tissue.

Fine-mesh gauze is the preferred dressing on these wounds because it inhibits the interweaving of granulation tissue into the gauze. Large-mesh gauze allows the interweaving to occur and may result in a hemorrhage when the dressings are changed.

Healing by second intention is prolonged, the wound is susceptible to further infection, and the scar is excessive. The consequence of this scarring is a contracture with loss of function and limited movement.

The nursing assessment should include observation of signs and symptoms of generalized infection and fluid and electrolyte imbalance. Attention should also be directed at a psychological assessment as the patient may be concerned with his or her altered body image or life-style. Due to prolonged hospitalization and multiple operations, these patients will require a support system. Consistently assigning the same circulating nurse to the patient will assist in fulfilling this need.

Healing by third intention, usually called delayed primary closure, is a combination of primary and secondary healing. It occurs when the wound is left open to heal by secondary intention. After 4 to 6 days, the granulation tissue covers the surface of the wound; the wound is then sutured closed. This procedure is used when the risk of infection is high, as the wound is less likely to become infected while open. The closed wound is most susceptible to infection in the first 4 days.

Healing of Incised Wounds

Wound healing begins immediately after injury and is the same process for all wounds. Variations in the process result from differences in the location, the severity, and the extent of the injury; the presence of pathogenic bacteria; and the regenerative capacity of the cells. The healing process can be divided into three phases that are interdependent and overlapping: inflammatory phase, fibroplasia phase, and maturation phase.

The inflammatory phase (also called the substrate, exudative, defensive, or lag phase) starts at the time of injury and lasts 4 to 6 days. This phase, as discussed in Chapter 6, prepares the wound for healing through hemostasis, inflammation, and biologic cleansing of the wound. During this phase, the tissues are held together by fibrin from blood clots and serum. The inflammatory reaction increases in degree and duration with the severity of the injury, the presence of foreign bodies, or contamination by bacteria. A prolonged inflammatory phase delays the formation of new tissue and results in the retarded development of strength in the wound.

The fibroplasia phase (also called healing, connective tissue, or proliferative phase) starts on the third or fourth day and continues for approximately 2 weeks. During this phase, the epithelial cells migrate along the cut edges of the wound to the base of the clot to form capillaries and lymphatics. The capillaries give a red appearance to the tissues and provide the blood flow for the delivery of oxygen and nutrients to the granulation tissue.

Fibroblasts synthesize a protein substance called *collagen*. The biochemical mechanism responsible for initiating collagen formation is unknown; however, it is thought to be similar to protein synthesis.[1] Collagen is the chief constituent of connective tissue and influences the tensile strength and the pliability of the wound. As the collagen content increases, so does the tensile strength.

Wounds in highly vascular areas, such as the head and neck, may regain sufficient tensile strength by the fourth day so that skin sutures can be removed. Wounds of the abdomen heal more slowly; therefore, skin sutures are removed about the seventh day.

The maturation or remodeling phase may last as long as 2 years. During this phase the strength of the scar increases despite a decrease in the number of fibroblasts and a net loss of collagen. The increase in wound strength is due to the restructuring of the collagen fiber network. Tensile strength is usually adequate to withstand normal activity in 3 to 4 weeks; however, wounds do not regain the strength of uninjured tissues. For example, the skin and the fascia achieve only about 80% of their normal strength.[2] The suture line continues to contract and decrease in size, and the color diminishes during the ensuing months.

Complications of Wound Healing

Wound Dehiscence. Wound dehiscence is the partial or total separation of the wound and occurs most often between the fifth and the tenth postoperative days. As an example, total dehiscence in an abdominal wound results in evisceration, a protrusion of the viscera through the abdominal incision. In this example, wound dehiscence may be preceeded by excessive coughing, vomiting, or straining; and the patient may state that "something gave way." The contour of the abdomen may change with marked bulging and the dressing becomes saturated with serosanguineous drainage. Additional causes of dehiscence may be infection, abdominal distention, malnutrition, poor surgical technique, improper selection or placement of suture, and poorly tied knots.

In the event of an abdominal dehiscence, nursing actions are to cover the abdomen with a sterile towel moistened with saline, monitor vital signs, and provide emotional support to the patient until he or she can be returned to the operating room.

Incisional Hernia. An incisional hernia results from incomplete wound dehiscence in which the peritoneum and the skin remain intact. This complication occurs most frequently in lower abdominal incisions because, anatomically, there is a deficit of the posterior fascial sheath beneath the rectus muscle in that region. Incisional hernias become apparent usually 2 to 3 months after surgery, and the defect must be treated surgically to avoid bowel strangulation.

Fistula and Sinus. During the fibroplasia phase of wound healing, a fistula or a sinus may develop. A fistula is a tract between two epithelium-lined surfaces and is open at both ends, whereas the sinus is open at only one end. This complication occurs most frequently in patients having surgical procedures involving the bladder, the bowel, or the pelvic organs. The primary symptom is drainage, not normally found, arising from a particular cavity. For example, in ureterovaginal or vesicovaginal fistulas, there is a constant drip of urine through the vagina. With a rectovaginal fistula, there is a constant escape of flatus and fecal material through the vagina. Surgery to repair fistulas may not be performed until the inflammation and the induration have subsided; this may take 3 to 4 months.

Sutures. On rare occasions there will be complications with suture material. Surgical gut does not always absorb appropriately; and nonabsorbable sutures, especially silk and cotton, may be a source of irritation and inflammation. When this occurs, the suture knots encapsulate and are surrounded by a serous fluid. The suture then migrates through the incision and is rejected from the body. This is usually referred to as "spitting." If the suture is not rejected, a sinus tract may eventually develop around the suture, and surgical removal of the suture may be required.

Keloid Scars. Alteration in the metabolism of collagen during the fibroplasia phase may result in the development of a keloid or hypertrophic scar. This dense, fibrous tissue grows outside the original incision. These scars may be revised; however, the condition tends to recur. In most patients, injections of corticoids directly into the scar will reduce the size. Keloids are found among blacks and dark-skinned Caucasians.

Hemorrhage. Hemorrhage is a serious complication that can occur during the first few days postoperatively. The bleeding may be evident or concealed. Fresh blood on the dressing or in the drainage device should be observed closely as it may indicate that there is some active bleeding within the wound. Skin discoloration suggests the accumulation of blood in the interstitial spaces and hematoma formation.

An internal hemorrhage will be accompanied by a fall in blood pressure; a weak, rapid pulse; rapid and deep respirations; restlessness; apprehension; thirst; cold, clammy skin; and cyanosis or pallor.

Postoperative hemorrhage may result from a suture sloughing off a vessel, a blowout of clots from a vessel, or faulty tying of a ligature. Any sign of an active postoperative hemorrhage or of the formation of a hematoma should be reported to the surgeon immediately.

Infection. Some degree of bacterial contamination occurs in all open wounds. However, only a small percentage becomes infected. Infection is the unfavorable result of the equation of the dose of bacteria multiplied by the virulence divided by the resistance of the host.[3]

Many of the factors that cause wound infection are in the direct control of the perioperative nurse and have been discussed in earlier chapters of the book. There are, however, nonmicrobial factors that influence the invasiveness of the bacteria in the wound and are important in determining if an infection develops.

Unhealthy, irritated, or dead tissue encourages the growth of bacteria, as such tissue is unable to resist bacterial invasion. Precautions should be taken to keep the tissue moist and to handle it as gently as possible. Excessive use of the electrosurgical machine and sutures tied too tightly result in necrotic tissue and increase the chance for infection.

Foreign bodies such as dirt, gravel, glass, and metal harbor microorganisms. Every attempt should be made to rid the wound of all foreign bodies prior to closing the wound.

The location, the nature, and the duration of the wound are significant factors in the development of an infection. Infection rates are relatively high in wounds involving large masses of tissue, gunshot wounds, compound fractures, and crushing injuries. Wounds of the abdomen, calf, thigh, buttock, and perineal area all have a high incidence of infection, whereas wounds of the head and the neck tend to heal with a few complications. Wounds that are not treated within 6 to 10 hours of the injury are more susceptible to infection.

Dead spaces due to the inadequate approximation of wound edges result in the trapping of air or serum between the layers of tissue; wound healing is delayed. This predisposes the wound to develop an infection.

Hemostasis is important in preventing postoperative wound infections. The accumulation of secretions or hematomas distend the tissue and compress the surrounding capillaries. This results in devascularization and impaired oxygen diffusion to the repairing cells and provides a favorable environment for the growth and the invasion of microorganisms.

Use of Drains

Drains can expedite the healing process. They are used to remove serosanguineous fluid, blood, and purulent material; to obliterate dead spaces; to prevent deep wound infections; and to drain anticipated secretions such as bile and intestinal contents. Drains function by gravitational flow or capillary action or are attached to a suction system.

Closed-wound suction drains maintain a constant negative pressure and are effective when pressure dressings cannot be applied. This system consists of a plastic tubing with multiple perforations connected to a portable self-contained suction unit that is compressed fully to create a negative pressure. This negative pressure evacuates tissue fluids and blood, promotes healing by reducing edema, prevents hematoma formation, and eliminates a media for bacterial growth. This system is frequently used in radical mastectomy, radical neck dissection, total hip replacement, and in the pelvic cavity after abdominoperineal resection.

If the patient with closed-wound suction is ambulatory, the drainage device should be placed dependent to the drainage site and free of tension on the wound, with the excess tubing coiled to prevent inadvertent dislodging.

Drains do not exit from the incision site. They exit from a separate stab wound and are taped or sutured into place to prevent excessive movement. The number of drains, their locations, and any drainage collected intraoperatively are documented on the intraoperative nurse's notes.

Systemic Factors Affecting Wound Healing

Nutrition. Adequate nutrition and balanced electrolytes are essential to the healing process. Mild to moderate nutritional deficiencies do not affect healing. However, major nutritional depletion does retard healing.[2]

Protein provides the essential amino acid, cystein, that is necessary for the fibroblasts to synthesize mucopolysaccharides and collagen.

Carbohydrates and fats are the major energy sources and are essential to prevent excessive oxidation of amino acids for caloric needs.

Vitamins A, B, and C are also necessary for repair. Vitamin A accelerates healing of skin incisions and the forming of granulation tissue. It is thought to promote the inflammatory response by inhibiting glucocorticoids.[4] Vitamin B is necessary for carbohydrate metabolism. Vitamin C (ascorbic acid) enhances capillary formation and permits collagen formation.

Trace metals—copper, iron, and manganese—are essential for collagen synthesis. Zinc is also necessary for repair, although its exact function is unknown.

General Physical Condition. Uremia, uncontrolled diabetes, malignancies, and cirrhosis make the wound more vulnerable to infection and abnormal healing. Anemia produced by hypovolemia can also delay the wound-healing process.[2]

Oxygen is a prime nutritional component in wound healing as it promotes collagen formation and fibroblast synthesis. Any respiratory dysfunction that results in an inadequate delivery of oxygen to the tissue will impair wound healing. An increased supply of oxygen can accelerate healing and appears to be effective in open, poorly healing, nonnecrotic wounds where an impaired blood supply is the major reason for inadequate healing.[2]

Smoking has an impact upon wound healing, as it reduces the amount of functional hemoglobin by 10% to 15%. This hemoglobin is therefore unavailable for oxygen delivery to tissues, and wound repair is prolonged.

The obese patient has a thick layer of subcutaneous fat requiring vigorous retraction that frequently causes trauma to the abdominal wall.[5] This excessive abdominal fat makes closure technically more difficult for the surgeon.

Obese patients have a tendency to breath shallowly due to thick, heavy chest walls, and increased intraabdominal pressure on the diaphragm. Therefore, oxygen delivery to the tissues is diminished, and wound repair is extended. Fatty tissue is relatively avascular and is therefore vulnerable to microbial invasion. Wound dehiscence is not uncommon in obese patients.

Drugs. Any antiinflammatory steroid will suppress the inflammatory response in wound healing. These drugs have the greatest impact when they are given in the first 3 days after injury. After 4 or 5 days, the effect is reduced; however, contraction and collagen synthesis will be delayed no matter when steroids are started.

In renal transplant patients who are taking steroids, primarily closed wounds heal in a reasonable time. However, if the wound is left open or opens up, the steroid effect becomes vastly more significant. The open wound requires more circulation and more energy expenditure for healing than does the primarily closed wound.[6]

Chemotherapeutic drugs such as nitrogen mustard, actinomycin D, 5-fluorouracil, and methotrexate also retard wound repair. When the wound is healing by primary intention, these drugs inhibit protein synthesis during the period of maximum cellular response, the second to the tenth days.[6]

Radiation Therapy. There is little effect on wound repair from a small dose of radiation given 24 hours before surgery. When larger doses are required preoperatively, surgery is usually delayed for 4 to 8 weeks. By this time, the inflammation from the radiation has subsided and the blood supply is still good. As more time passes, the blood supply to the irradiated tissue is decreased and the risk of poor repair is increased.

The Aged Patient. Studies have shown that there are delays in the healing of wounds in older individuals. The wounds contract more slowly, and incised wounds gain strength more slowly.[7] Clinically, wound failure is more frequent in elderly patients. The cellular responses reported to account for delayed wound repair include: (1) increased number of autoantibodies; (2) mutation in lymphocytes and fibroblasts with production of altered proteins; and (3) decrease in the synthesis of collagen, elastin, and structural glycoproteins by cells within the connective tissues.[8]

Whenever possible, the patient's nutritional status must be evaluated preoperatively and nutritional deficiencies corrected prior to surgical intervention.

The elderly patient also experiences compromised wound healing as a result of decreased pulmonary function. The forced vital capacity, the inspiratory reserve volume, and the maximum breathing capacity decrease progressively with age.[9] Preoperative instruction in coughing and deep breathing exercises to facilitate lung expansion will assist in improving gaseous exchange.

DRESSINGS

Dressings are applied after the surgeon removes his or her gown and gloves. Dressings have several functions. They

1. Protect the incision from contamination
2. Absorb drainage
3. Give support to the incision
4. Provide pressure to reduce edema
5. Assist in achieving hemostasis
6. Maintain an optimal (moist) environment
7. Serve as an esthetic measure

Nearly all surgical wounds should be covered with a dressing for the first 24 to 48 hours for optimal resurfacing and more rapid healing.[10] Generally, a moist environment promotes the best epithelial migration and protects the wound from invading microorganisms.[11] Currently, there are several dressings designed for specific purposes and each one has specific advantages.

Various polyurethane dressings can be used for a one-layer dressing. Optimal resurfacing of superficial wounds using polyurethane dressings occur when the dressing is applied within 2 hours after the incision is made and left in place for at least 24 hours.[10] These occlusive materials maintain a moist wound environment, inhibit crust formation, decrease pain and inflammation, prevent bacterial contamination, and produce epithelialization of superficial wounds 30% to 45% faster than air exposed wounds.[10]

On a moist surface, new cells can slide easily from the edge of the wound where they are produced, to create "islands" of epithelial covering. In dry wounds, these new cells cannot move as readily and the body uses energy attempting to move them. In addition, the dry environment damages or destroys many of the cells. Pain is relieved because occlusive and semiocclusive dressings protect exposed cutaneous nerve endings.[12]

The three-layer technique is used for primarily closed wounds that may have drains present, secondary or tertiary healing wounds that are full thickness and have moderate to heavy drainage, and dressings that will be in place longer than 48 hours. The three-layer dressing consists of a contact layer, absorbent or intermediate layer, and a securing layer.[11]

The surface of the material in contact with the wound may be occlusive, semiocclusive, or nonocclusive. Occlusive dressings prevent drying of the wound and are impermeable to air and water. Semiocclusive dressings include hydroactive dressings such as those used for chronic wounds. Nonocclusive dressing material facilitates removal of excessive drainage and should be nonadherent for painless removal.

The layer beneath the surface dressing must be absorbent and easily molded to the contour of the body. The dressing is held in place by tape or a binder. Montgomery straps may be used when frequent dressing changes are anticipated. Tincture of benzoin applied around the dressing will assist in securing the tape. On patients having an allergy to tape, nonallergenic paper tape is used.

Pressure dressings are used to obliterate dead spaces and to prevent capillary oozing, serum accumulation, and hematoma formation. The area around a pressure dressing must be checked for adequate circulation. Any discomfort or change in sensation around the dressing may indicate that the dressing is applied too tightly. Materials used for pressure dressing are fluffed gauze, bulk dressing, cotton rolls, foam rubber, and abdominal pads.

For burns and large pressure sores, biologic dressing may be used. Biologic dressings include cadaver skin, pigskin, and human amniotic membranes. These dressings reduce fluid loss, minimize local bacterial growth, and help granulation tissue to form. This ensures that the wound will be in the best possible condition for retaining an autograft.[12]

Research is being conducted to improve wound healing. For example, researchers have found indications that macrophages and blood platelets may be responsible for stimulating collagen synthesis. In addition, transforming growth factor beta, vaccinia growth factor, platelet-derived growth factor, epidermal growth factor, and fibronectin are currently being investigated as factors that might enhance wound healing. In the future, these biologic materials may be applied locally to the wound or incorporated into a synthetic wound dressing material designed specifically for compromised wounds or for wounds with specific liabilities.

REFERENCES

1. Hunt TK et al. Anaerobic metabolism and wound healing: A hypothesis for initiation and cessation of collagen synthesis in wounds. *Am J Surg.* 1978;135:328–332

2. Way LW, ed. *Current Surgical Diagnosis and Treatment*. Los Altos, Cal: Lang Medical Publications; 1985:91, 94–95
3. Altemeier WA et al. *Manual on Control of Infection in Surgical Patients*. Philadelphia: J. B. Lippincott; 1976:124
4. Ehrlich HP, Hunt TK. Effect of cortisone and vitamin A on wound healing. *Ann Surg*. 1968; 167:325
5. Strauss R, Wise L. Operative risks of obesity. *Surg Gynecol Obstet*. 1978;146(2):289
6. Hunt TK. *Fundamentals of Wound Management in Surgery*. South Plainfield, NJ: Chirurgecom; 1976:10, 39.
7. Goodson WH, Hunt TK. Wound healing and the aging. *J Invest Dermatol*. 1979;73:90
8. Greenfield L. *Surgery of the Aged*. Philadelphia: W. B. Saunders; 1975:28–29
9. Campbell EJ, Lefrak SS. How aging affects the structure and function of the respiratory system. *Geriatrics* 1978;33(6):73
10. Eaglstein W et al. Optimal use of an occlusive dressing to enhance healing. *Arch Dermatol*. 1988;124:393–394
11. Wysocki A. Surgical wound healing. *AORN J*. 1989;49(2):511, 514
12. Reckling J. Wound care what's clear what's not. *Nursing 87*. 1987;17(2):34–37

PART FIVE

Postoperative Care
of the Surgical Patient

Chapter 15

Immediate Postoperative Nursing Care

Lillian H. Nicolette

The perioperative nurse functioning in the circulating role accompanies the patient to the postanesthesia care unit (PACU) where he or she will give a report to the postanesthesia care nurse (Fig. 15–1). Information that the perioperative nurse should relay includes the patient's psychological status prior to the induction of anesthesia; type of surgical procedure; location of tubes, drains, catheters, packing, dressings; condition and color of the skin; actual or potential impairment of skin integrity; joint or limb mobility or impairment; primary language (if the patient speaks other than English); respiratory function or dysfunction, including whether the patient has a history of smoking; any special requests the patient may have verbalized preoperatively (i.e., replacement of prosthetic devices, warm blankets, location of family and spouse, wedding rings); and all pertinent intraoperative occurrences and complications.

The anesthesiologist's responsibility includes reporting the type and extent of the surgical procedure, and the anesthetic agents used (type of anesthesia technique—fluid therapy, location of IV/CVP lines, type and amount of solutions infused, including blood); estimated blood loss; level of consciousness; level of comfort; muscular response; and any complications occurring intraoperatively (Table 15–1).

PHYSICAL ENVIRONMENT

Achieving the ideal physical design for a PACU is not always possible. The PACU must be located as close to the surgical suite as possible to allow uninterrupted transfer of patients and direct access to the services of the perioperative nurse, anesthesiologist, and nurse.

The size of the PACU needed in each hospital must be based on the volume of surgery, types of surgical procedures performed, and directly related to the number of operating rooms. The norm is $1\frac{1}{2}$ to 2 recovery areas per operating room.

The area is usually one large room with cubicles; there should be at least 4 feet of maneuvering space on both sides of each bed and a stretcher radius of approximately 38.5 square feet in the open areas.[1] There should be a separate PACU area for isolation patients (i.e., burn patients) or for loud, combative patients. The presence of a large,

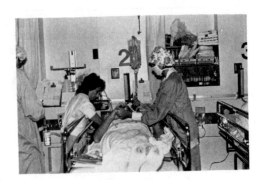

Figure 15-1. The circulating nurse accompanies the patient to the recovery room where a report is given to the recovery room nurse.

TABLE 15-1. STANDARDS OF CARE FOR POST ANESTHESIA CARE UNIT: BASIC ASSESSMENT FACTORS

Physical status and physiological response
- Vital signs
    - Temperature
    - Pulse rate, volume, regularity, and cardiac monitor pattern, if applicable
    - Respiratory rate, depth, symmetry of chest expansion; breath sounds; color of mucous membranes; patency of airway and type of artificial airway; if applicable, mechanical ventilator, oxygen, tidal volume, PEEP, compliance
    - Pressure readings including arterial (direct and indirect), CVP, pulmonary artery
- Level of consciousness
- Pupillary response, if applicable
- Position of individual
- Skin color, temperature, integrity, turgor, presence of rash, abrasions or burns
- Circulation (peripheral pulses) and sensation of extremity(ies); if applicable
- Presence, type and condition of dressing
- Condition of suture line if dressing is absent
- Presence, type of tubes and catheters
- Amount and kind of drainage (quantity and character)
- Muscular response and strength
- Ability to communicate
- Fluid Therapy
    - Amount of output in OR including blood loss
    - Amount of intravenous fluid (IV) including blood in the OR IV and blood infusing
- Laboratory results
- Emotional status and response

Current medical diagnosis, drug allergies, disabilities, impairments, mobility limitations, prosthesis
Operative procedure performed and rationale, length of surgical procedure
Type of anesthesia (general, regional, local)
Anesthetic agents, narcotics, muscle relaxants, antibiotics and drugs used for reversal of muscle relaxants
Complications encountered during surgery and treatment
Previous response to surgery and anesthesia

From Cramer C. ASPAN Newsletter. Summer 1985, with permission.

clean storage area and utility room with a sink adjacent or within the PACU is recommended.

The provision of quality care in the PACU requires strong, knowledgeable leadership and excellent management. Particular attention must be paid to developing the organizational structure of the unit and maintaining the best possible nursing staff.[1]

Postanesthesia nursing is a specialty requiring that the practitioner have an indepth knowledge of the process of anesthesia, anesthesia types, actions, emergency drugs, potential complications, and emergency treatment for complications. The medical director of the PACU is usually an anesthesiologist; however, in some circumstances it may be a surgeon.

In ambulatory surgery centers and some rural health care institutions, the perioperative nurse may serve a dual role, also acting as the postanesthesia nurse. This chapter offers basic information on providing quality care for the surgical patient.

NURSING CARE OF THE PATIENT IN THE POSTANESTHESIA CARE UNIT

Maintenance of Respiratory Function

As soon as the patient arrives in the PACU, he or she is checked for a patent airway and adequate respiratory exchange.

To determine the patient's respiratory exchange, place the hand lightly over the nose and mouth.

The administration of oxygen to the patient in the PACU is an important facet in the emergent phase of anesthesia. Oxygen is given primarily because the patient has a blunt or depressed response to carbon dioxide and low lung volumes.[1]

A patent airway must be maintained throughout the administration of oxygen. The patient should be encouraged to cascade cough and to perform the sustained maximal inspiration (SMI). Oxygen should be administered, according to the patient's needs: if a nasal catheter system is used (6 liters per minute) or a full mask (10 liters per minute). The patient should be observed for the following signs of anoxia:

1. Color of the skin, lips, and nail beds (if pigmentation prevents an accurate evaluation of skin color, inspection of the oral mucosa would be done)
2. Rapid, shallow breathing, rhythm of breathing, respiration with intercostal/diaphragmatic effort
3. Rapid apical and radial pulses
4. Capillary filling of the fingers and toes
5. Restlessness and apprehension

It is important when obtaining a history on the patient to note whether he or she chronically retains carbon dioxide, as in chronic obstructive pulmonary disease. The patient with CO_2 retention who is receiving oxygen should be closely monitored for signs of hyperventilation, confusion, or becoming semicomatose.

If a partial airway obstruction occurs, it may be the result of muscle relaxants, narcotics, mucous accumulation, or the position of the patient on the OR or PACU bed.

When the patient's tongue falls toward the back of the mouth and prevents the free passage of air, the head can be hyperextended and the chin brought forward, or the patient can be positioned laterally on the bed to facilitate appropriate respiration/breathing.

Pulse Oximetry. The use of pulse oximeters has become a standard of practice in the operating room as well as the PACU. Pulse oximetry is widely used, as it shows trends in the patient's oxygenation and helps to detect states of hypoxia more quickly than such subjective signs as skin color, blood color, and respiratory and cardiac rates.[2] In some hospitals, the circulating nurse may be asked to assist the anesthesia personnel in attaching the oximeter probe and monitoring the display readout. In the PACU, the pulse oximeter is another aid to using subjective assessment data when caring for the patient.

If pulse oximetry equipment is used, the PACU nurse must be able to interpret the data from the monitoring equipment. How to deduct PO_2 from the pulse oximeter is important (Fig. 15-2).

The percentage of oxygen saturation is not a measurement of arterial PO_2. There is not a straight correlation between the two figures. When plotted on the oxyhemoglobin dissociation curve, minor changes in O_2 saturation may result in significant changes in PO_2 levels[2] (Fig. 15-3). The nurse must not think that an acceptable PO_2 of 70 mm Hg is reflected by an advanced stage of hypoxia with an oxygen saturation of 70%. The

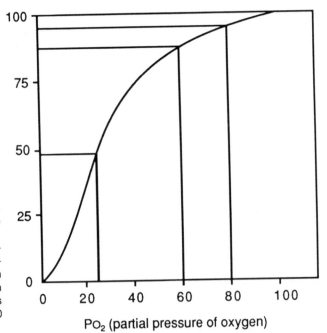

Each molecule of hemoglobin (Hb) is capable of binding 0–4 oxygen molecules. If a Hb molecule is binding 4 O_2 molecules, it is 100% saturated; if it is binding 3 O_2 molecules it is 75% saturated. O_2 saturation in the blood is determined by averaging the O_2 saturation of all the individual Hb molecules. The oximeter measures O_2 saturation.

The partial pressure of oxygen (PO_2) can be derived from the oxygen saturation curve. Choose the oxygen-saturation value from the vertical axis and draw a line across to the curve. Then draw a line down to the horizontal axis to determine the PO_2 value.

Remember that oxygen saturation is not equal to the partial pressure of oxygen. As you can see from the graph, a small drop in oxygen saturation, from 96% to 90%, yields a big drop in the PO_2—from 80 to 60 mm Hg.

Figure 15-2. How to deduce PO_2 from pulse oximetry. (*From Schultheis AH. When and how to extubate in the recovery room. Am J Nurs. August, 1989; 1042, with permission.*)

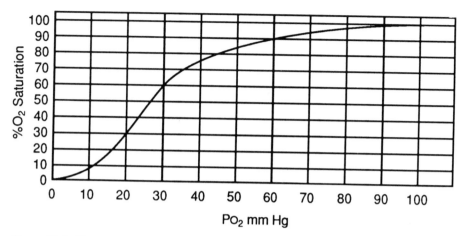

Figure 15–3. The oxyhemoglobin dissociation curve demonstrates that seemingly minor changes in oxygen saturation may result in significant changes in Po₂ levels. (*From Jones M. Pulse oximetry: the numbers behind the numbers. Point of View. 1988; 25 (3):10, with permission.*)

PACU nurse needs to know the specific pulse oximeter measurement and what that measurement means in terms of the patient's status.[2]

Caution must be taken with patients having ventilatory depression, chronic obstructive pulmonary disease, and other pulmonary pathologies, as a decrease in ventilation occurs when the patient is positioned laterally. However, these patients may be turned from side to side for short intervals. If the patient remains supine, the head should always be turned to one side to avoid aspiration of secretions. This procedure should also be done while suctioning a patient. If the air exchange does not improve, the administration of reversal agents for narcotics and muscle relaxants may be indicated. In some patients, the insertion of a nasopharyngeal or oropharyngeal airway may be indicated.

If the patient is responsive, he or she should be encouraged to breathe deeply and cough to promote gas exchange and assist in the elimination of inhalation anesthestic agents.

MAINTENANCE OF ADEQUATE CIRCULATION

The PACU nurse needs to be astute to the signs of patient anxiety, arrythmias, shock, left ventricular failure, pulmonary embolism, and systemic embolism.[1] Vital signs should be checked every 10 to 15 minutes and compared to the preoperative and intraoperative readings. If a large variation exists, the anesthesiologist and surgeon should be notified immediately so that a medical evaluation can be accomplished.

Postoperative patients should be observed for shock. Shock indicates the inability of the circulatory system to meet the oxygen demands of the body. The most common postoperative causes of shock are:

1. Vasomotor collapse caused by deep anesthesia or overdoses of narcotics
2. Hypovolemia caused by excessive loss of blood or plasma
3. Toxemia due to a bacterial infection

The signs and symptoms of shock are restlessness; pallor; rapid, thready pulse; cyanosis of lips and fingernails; low blood pressure; cold, moist skin; rapid, shallow respiration; decreased body temperature; and decreased urinary output.

The treatment of shock is based on the cause. In hypovolemic shock, the treatment is to restore the blood volume by administering whole blood, plasma, or plasma substitutes. Oxygen may be administered to increase the oxygen saturation of the blood and the tissues. When shock is caused by vasoconstricting drugs, phenylephrine hydrochloride (Neo-Synephrine) or levarterenol bitartrate (Levophed) may be administered.

Fluid therapy and urinary output should be monitored closely to prevent fluid overload. A Swan-Ganz catheter or central venous pressure monitor can be used to determine fluid replacement with reduced intravascular volume and hypotension.

MONITORING THE PATIENT'S LEVEL OF CONSCIOUSNESS

The patient's level of consciousness should be assessed and documented every 5 to 10 minutes while the patient is in the PACU. During emergence from general anesthesia, the patient will first react to painful stimuli, such as pinching the earlobe, and to motor or reflex activity if the nurse touches the eyelashes or eyelid. When the patient is semiconscious, he or she may respond to verbal stimuli but drifts off to sleep easily. During this phase, he or she also responds to commands slowly. The conscious patient will be drowsy, but awake and alert, oriented to time, place, and person. The exception is the patient who has had a ketamine anesthetic; such a patient must have *no* nystagmus when released from the PACU.

ASSESSMENT OF DRESSINGS, DRAINS AND CASTING MATERIALS

Postoperative dressings need to be checked every 10 to 15 minutes in the PACU for the type of drainage (if any), the amount, the color, consistency, and the odor. Many surgeons currently use a spray that seals off the surgical site from outer lying materials, (i.e., Nu Skin Spray). PACU documentation of all assessments of dressings should be noted on the PACU record.

All surgical drains, such as hemovacs, sump drains, J-vacs and Pleur-vacs should be connected to the appropriate drainage apparatus and checked for patency every 15 minutes from the immediate postoperative period until discharge from the PACU. Materials excreted into the drainage apparatus should be noted for amount, color, consistency, and any odor. This information needs to be documented on the patient's record.

Casting materials for patients undergoing orthopedic or podiatric procedures should be assessed every 10 to 15 minutes for signs of circulatory impairment. Clinical manifestations of circulatory impairment include swelling and a decreased return of color after pressure has been applied to the exposed distal portion of the extremity. The patient's skin may also "feel cold" and be cyanotic in color. If circulatory impairment is imminent, the surgeon should be notified immediately. If during the physical assessment blood is noted seeping through the cast from the incision, the boundaries need to be identified and the time noted so that excessive bleeding can be readily determined.

PROMOTION AND MAINTENANCE OF PHYSICAL AND EMOTIONAL SAFETY AND COMFORT

Physical and emotional safety are always important aspects of care, specifically when the patient is either semiconscious or in an unconscious state. The nurse's responsibility includes ascertaining that all bed or stretcher rails are in the up position and that the bed or stretcher is in the locked position. It is recommended that an armboard or arm protector be used to ensure that IV lines do not become dislodged, uncapped, and cause injury.

Frequently after anesthesia, patients develop excessive restlessness. The periopera-tive nurse in the PACU needs to do a nursing assessment of underlying or causative factors involving this symptom. As discussed previously, restlessness may be caused by hypoxia, carbon dioxide retention, hemorrhage, discomfort due to a full bladder, or incisional pain. The application of restraints should only be applied to protect the patient from self-injury and only after nursing interventions have been implemented. A thorough nursing assessment and formulation of a nursing diagnosis related to possible injury should be made and documented on the care plan and nursing record.

Providing emotional support is an important aspect of PACU care. A warm, quiet environment should be provided so that the patient can emerge from anesthesia without obtrusive external stimuli. After the patient is fully conscious, he or she may want to discuss the surgical procedure. The nurse should allow the patient to express such feelings and should provide the emotional support necessary.

DOCUMENTATION

The nursing process is the essential key in documenting nursing care. Development of a comprehensive nursing record should be the objective of each PACU. The American Soci-ety of Post-Anesthesia Nurses, Guidelines for Standards of Care in the Post-Anesthesia Care Unit,[3] suggest a formalized system of reporting and recording the care given to each anesthetic patient. The record should include the following[3]:

1. Assessment of the:
   a. Preoperative status including: ECG, vital signs, radiology findings, laboratory values, allergies, disabilities, drug use, physical or mental impairments, mobil-ity limitations, and prostheses (i.e., dentures, hearing aids, contact lenses)
   b. Anesthesia techniques (i.e., general, regional, local) (Table 15-2)
   c. Anesthetic agents

TABLE 15-2. POSTANESTHETIC ASSESSMENT CHECKLIST

Criteria
  Responds appropriately to directions
  Responds verbally and appropriately

  Requires no airway assistance: patent
  Requires chin lift or hyperextension of neck to maintain airway patency
  Requires oral/nasal airway or nasotracheal/endotracheal tube: Dc'd @ (document specific time)
  Respirations deep, rhythmical without effort
  Respirations shallow, rhythmical without effort
  Respirations with intercostal/diaphragmatic effort or:
    Breath sounds clear to auscultation
  Regular apical and radial pulses or:
    Capillary filling of fingers and toes ≤ 3 seconds
    Capillary filling of fingers and toes > 3 seconds
  Palpable/Doppler peripheral pulses:
    Absence of edema or hematoma of surgical site
    Dressing dry without evidence of drainage
    Surgical drains patent without excessive drainage
  Absence of nausea or emesis
  Absence of pain or discomfort
  Absence of palpable bladder distention
  Epidural or spinal sensory level

From Cramer, C. ASPAN Newsletter. Summer 1985, with permission.

    d. Length of anesthesia time
    e. Type of surgical procedure
    f. Estimated fluid/blood loss and replacement therapy
    g. Complications occurring during anesthesia course of care
  2. Documentation should include:
    a. Vital signs
      1) Respiratory rate: patency and types of artificial airways, mechanical ventilators
      2) Blood pressure: cuff and/or arterial line
      3) Pulse: apical–peripheral and cardiac monitor patterns
      4) Temperature: oral/rectal/axillary (whichever is appropriate)
    b. Pressure readings (CVP; arterial lines; pulmonary wedge)
    c. Position of the patient
    d. Condition and the color of skin
    e. Circulation—peripheral pulses and sensation of extremities as applicable
    f. Condition of dressing
    g. Condition of suture line
    h. Type and patency of drainage tubes and catheters
    i. Amount and type of drainage
    j. Muscular strength
    k. Fluid therapy, location of lines, type and amount of solutions including blood

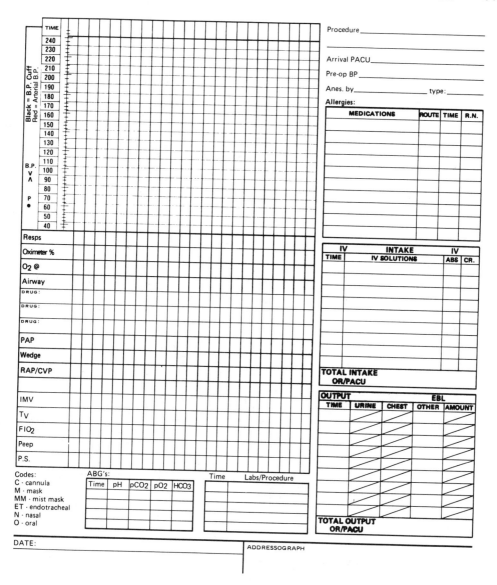

Figure 15-4. Post-anesthesia nursing notes. (*Courtesy, Saddleback Memorial Hospital and Health Center, Laguna Hills, California.*)

MEDICAL HISTORY
Cardiac:
Respiratory:
Neurologic:
Endocrine:

● ● ● ● ● ● · · ·
9mm 8mm 7mm 6mm 5mm 4mm 3mm 2mm 1mm

Professional Assessment √ Assessed &/or Completed ∗ Assessed — Narrative	Time											Nursing Diagnoses upon Discharge
COGNITIVE PERCEPTUAL Neurological Assessment												☐ Thought processes, alterations in
Alert/Oriented												☐ Communication, impaired verbal
Speech clear & appropriate												☐ Sensory-perceptual alterations
PERL R: L:												☐ Alteration in comfort pain
Follows commands												☐ Alteration in level of consciousness
Comfort level												☐ Potential for physical injury
ACTIVITY/EXERCISE Cardiovascular assessment												
Heart sounds assessed												
Extremities warm & pink												☐ Airway clearance, ineffective
Peripheral pulses present & strong bilat.												☐ Breathing patterns ineffective
IV site checked ☐site:_____size:												☐ Cardiac output-decreased (CP)
S.G. bal/cal ☐site:_____checked☐												☐ Gas exchange, impaired (CP)
Artline bal/cal ☐site:_____checked☐												☐ Tissue perfusion, alterations in (CP)
												☐ Mobility impaired, physical
Respiratory assessment												
Respirations regular, symmetrical												
Breath sounds equal & clear all lobes												
Neuromuscular assessment												
Able to raise head												
Move all extremities equally												
Spinal level assessed												
Position												
NUTRITIONAL/ METABOLIC Nutritional/Metabolic assessment												☐ Alterations in body temp
Skin warm and dry												☐ Skin integrity, impairment of
Dressing dry & intact site:												☐ Infection, potential for
Surgical drains patent												☐ Fluid volume, deficit☐ or excess☐(CP)
Type drain: drainage:												
ELIMINATION GI assessment												☐ Bowel elimination, alterations in
Abdomen soft, non distended												
NG tube patent to low cont. suction												
Type of drainage												☐ Urinary elimination, alteration in pattern of
GU assessment												
Foley catheter present and patent												
MISC. Elastic/sequential Ted hose on												
Side rails up at all times												
Warm blankets applied												∗CP Collaborative Problem

Figure 15-4. Continued.

Admission Rhythym Strip Interpretation: _____ PR. _____ QRS. _____ Q.T. _____

Date	Time	Post Anesthesia Narrative Nursing Notes

PT. TRANSPORTED:
  Via Guerney ☐
  Via Floor Bed ☐
  Other_____ ☐

PT. TRANSPORTED:
  Oxygen/Mode_____
  Cardiac Monitor ☐
  Time_____ Room_____

DOCTORS ORDERS:
Patient may be transferred from PACU when discharge criteria are met, and/or upon order of anesthesiologist/surgeon.

_____ M.D.

TIME	PACU NURSE SIGNATURE	INITIAL

FLOOR NURSE
RECEIVING REPORT: _____

FLOOR ADMISSION VITAL SIGNS: BP_____ HR_____ R_____

ADDRESSOGRAPH

Figure 15-4. Continued.

    l. Level of consciousness
    m. Level of comfort

See Figure 15–4 for an example of a PACU record.

    When the patient is conscious and ready for discharge to the nursing unit, he or she should be accompanied to the unit by the PACU nurse and a hospital assistant. A full report on the patient's perioperative course of care is given to the unit nurse, including: the surgical procedure performed, the type of anesthesia, vital signs, the surgical dressings and exudate (if present), drains and tubes, urinary output, fluid therapy, results of laboratory values, radiology reports, ECG interpretations, levels of consciousness, any medications administered in the PACU and any emotional responses the patient may be experiencing.

REFERENCES

1. Drain CB, Christoph SS. The Recovery Room—A Critical Approach to Post-Anesthesia in Nursing, 2nd ed. Philadelphia: W.B. Saunders; 1987:4, 9, 72
2. Jones M. Pulse oximetry: The numbers behind the numbers. *Point of View.* 1988;25(3):10, 11
3. ASPAN. Guidelines for standards of care. In: The Recovery Room—A Critical Approach to Post-Anesthesia Nursing, 2nd ed. Philadelphia: W. B. Saunders; 1987:18, 19

PART SIX

Other Professional Concerns

Chapter 16

Assuring Quality of Care

One of the first individuals to express concern regarding the adequacy of medical and nursing care was Florence Nightingale. She compared the mortality experience in the British Armed Forces during the Crimean War with mortality experience in the civilian population. In her *Notes on Matters Affecting the Health, Efficiency and Hospital Administration of the British Army,* published in 1858, Nightingale brought to the attention of the government and the public the atrocious standards of care for military personnel. Although by today's standards the data were crude, the report was instrumental in bringing about basic reforms in the living standards and the health services for the armed forces.

Again, in 1863, Nightingale proposed keeping a log of circumstances surrounding surgical procedures for the purpose of improving the morbidity and mortality of surgery.[1]

Despite these efforts, little emphasis was given to assessing quality in health care until the early 1970s. Since that time, the concept of assuring quality has gained momentum from governmental agencies, accrediting bodies, and consumers. Through the news media, consumers have become more knowledgeable about health care and the increasing cost of that care. As a result, consumers are demanding that the health care profession be more accountable for the quality and the quantity of the services delivered.

One method of increasing accountability by the health care profession to the consumer is through the development of quality assurance programs. A quality assurance program is a system organized to assess the quality of care as compared to standards and to verify that all variations are reviewed and all deficiencies are corrected and reassessed.

BACKGROUND OF QUALITY ASSURANCE PROGRAMS

One of the first proponents of the concept of quality assurance in health care was the federal government, which required, as part of the 1972 amendments to the Social Security Act, that a Professional Standard Review Organization (PSRO) be created. The PSRO was designed to involve practicing physicians in the ongoing review of the quality and the cost of care received by clients of Medicare, Medicaid, and maternal and child health programs. All facilities receiving these funds were to have state and local PSROs developed by July 1, 1978.

The legislation was based on two concepts:

1. Health professionals are the most appropriate people to evaluate the quality of health care services.
2. An effective peer review at the local level is the soundest method for assuring appropriate use of health care resources and facilities.

In 1973, the Joint Commission on Accreditation of Healthcare Organizations (JCAHO) included medical and nursing audits as a requirement for accreditation. The standard directed the professions to formulate criteria and to implement a systematic evaluation system to assure that optimal quality care was delivered.

CURRENT REGULATIONS

During the past 8 years, the focus of JCAHO has evolved from requiring a specific number of audits that focused on retrospective chart reviews to the current standard that promotes the monitoring and evaluation of the quality and appropriateness of care.

The 1989 JCAHO standard states that:

> There is an ongoing quality assurance program designed to objectively and systematically monitor and evaluate the quality and appropriateness of patient care, pursue opportunities to improve patient care, and resolve identified problems.[2]

Each institution must establish, maintain, and support an ongoing quality assurance program that includes an effective mechanism for reviewing and evaluating patient care as well as an appropriate response to the findings. The plan must be defined in writing and include a mechanism for assuring the accountability of the medical and other professional staffs for the care they provide.

The responsibility of administering or coordinating the institution's quality assurance program is through an individual. However, each clinical discipline is responsible for developing a quality assurance program and for reporting the findings through the designated mechanism. To the extent that integration is possible, multidisciplinary audits are encouraged. This should minimize duplication and enhance communication and has the potential for cost savings to the institution.

In 1986, the JCAHO introduced the "Agenda For Change" that identified the ten-step process by which monitoring and evaluation was to occur in health care institutions. It included the following steps:

1. *Assign Responsibility.* The manager of the department is ultimately responsible for the quality assurance program. However, the responsibility can be delegated to a member of the department. A written departmental plan is not required but it will assist in planning the activities.

2. *Delineate the Scope of Care.* Identify the service provided in the department, the types of patients cared for, the times that services are available, and the types of health-care professionals providing the services. The monitoring and evaluation activities must encompass the major services provided by the department.

3. *Identify Important Aspects of Care.* After the scope of patient care is defined, the next task is to identify the activities that are considered most important to the quality and appropriateness of the service. These should include the following situations:

- Aspects of care that occur frequently and affect large numbers of patients
- Aspects of care that would result in serious consequences or when the patient would be deprived of substantial benefit if the care was not provided correctly, in a timely fashion, or on proper indication
- Aspects of care that have tended to produce problems for the staff or patients

This means that high volume, high risk, or problem-prone aspects of care should be the highest priority for monitoring and evaluation, for example, monitoring local patients, skin integrity, and patient positioning.

4. Identify Indicators. An indicator is a well-defined, objective variable used to monitor the quality and appropriateness of an important aspect of patient care. The indicator can be a resource, process, clinical event, complication, or the outcome of care. The indicators should be based on the department's standards of care as determined in policies, procedures, and models of care. The indicators may relate to the structure, process, or outcome of care (Table 16–1).

5. Establish Thresholds for Evaluation. A threshold is a predetermined level of compliance to a specific indicator. This should be stated as a percent and can be stated either positively or negatively. For example, the threshold for needle counts could be identified as:

- Needle counts will be accurate 95% of the time.

  or
- Needle counts will not be accurate 5% of the time.

The thresholds should never be lower than 90%; however, some activities are so important that nothing less than 100% is acceptable. These activities or outcomes are referred to as "sentinal events."

Both indicators and thresholds for evaluation pertain directly to patient care and are derived from reviewing the available clinical and quality assurance literature, discussions with the staff, reviewing the community norm, and examining past experience (see Table 16–1).

It is important that the staff agree with both the indicators and the thresholds for evaluation. Involving the staff adds to the credibility of the review and contributes significantly to their commitment to improve the quality of care.

6. Collect and Organize Data. The quality assurance committee should determine the following for each indicator:

- The data sources
- The data collection method (concurrent or retrospective)
- The appropriateness of sample size
- The time frame for data collection
- The process for comparing level of performance with the thresholds for evaluation

TABLE 16-1. OPERATING ROOM DEPARTMENTAL QUALITY INDICATORS

Quality Indicators	Thresholds (time, % or $)	Method of Collecting Data
Transportation delays	No more than 1% of total monthly delays in surgery are attributed to transportation delays	Data collected by preop and reported quarterly to Quality Assurance Chairman
Preop lab work	100% compliance before anesthesia induction	Collected by circulating nurse and given to QA chairperson every 2 weeks
Case delay (turnaround time)	No more than 15 min. between one patient leaving and next entering OR suite. First patient of the day on table at start time	Data sheet completed by circ. nurse giving reason for delay, amount of delay. Monitored every 3 months by QA committee
Surgery consents	Complete 100% with procedure, patient name, date, time, signature (proper) and a witness, and explanation for other signature	Data sheet by circulator to QA every 2 weeks
History and physical	100% on chart prior to induction or progress note if dictated with all parameters covered, none older than 72 hr	Data sheet by circulator to QA
Intraop		
Completed blood transfusion record	98% Completed	Data collected by OR personnel for period of 1 month. Results reported to QA committee

Properly assembled equipment	95% Assembled	Data collected by verbal and written complaint.
Completion (documentation) of OR records	95% Completed	Data collected by OR personnel and reported to QA committee.
Disposition of specimens and cultures	98% Documented	Data completed by OR staff, pathology, lab personnel.
Intraoperative x-ray technician delay	Negotiate with x-ray 10 min. to OR	Data collected by OR staff and reported to QA committee.
Postop		
Documentation of wound classification	96% Documented	Retrospective chart review by QA department
Documentation of postop complications	98% Documented	Retrospective chart review by QA department
Clean wound infections	Less than 4% of cases are infected	Review of chart by QA department
Number of admissions of outpatients	Less than 1%	Recovery room admission log information
Come and go patients discharged according to procedure	95%	Ambulatory nurses notes
Timely recovery room discharge	95%	Recovery room log
Postop calls are completed	100% placed; 50% contacted	Recovery room log

Current sources of data include:

- Staff concerns
- Patient records
- Log books
- Incident reports
- Committee reports/meetings
- Patient satisfaction questionnaires
- Infection control reports
- Direct observation of staff and patients

In addition, specially designed tools can assist with a specific monitor. These tools should be designed to make it easy to collect data by using a checklist or a yes/no response (Table 16–2).

For each indicator, the committee determines what the appropriate sample size should be to provide a representative sample. Adequate sample size is important in making inferences in regard to the quality of care delivered. Reasonably homogeneous patient populations require a small sample size to be representative of the population.

One of the best methods of sampling techniques is random sampling. This ensures that all patients in the population have an equal chance to be included in the sample size. Random sampling can be conducted by drawing patients' numbers or names out of a large container until a predetermined sample size is chosen. A table of random numbers available in any statistic book may also be used to assist in random sampling.

Systematic sampling consists of selecting every Nth patient. For example, if the goal is to audit 10% of the population, every tenth patient would be audited.

To adequately evaluate patients from all surgical specialties, stratified sampling

TABLE 16–2. BLADDER CATHETERIZATION MONITOR

Patient Register Number   Sex/Age
OR Bldg and Room
Operation   Auditor
Date/Time

	YES	NO	N/A
1. Supplies available and ready for immediate use	( )	( )	( )
2. Permission obtained from anesthesia to catheterize the patient (if patient under anesthesia)	( )	( )	( )
Procedure explained to patient, if local anesthesia is used	( )	( )	( )
3. If patient is female, legs are placed in the frogleg position	( )	( )	( )
4. Appropriate light is available to facilitate accurate placement of the catheter	( )	( )	( )
5. The catheter tray and table are prepared and maintained sterile using aseptic technique	( )	( )	( )
6. The catheter balloon has been tested (via inflation using sterile solution) prior to insertion	( )	( )	( )

7. The urethra and labial folds on the female patient are cleansed according to OR policy
   a. Labia spread apart correctly ( ) ( ) ( )
   b. Area cleansed using antiseptic-soaked cotton balls in a forceps, employing a downward-motion stroke ( ) ( ) ( )
   c. Cotton balls are discarded after each use; new cotton ball obtained ( ) ( ) ( )
8. The external urethra meatus on the male patient is cleansed accordingly:
   a. If the patient is not circumcised, the foreskin is retracted and the meatus is cleansed, using antiseptic-soaked cotton balls, each discarded after use ( ) ( ) ( )
   b. If the patient is circumcised, the meatus is cleansed using antiseptic-soaked cotton balls, each discarded after use ( ) ( ) ( )
9. The catheter is gently placed in the meatus, inserted until urine begins to flow
   a. About 3 inches for female ( ) ( ) ( )
   b. Full length for male ( ) ( ) ( )
10. If catheter is placed in incorrect orifice
   a. The misplaced catheter is left in place—not reinserted ( ) ( ) ( )
   b. New catheter inserted ( ) ( ) ( )
11. a. The catheter balloon is inflated according to manufacturer's guidelines ( ) ( ) ( )
   b. Catheter is drawn back to the base of the bladder ( ) ( ) ( )
   c. The catheter is connected to straight drainage (tubing with bag), if indicated ( ) ( ) ( )
   d. For occlusion of tubing, catheter plug is used ( ) ( ) ( )
   e. While connecting the catheter to the bag, careful attention is given to preserving sterility ( ) ( ) ( )
12. On male patients, if applicable, the foreskin is returned to original position ( ) ( ) ( )
13. a. The patient is dried ( ) ( ) ( )
   b. Wet material is discarded ( ) ( ) ( )
   c. Legs repositioned ( ) ( ) ( )
   d. Safety strap is reapplied ( ) ( ) ( )
14. a. The catheter is taped and/or secured in place ( ) ( ) ( )
   b. The tubing is placed under the knee ( ) ( ) ( )
15. Procedure recorded in the nursing notes to include:
   a. Catheter type ( ) ( ) ( )
   b. Urine return, color, and amount ( ) ( ) ( )
   c. Name of person who inserted the catheter ( ) ( ) ( )
16. Drainage bag is kept below the level of the bladder
   a. While in the room ( ) ( ) ( )
   b. During transportation ( ) ( ) ( )

TOTAL:

Comments: Document the reason for all "no" responses and include staff comments when applicable.

1. Criteria number _____   Indication letter _____
   Reason:
2. Criteria number _____   Indication letter _____
   Reason:
3. Criteria number _____   Indication letter _____
   Reason:

may be required. After establishing the percentage of total cases to be monitored, the number of cases to be assessed in each surgical specialty is identified and the cases are numbered and then randomly selected from the random sampling distribution chart (see Tables 16–3 and 16–4). This identifies the day of the week each audit is to be performed. The committee should also discuss the relevance of auditing procedures on the evening and the night shifts so that a representative sample is obtained.

7. Evaluate Care. Once the monitor is complete, the committee must analyze the degree of variation between the established threshold and the current level of nursing practice. The strengths as well as the deficiencies of the monitor should be discussed with the nursing staff. Discussion of the strengths will increase staff morale, provide greater job satisfaction, and induce the staff to continue to strive for a high quality of care.

If the threshold was not achieved, the committee should analyze patterns or trends of care. Patterns or trends could be related to specific shifts, units, personnel, and skills, or segments of the patient population. If it appears that a single practitioner is of concern, the issue should be referred to a supervisor or the peer review committee.

The Joint Commission indicates that a "problem" is present when a deficiency in care is serious, repeated, or widespread. An "opportunity for improvement" is present when a level of quality is acceptable but, given the resources available, could be improved. It is expected that there will be some areas for improvement identified in all departments.

8. Take Actions To Solve Identified Problems. If the data collection indicates that the threshold was reached, the monitor should be evaluated as to whether it should be continued.

When the evaluation identifies a deficiency, the reason for the deficiency must be determined, possible courses of action explored and, finally, a recommendation for cor-

TABLE 16-3. STRATIFIED SAMPLING TABLE

Service	6% Per Year	Monitors Per Month	Case Numbers
Cardiothoracic	30	3	1–3
Cystoscopy	78	7	4–10
General	124	10	11–20
Gynecology	48	4	21–24
Neurosurgery	50	4	25–28
Orthopedics	62	5	29–33
Kidney transplant	14	1	34
Urology	13	1	35
Vascular	41	3	36–38
Ophthalmology	33	3	39–41
Ear, nose, throat	55	5	42–46
Oral surgery	26	2	47–48
Plastic	26	2	49–50
Total	574	50	

TABLE 16–4. SAMPLE MONITOR SCHEDULE

	Oral	Oral	Gyn	Ent	Eye	Gen	Gyn	Gen	Cysto	Gyn
Monday	48	47	23	44	39	14	21	17	6	22
	Cysto	Ct	Cysto	Kid	Cysto	Ent	Cysto	Ent	Gen	Plastic
Tuesday	10	1	4	34	7	45	5	43	16	49
	Eye	Ct	Gen	Neuro	Gyn	Ortho	Eye	Ortho	Neuro	Ent
Wednesday	41	2	12	25	24	31	40	30	28	46
	Gen	Gu	Vas	Vas	Gen	Gen	Ortho	Cysto	Vas	Plastic
Thursday	13	35	36	37	19	20	29	8	38	50
	Cysto	Gen	Ct	Neuro	Ortho	Ent	Gen	Ortho	Gen	Neuro
Friday	9	18	3	27	32	42	13	33	11	26

rective action be made. If a cause cannot be located through analysis, the solution should be sought through research.

The plan of action should be developed and should indicate what is expected to change, how the change will occur (what method will be used), who is responsible for implementing the action plan, and when the change will be achieved.

Reasons for not meeting the threshold can usually be related to one of three factors:

1. Insufficient knowledge
2. Defect in the system
3. Deficient behavior or performance

Insufficient knowledge can be addressed through educational/training programs and additional reference material.

Defects in the system can be changed by reviewing departmental policies and procedures, redistributing staff, supplies, and equipment, and correcting communication problems. Behavior or performance deficiencies may be corrected through coaching and counseling.

9. Assess the Actions and Document Improvement. To assess whether the corrective action was implemented successfully and nursing care improved, another monitor utilizing the same monitoring evaluation methods employed originally should be conducted within 3 to 4 months. Those changes that do occur should be documented and reported back to the nursing staff, as this will assist in developing credibility for the audit process. If this assessment indicates that there is improvement, no further action is required. The monitor should be slated for reassessment at some point in the future to ensure that the problem does not recur and that improvement is sustained. If the monitor does not show improvement, the problem, its cause, and the action taken to solve it should be reassessed. A new action plan should be developed and, once again, the problem monitored and evaluated.

10. Communicate Relevant Information to the Organization Quality Assurance Program. The departmental chairperson is responsible for reporting the QA committees findings and activities to the institutional committee at specified times. The committee also has a responsibility to communicate the findings to the staff via inservice sessions, departmental newsletters, and communication book.

DEVELOPING A QUALITY ASSURANCE PROGRAM

As stated in the JCAHO standards, each clinical department is responsible for developing a quality assurance program. Due to the complex nature of perioperative nursing, it is imperative that this department develop a quality assurance program that assesses the level of care delivered to the surgical patient. Results of the quality assurance program in the operating room should be shared with other departments by representation on the institutional committee.

To assist in developing a quality assurance program, a departmental committee should be formed to establish the criteria and to determine the process to be used in conducting the program. Ideally, the committee should consist of five to seven members and have the representation of staff nurses, head nurses, the clinical specialist, and the staff development instructor. The chairperson should be committed to the concept of quality assurance and to facilitating progress toward developing the program.

The committee should review the institutional plan for quality assurance and then develop a departmental program consistent with that plan. The departmental program should include a statement regarding the purpose of the committee, composition of the committee, tenure of committee members, frequency of meetings, and confidentiality of committee findings.

Specific objectives of the committee will include:

1. To review current standards of nursing practice
2. To identify actual or potential patient problems
3. To collect and assess data regarding the quality of care delivered
4. To report findings to appropriate individuals (i.e., director of department, supervisor)
5. To make recommendations to eliminate identified problems and to improve the quality of care
6. To reevaluate the identified problems and assess the effectiveness of the interventions
7. To maintain documentation regarding quality assurance activities
8. To annually assess the effectiveness of the quality assurance committee

Committee members should review the literature to assess "the state of the art" and to develop an understanding of quality assurance and nursing audits.

This review will assist the committee in identifying the standards and criteria that have been developed by other institutions and national associations. Since the development of standards is a costly process, the committee can use these standards as guidelines to develop specific criteria that are applicable to the individual institution. Using established standards encourages identification with national standards of practice and thereby with nursing as a profession.

During this process, the nursing staff should be kept informed about the committee's progress. The rationale for the program, as well as the advantages and disadvantages, should be openly discussed to assist the staff in reducing any anxiety they may be experiencing. The focus of these discussions should stress that the desired outcome of the monitoring process is the improvement of the quality of nursing care through the resolution of actual or potential problems.

To assist in understanding the essential components of a quality assurance program, Norma Lang developed a model for quality assurance in nursing. Figure 16–1 includes the following components of a quality assurance program:

1. Identify values.
2. Identify structure, process, and outcome standards and criteria.
3. Measure current level of nursing practice and compare to the established standards and criteria (this process is referred to as auditing).

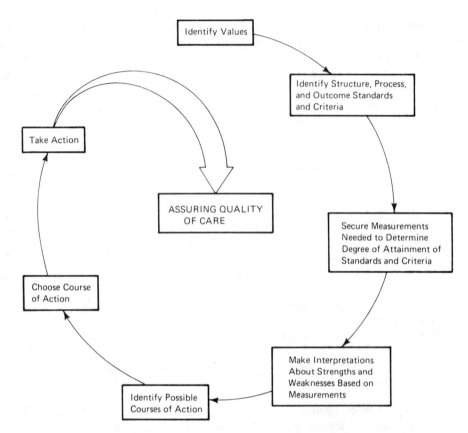

Figure 16-1. ANA model for quality assurance. *(Adapted from N. Lang, "A Model for Quality Assurance in Nursing," in American Nurses Association:* A Plan for Implementation of the Standards of Nursing Practice. *Kansas City, MO: American Nurses Association, 1975, with permission.*

4. Make interpretations about strengths and weaknesses based on measurements.
5. Identify possible courses of action.
6. Choose course of action.
7. Take action.

The circular model indicates that measuring quality is a continuous, dynamic process.

The reaudit will determine if the appropriate action was taken and if the level of care measures up to or exceeds the identified standard.

Identifying Values. To clarify values, the committee will review professional and societal values in relation to the delivery of health care. Professionally, the review will appropriately begin with the departmental philosophy of nursing care. Does it include independent nursing judgments and promote collegial relationships with physicians?

Will the quality of nursing care delivered meet minimal or optimal standards? How do the institutional and departmental philosophies relate to the individual nurse's philosophy of his or her role in the health care profession?

Societal values have an impact on the delivery of health care. What expectations do the patient, the family, and significant others have of the nurse and of their right to participate in decisions regarding health care? What level of health care is society willing to pay for?

These values and beliefs will be incorporated into the standards and the criteria for nursing care.

Developing Standards and Criteria. Standards are established by authority, general consensus, or theory, and establish a level of performance that is acceptable. Standards are either voluntary or mandatory. Voluntary standards serve as guidelines for the profession in establishing policies and procedures. These standards represent the ideal to strive for. Regulatory or mandatory standards such as those developed by accrediting and licensing bodies establish minimum expectations and must have 100% compliance.

A standard, as identified by ANA,[3]

1. Is based on principle
2. Is a statement of a positive objective
3. Gives direction toward achieving the objective
4. Is specific, reasonable, attainable, measurable, time limited, predetermined, and acceptable to those for whom it is formulated
5. Is flexible to permit creativity without the sacrifice of an ideal
6. Is based on current theory and practice but should describe a state of improvement
7. Includes assessment factors by which it can be measured
8. Is subject to continued evaluation and revision

Criteria are specific statements that can be used to assess the extent to which the standard is met. They must identify one behavior and be realistic, understandable, measurable, and achievable, as for example:

1. Standard—Sharps should be counted on all procedures[4]
2. Criteria—Sharps are counted in the operating room by the scrub person and the circulating nurse
   a. Prior to the beginning of the operating
   b. When closure is started
   c. When skin closure is started

Donabedian[5] and Bloch[6,7] have outlined and defined three major criteria for assessing the quality of care—structure, process, and outcome. Each of these measures a different aspect of patient care.

Structure standards and criteria are concerned with the physical facilities; the equipment; the philosophy and objectives; the organizational characteristics; the management of human, material, and fiscal resources; and the status of the department in regard to certification, accreditation, and licensure as for example:

- All local cases will have two circulating nurses.
- Electrical safety is monitored by the biomedical technician and is consistent with the institutional and national standards.

The structure of the hospital or department may meet the designated standards, but the quality of the care delivered may be suboptimal.

Process standards and criteria are concerned with all the activities performed by the nurse in the delivery of nursing care. Of critical importance is how the activities are performed and in what sequence. Evaluation of the structure and process audits may lead to the prediction of quality but not to its assurance.[1] Evaluation of outcome is the most reliable means of auditing patient care.

Outcome standards and criteria focus on what happens to the patient as a result of nursing intervention. In identifying patient outcomes, the nurse must predict before delivering care what the desired outcome is and then measure results against that criteria. Failure to meet the desired outcome results in examining the process and structure standards to identify areas of deficiency. This method of assessing the quality of care provides for input from the patient and the family and therefore has the most relevance in measuring the quality of care delivered. The following are examples of outcome criteria:

- Integrity of skin is maintained
    - No burns
    - No blisters
    - No redness
- No musculoskeletal discomfort postoperatively
- Fluid and electrolyte balance maintained

APPROACHES TO AUDITING PATIENT CARE

Concurrent evaluations are accomplished during the patient's hospitalization and may result in improved outcomes. This method of monitoring care includes mechanisms other than the patient's record such as input from the patient, the family members, and other members of the health care team. Data obtained from the patient or the patient's environment provide for greater reliability in assessing the quality of care than does the health record, a secondary source.[8]

Sources of information for concurrent evaluations are observations of the staff while performing patient care activities (process audit), physical assessment of the patient, open-chart audits, staff interviews, patient interviews, or surveys and group conferences that include patient, family, and staff.

The retrospective monitors are designed to measure the quality of nursing care received by a patient after the care has been completed and the patient is discharged.

This method uses closed-chart reviews, patient care plans, postcare interviews, or questionnaires. One of the disadvantages of the retrospective chart review is that the quality of the record may be assessed rather than the care that was actually delivered.

Skillful recording may give a false impression of quality. When omissions from the record occur, it is assumed that the care was not delivered and therefore may also result in a false assessment of the quality of care.

Since the principle of quality assurance is to deliver optimum patient care, a combination of concurrent and retrospective audits is appropriate to be included in the committee's repertoire of audit skills.

Selecting an Audit Topic

Several instruments have been developed and can be used as guidelines in developing a measurement tool. Maria Phaneuf designed a tool to be used in retrospective chart reviews. The focus of this tool is on the outcome of nursing interventions. The tool consists of 50 items divided into the seven legal dependent and independent nursing functions. These functions are

1. Application and execution of the doctor's orders
2. Observation of symptoms and reactions
3. Supervision of the patient
4. Supervision of care givers
5. Reporting and recording
6. Execution of nursing procedures and techniques
7. Promotion of health by direction and teaching

The focus of Phaneuf's tool is on the patient and the care he or she received. The care is rated as excellent, good, incomplete, poor, or unsafe.[9]

The process audit requires the presence of an observer. This may influence the behavior of the nurse, resulting in delivery of a higher level of care and in the distortion of the data. Some observations can be difficult to record; therefore, the tool used in process audits must be specific and provide an option for additional comments. These audits are subject to the biases of the observer, and the results may vary between observers. Consequently, the selection and the training of observers are of prime importance in producing valid process monitoring.

Developing models of patient care (standard care plans) can assist in monitoring outcomes of patient care (see Chapter 5). Models of patient care are developed for specific patient populations that can be expected to have the usual predictable problems as a result of existing similar conditions. Model care plans can be developed by surgical procedure, medical diagnosis, age of patient, nursing diagnosis, and position of the patient.

Analysis of incident reports related to both individual safety and clinical care, as well as findings of committees, may serve as important data in identifying problems and thus serve as topics requiring quality assessment activities. For example, if the infection control committee notes an increased incidence in urinary tract infections, an audit of bladder catheterization would be appropriate (see Table 16–2).

Subjects for structure audits may include the turnover time between surgical procedures and a random sampling of patient charges to determine the appropriateness of those charges.

Interviews and Questionnaires

Interviews with the patient and his or her family offer an excellent way to obtain information regarding their perception of the care delivered. The interview can be used on a wide variety of patients, and the interviewer can minimize misunderstandings by probing or clarifying a topic in detail. The interview may be structured—the interviewer asks routine questions of all patients, or unstructured—the interviewer asks random questions and the interview is directed by the patient's responses. The interview method is expensive and may elicit answers from the patient that he or she thinks the interviewer wants to hear. To minimize subjectivity, the nurse who conducts the interview should not be the one who delivered care to the patient.

Questionnaires are less time-consuming and offer anonymity to the patient; consequently, there is less pressure on the patient and his or her responses. The use of questionnaires requires that the patient be literate and that the language of the questionnaire be geared to the various socioeconomic and ethnic groups that the institution serves. The questions should be short and contain only a single idea. The questionnaire should be field tested with an appropriate sample size prior to being implemented. Routinely, only a small percentage of questionnaires are returned; however, the use of a personalized covering letter explaining the project and a self-addressed return envelope or postcard are excellent inducements that frequently result in an increased rate of return.

Interviews and questionnaires cannot measure quality, but they can assist the nursing staff to improve care and interactionary skills.[10]

Selection and Training of Auditors

The selection and the training of observers are of prime importance to the success of the audit program. It is essential that the auditors be competent practitioners and that the number of auditors be realistic in relation to the identified sample size. Specific criteria for selecting auditors are

- Sound base of knowledge regarding perioperative nursing
- Consistency in performance and application of accepted standards of practice
- Flexible and adaptable in applying the standards of practice
- Observant and perceptive
- Tactful, diplomatic, and objective
- Assertive and willing to indicate findings

The use of 16 mm slides depicting the institutional standards or action shots of nurses delivering care can be useful tools in training monitors for process audits. It is important to give detailed instructions so all monitors have the same understanding of the process, the terminology, and the audit tool. This will assist in overcoming biases and in achieving greater consistency between auditors.

Once the initial group of monitors is trained, a buddy system to train additional monitors is helpful. This method provides the opportunity for comparison and immediate feedback.

One of the greatest problems in quality monitoring is that of observer reliability. Periodically, two observers should be assigned to the same audit to test for interobserver reliability. Results of this monitor should then be used for discussion with the monitors and to assess the reliability of the criteria statements.

If a cause cannot be located through analysis, the solution should be sought through research.

NURSING MANAGEMENT AND ASSURANCE OF QUALITY CARE

Inherent in the nurse manager's responsibilities is the establishment of a viable quality assurance program. By allocating the necessary human and fiscal resources, the nurse manager will demonstrate a commitment to quality assurance and will establish an environment conducive to such a program.

After determining the kind of monitors to be conducted on a yearly basis, the following formula* can be utilized to determine the number of full-time equivalents required for quality assurance activities:

$$\frac{a}{b} \times \frac{c}{d} = z$$

$$\frac{z}{e} = v$$

$$v \times f = w$$

The formula requires the following information:

a = Number of monitors to be conducted in 1 year
b = Number of days monitors are to be conducted during the year
c = Time required to perform monitors
d = 60 minutes (equivalent to 1 hour)
z = Employee hours of effort required to conduct monitors
e = 8 hours per working time period
v = Number of monitors required on a daily basis
f = 1.6 (relief factor suggested by the JCAHO)
w = Total staffing requirements

An example of the formula is as follows:

$$\frac{1000 \text{ monitors per year}}{240 \text{ days per year}} \times \frac{60 \text{ minutes to perform}}{60 \text{ minutes}} = \frac{60,000}{14,400} = 4.17 \text{ hours per day}$$

$$\frac{4.17}{8} = 0.5$$

$0.5 \times 1.6 = 0.8$ full-time equivalents to conduct monitor

---

*Formula adapted from Sharon Van Sell Davidson, Editor, "Staffing Requirements for Concurrent Review Activities," in *PSRO Utilization and Audit in Patient Care* (St. Louis: C. V. Mosby Co., 1976), 193.

The nurse manager should guide the committee in developing protocols and assist in developing the standards and the criteria. The approach to the program should be realistic and the usefulness of the program not oversold as the credibility of the program is at stake.

Results of the findings and the recommendations should be discussed with the committee chairperson. Following any necessary negotiations, the recommendations should receive the full support of the nurse manager. If the corrective action requires administrative action (i.e., policy changes, budget implications), the manager should prepare a realistic schedule for completion and report to the committee at intervals regarding the status of those changes.

Quality assurance programs can be synonymous with cost containment. It is the responsibility of the nurse manager to evaluate the program and to conduct a cost-benefit analysis. Results of such an analysis may reveal that the value to the patient and to the department exceeds the value of the resources allocated to conducting the program.

CREDENTIALING AND ASSURANCE OF QUALITY

As a profession matures, it recognizes the need to be accountable and to ensure the competence of the practitioners. Credentialing and its components of accreditation, certification, and licensure are formal methods of recognizing professional and technical competence. The purpose of credentialing in nursing is to assure the consumer that quality care is being provided by identifying the members qualified to practice through the issuing of a license. This process controls the practice by establishing parameters of practice and minimal standards of performance for all members of the profession. Therefore, the consumer is protected from the practice of unqualified individuals.

The JCAHO standard indicates the "the governing body requires a process or processes designed to assure that all individuals who provide patient care services, but who are not subject to the medical staff privilege delineation process, are competent to provide such services."[3] AORN developed a Perioperative Nursing Credentialing Model to assist with the credentialing of nurses practicing in the operating room (Fig. 16–2). Files should be maintained on each individual that includes the following information:

1. Educational preparation
2. Verification of licensure
3. Certification
4. Professional development
    a. Professional associations
    b. Continuing education
    c. Research, publications, seminars
5. Institutional requirements
    a. Verification of orientation
    b. Job description
    c. Performance appraisal
    d. Verification of skill level by surgical specialty

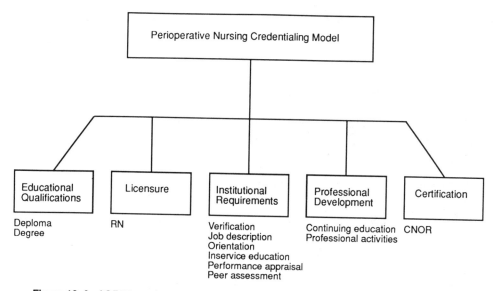

Figure 16-2. AORN's perioperative nursing credentialing model. *(Reprinted from Periop- erative Credentialing Model. AORN J 1986;43(1):262, with permission.)*

To maintain clinical competency by surgical specialty, the number and type of cases should be defined for each service, the staff should then be responsible for scrubbing and circulating on these cases throughout the year. Failure to meet this requirement should result in a "mini rotation" through that service.

The accreditation component assures the consumer that the institution or program of study meets certain predetermined criteria or standards (for example, those of the JCAHO and the National League for Nursing whose focus is on accrediting educational programs for nurses).

The process of certification in nursing was developed as a mechanism to provide formal recognition for excellence in the practice of nursing. The ANA and the AORN are currently certifying individuals who achieve a level of performance based on prede- termined standards relating to an area of specialty practice.[11]

Accountability for assuring quality is no longer a philosophic concept. It is de- manded by consumers of all health care services. It is required by federal legislation and the JCAHO and is mandated by the profession.

Nursing has the opportunity and is faced with the challenge to demonstrate that it can control its practice by implementing professional nursing standards, assessing those standards, and changing the practice that does not meet the established levels of care. Self-regulation is the authentic hallmark of a mature profession.[12]

REFERENCES

1. Van Sell Davidson S. ed. *PSRO Utilization and Audit in Patient Care.* St. Louis: C. V. Mosby; 1976:8–9

2. *Accreditation Manual for Hospitals.* Chicago: Joint Commission on Accreditation; 1989:219–223

3. *American Nurses Association: Standards of Nursing Practice.* Kansas City, Mo: American Nurses Association; 1974

4. Recommended Practices for Sponge, Sharp and Instrument Counts. *AORN J.* 1984; 39(4):699

5. Donabedian A. Evaluating the Quality of Medical Care. *Melbank Memorial Fund Q.* 1966; 44:166–206

6. Bloch D. Evaluation of nursing care in terms of process and outcome: Issues in research and quality assurance. *Nurs Res.* 1975; 24(1):256–263

7. Bloch D. Criteria, standards, norms—Crucial terms in quality assurance. *Nurs Admin.* 1977;7:20–30

8. Stevens BJ. Analysis of trends in nursing care management. *J Nurs Admin.* 1972; 2:12

9. Phaneuf MC. *The Nursing Audit: Self-Regulation in Nursing Practice,* 2nd ed. New York: Appleton-Century Crofts; 1976:40

10. Daefflen RJ. Patients' perception of care under team and primary nursing. *J Nurs Admin.* 1975; 5(3):26

11. Hercules P, Kneedler J. *Certification Series Unit 1: Certification Process.* Denver: Association of Operating Room Nurses; 1979:13

12. Phaneuf MC. *The Nursing Audit: Profile for Excellence,* Foreword by A. Donabedian. New York: Appleton-Century-Crofts; 1972:5

Chapter 17

Developing a Postgraduate Curriculum and Experience

Traditionally, the operating room experience was part of the basic educational preparation for professional registered nurses. As ideologies in nursing education underwent modification, the hospital apprenticeship type programs began to disappear. Concurrently, nursing education has moved out of these schools and into the mainstream of higher education.

Movement of nursing education from the diploma school to the collegiate environment has resulted in elimination of the operating room experience and, therefore, in a lack of qualified entry-level nurse practitioners for this speciality. In an effort to ensure that there are qualified practitioners in the operating room, postpreparatory or postgraduate courses have been instituted. These courses are more cost effective than the time-consuming, one-on-one orientation many institutions, by necessity, have formulated.

There are four groups of students who will be seeking a postpreparatory course. They are

1. Professional nurses with minimal or no previous operating room experience
2. Professional nurses who are reentering the work force and require updating before obtaining a position
3. Professional nurses who want to change their area of specialization
4. Experienced operating room nurses who desire to expand their skills into management

The contents of this chapter will focus on developing a postgraduate course for the professional nurses identified in the first three groups.

COMMUNITY REVIEW

Before the decision to design a postgraduate course is made, the programs currently available should be reviewed. Is there a need for a postgraduate course? What is the supply and demand for operating room nurses in the community? How is the current supply being met? Is there a college or university in the area interested in collaborating in the development of such a program?

If the didactic aspects of the course are to be offered outside the hospital premises, the clinical faculty must be identified. However, this should occur only after the hospital and departmental philosophy, objectives, and goals have been carefully scrutinized, defined, and aligned with the external educational channels to be utilized. In addition, the scope of the clinical facility's surgical case load should be reviewed for suitability and consistency. In these situations, a written contract should be developed between the educational institution and the hospital. It should contain clearly defined objectives of the affiliation, policies to be followed, and the names of the individuals responsible for implementation of the contract. In most settings, this will be the operating room manager and a representative of the educational institution. Once established, the relationship of the affiliated constituents is ongoing.

INSTITUTIONAL REVIEW

In surveying characteristics of an institution as a resource for the clinical experience several factors must be considered:

1. The size of the hospital
2. Number of operating rooms available for student assignments
3. Turnover rate of departmental staff
4. Institutional and departmental hiring policies
   a. Experienced versus inexperienced RNs
   b. Clinical competence criteria
5. Ratio of professional registered nurses to operating room technicians
6. Departmental commitments to existing programs (i.e., nursing, medical students)
7. Confirmed willingness of the professional nursing staff to participate actively as preceptors

In conjunction with the cited appraisal, a comprehensive census analysis depicting predominant trends and characteristics of the surgical case load must be prepared. Inclusive features are case consistency, variety, and the scope of technical complexity.

Following the community and institutional survey, a decision should be reached on what kind of end-product the program is anticipated to produce. Will it be an entry-level practitioner able to function in a community institution where less complex and routine procedures are performed; or a practitioner whose intraoperative skills are more advanced due to clinical experience in the highly complex surgical specialities?

Determination as to the desired competence level of practitioners will influence the length of the program and will assist in determining course objectives. A 3-month course in a hospital with a routine surgical case load, may produce an acceptable entry-level practitioner; however, 6 months, or longer, may be required in the hospital where extremely technical and involved procedures dominate the surgical schedule.

FINANCIAL IMPLICATIONS

It is essential that the financial resources for a postpreparatory course be identified and confirmed by the appropriate individuals early in the planning stage. Those concerned should include a member of the hospital administration, the operating room manager, the course instructor, and, when pertinent, a representative of the affiliating educational institution.

Paramount to this discussion is the determination of the kind of credit the course will grant. The choices are nondegree academic credit, degree academic credit, continuing education unit (CEU) contact hours, or a certificate.

A community-college or university-affiliated program may grant nondegree academic credit that, in some institutions, may be used to satisfy elective requirements. Hospital-based programs may award continuing education units,* according to the American Nurses Association guidelines, or a certificate attesting to satisfactory completion of the course.

Determination as to the type of credit awarded will assist in resolving the financial issues. Suggested options for fee structures are

1. The student pays a fee consistent with the rate per hour of course instruction established by the academic institution.
2. The student receives a stipend from a grant procured by the educational institution or the hospital.
3. The hospital establishes an internship program that provides a portion of the entry-level practitioner's salary for the duration of the course.
4. The student neither pays a fee for the course nor receives any monies for the training period. At the program completion however, the student is committed to remain on the departmental staff for a specific period of time.

Following the resolution of the economic issues, emphasis should be focused on developing the course philosophy and objectives.

RESPONSIBILITY FOR THE PROGRAM

The success of an implemented postpreparatory course is predetermined by the caliber of the institution and the individual selected as the course coordinator. It follows, therefore, that extreme care should be exercised in establishing appropriate criteria for the process. The minimal basic educational requirement should include credentials as a registered nurse, preferably with a baccalaureate or master's degree,** and extensive experience and knowledge of perioperative nursing. He or she should be articulate and enthusiastic, and demonstrate excellent professional and technical skills, as well as good interpersonal skills. It is preferable that the individual have knowledge of the principles of adult learning, curriculum development, methods of program evaluation and the methods of testing.

One of the most important factors in the adult learning process is how the educator views the student. Table 17–1 identifies five basic assumptions Knowles[1] makes between children and adults in the areas of:

---

*In states requiring continuing education for relicensure, the course must be approved by the State Board of Nursing.
**This requirement is predominately for a course affiliated with a university. Individuals capable of assuming the responsibility and the accountability of the course should not be overlooked due to a lack of educational achievement.

TABLE 17-1. CONCEPTS OF EDUCATION: ADULTS VERSUS CHILDREN

	Assumptions	
	Children	*Adults*
1. Self-concept	Dependence	Increasing self-directiveness
2. Experience	Of little worth	Adults are a rich resource for learning
3. Readiness	1. Biological development b. Social pressure	Developmental tasks of social roles
4. Time perspective	Postponed application	Immediacy of application Need to cope with person centered
5. Orientation to learning	Subject centered	Problem centered

	Process Elements	
	Children	*Adults*
Climate starts with first contact Quality is influenced by each contact	Authority oriented Formal Competitive	Mutuality Respectful Collaborative Informal
Planning	By teacher	Mechanism for mutual planning
Diagnosis of needs	By teacher	Mutual self-diagnosis
Formulation of objectives	By teacher	Mutual negotiation
Design	Logic of the subject matter Content units Transmittal techniques	Sequenced in terms of readiness Problem units Experiential techniques (inquiry)
Activities	By teacher	Mutual rediagnosis of needs
Evaluation	By teacher	Mutual measurement of program

Courtesy Malcolm S. Knowles, Boston University, with permission.

1. Self-concept
2. Previous experience
3. Readiness to learn
4. Time frame for application of new knowledge
5. Orientation to the learning process

If the educator views the teaching–learning process as participative, the student will have a greater commitment to the process. Collaboration and mutual goal-setting allow the student to become actively involved in this process. The educator must be sensitive to those individuals who will require a judicious combination of the process elements in teaching children and adults.

CANDIDATE SELECTION

Specific criteria should be developed for the selection of the candidates and should be confirmed during the interview process. Areas of consideration are

1. Graduate of an accredited school of nursing
2. Current state licensure
3. Good physical and emotional health
4. Desire to attain competence in perioperative nursing

PROGRAM DESIGN

The course philosophy should be developed collaboratively with members of the administrative staff and closely aligned with the philosophy of the clinical setting. The course philosophy should be reviewed annually and revised to reflect changes as they occur in perioperative nursing, the philosophy of the educator, and concepts of teaching and learning.

OBJECTIVES

An objective is a statement that is written clearly and concisely to include what is to be achieved and the time frame in which it is to be accomplished.

Objectives are useful because they describe the expected outcome for the student; are measurable and, therefore, can be evaluated; and allow flexibility to reflect the needs of the situation, the student, and the educator.

Objectives are classified as cognitive, psychomotor, and affective.

Cognitive objectives are concerned with the perception of factual knowledge and focus on the understanding of new material or ideas. Psychomotor objectives concern actions proceeding from mental activity, ranging from the simple reflex to the performance of highly complex skills. Affective objectives are the most difficult to measure due to their emotional basis, which is reflected through less than tangible attitudes and feelings.

Postgraduate Program Purpose and Objectives

Purpose. The purpose is to enable the clinician to assume responsibility for meeting the physical and psychologial needs of patients in each phase of the perioperative role by providing appropriate theory and clinical experience.

Objectives. Learning experiences selected collaboratively throughout the program will enable the clinician to:

1. Demonstrate a repertoire of clinical skills and knowledge pertinent to the operating room
   a. Practice selected clinical skills as a scrub and circulating nurse in general surgery and practice the less complex aspects of the surgical specialities
   b. Demonstrate progressive competency in performing these skills
   c. Modify approach to meet the specific needs of each patient
   d. Demonstrate progressive ability to safely use the equipment in the operating room
2. Apply principles of aseptic technique and state how this knowledge will apply to other areas of clinical practice
3. Demonstrate behavior commensurate with the entry-level practitioner in the operating room
4. Assess, plan, implement, and evaluate comprehensive individualized nursing care plans for the surgical patient that take into consideration life variables, namely, cultural, ethnic, socioeconomic, and sexual
5. Identify and explain to the patient appropriate nursing functions that are frequently performed during the perioperative period
6. Identify and explain the implications of possible changes in anatomical and physiological functioning that may occur following an operative procedure
7. Use a systematic method of inquiry to identify subtle and complex health problems that may have an impact on the patient's surgical experience
8. Provide information to the patient, family, and significant others in relation to the perioperative period
9. Identify the legal responsibilities involved in administering care to the patients undergoing surgical intervention
10. Participate and contribute effectively as a member of the health team
11. Identify the departmental and professional hierarchies present in the clinical setting
12. Demonstrate an ability to use the social system of the clinical setting for the benefit of the patient
13. Identify behavioral manifestations of individuals under stress
14. Recognize one's own reaction to stressful situations
15. Determine methods of incorporating knowledge gained from operating room experience into diverse patient care situations
16. Use current selected research to identify trends that influence the role of the nurse practitioner in the operating rooms

17. Demonstrate potential leadership ability in relation to goals of the operating rooms

COURSE CONTENT

The content of the course developed should be consistent with the list of objectives and its predetermined length. Accordingly, the educator must determine the magnitude of theory required to achieve the anticipated assimilation of student knowledge as well as the most appropriate sequence for presentation of the material.

If the participants differ in background and experience, they should be required to submit a current self-assessment of clinical practice. This will assist the educator in ascertaining individual and collective levels of competence. An analysis of the submitted data will provide the educator with valid documentation for adjusting the course content within the scope of a structured course curriculum.

The course content should include:

1. Introduction to:
   a. Course overview
   b. Clinical experiences
   c. Educator expectations
      1. Attendance
      2. Assignments
      3. Method of evaluation grading
2. Institutional–departmental
   a. Philosophy
   b. Organizational structure
   c. Personnel policies
3. Perioperative nursing—a historical perspective
4. Operating room design and construction
   a. Environmental orientation
   b. Hazards
   c. Safety measures
   d. Maintenance-housekeeping
   e. Related hospital departments
5. Identify the roles of the team members
   a. Introduction
   b. Job descriptions
6. Perioperative role
   a. Nursing assessment
   b. Planning
   c. Implementation
   d. Evaluation
7. Principles of operating room technique
   a. Asepsis
      1. Microbiology

2. Infection control
3. Sterilization
4. Disinfection
5. Preparation of the skin
6. Surgical hand scrub
7. Gowning and gloving
b. Anesthesia
1. Types
2. Methods of administration
3. Complications
4. Cardiac arrest and resuscitation
5. Care of anesthesia equipment
c. Positioning
d. Draping
e. Methods of maintaining homeostasis
1. Sutures
2. Electrosurgery
3. Synthetic agents
4. Tourniquets
f. Wound healing
g. Terminal cleaning of
1. Operating room
2. Instruments
3. Supplies
4. Equipment
8. Care of the patient during the immediate postoperative period
9. Review of basic sciences and operative procedures
10. Professional responsibility
a. Personal attitudes and attributes
b. Hygiene
c. Ethics and legal responsibility
d. Continuing education
e. Current issues affecting nursing
f. Legislative action
g. Nursing research
h. Professional organization involvement
11. Operating room management
a. Functions of the nurse manager
1. Fiscal
2. Interpersonal
3. Technical

Additional information and guidelines regarding course content may be found in Speciality Nursing Courses: OR,[2] and Surgical Experience Model for Professional Practice in the OR.[3]

TEACHING METHODOLOGIES

There is a wide variety of teaching methods available to the educator. The method selected should meet the identified objectives, be compatible with the resources available, and be able to be used effectively by the educator.

Lecture

The lecture is a formal discourse of facts usually presented by a member of the surgical team. In addition to members of the surgical team, a wide variety of resource people are available in the health care facility and in the educational setting who can contribute in this capacity (i.e., infection control nurse, hospital attorney, chaplain, dietician, and social worker). Use of these resources adds interest and depth to the educational experience.

Demonstration

The demonstration is the best method for students to learn psychomotor skills. In this method, the educator identifies the objective of the procedure, describes each step while demonstrating it, and relates each step to a relevant principle. The student repeats the demonstration to verify comprehension and dexterity. Evidence of student error during the repeat demonstration is an indication for corrective instructional measures.

Observation

Identification of specific objectives followed by observation in the clinical setting can be an asset to the teaching–learning experience. For instance, following a lecture on stress, the specific objective for observation might be, "Observe interactions of surgical team members to identify symptoms of stress."

Role Playing

Role playing is the method of choice to build skills in learning to use interviewing techniques or in using effective listening skills. In this method, a situation is described and the students are assigned parts without a script. Role playing provides for trial use of interventions in a nonthreatening environment. A discussion follows the dramatization and culminates in a critique by the observers. This method is useful in teaching preoperative assessments.

Programmed Instructions

The educator may develop programmed instruction modules to teach a variety of subjects such as the principles of aseptic technique, patient prepping, and draping. This method allows the student to progress at his or her own rate and may be in a written or audiovisual format.

The programmed instruction[4]:

1. Presents information and requires frequent responses from the student
2. Provides immediate feedback to the student with information on whether or not the response is appropriate

3. Allows the student to work individually and adjust his or her own rate of progress to personal needs and capabilities

Educational Media

There is a wide variety of educational media available to aid in the teaching–learning process. Those used most frequently are

1. Audio tape recorders
2. Direct circuit television
3. Educational television
4. Film strips
5. Motion pictures
6. Slides
7. Transparencies

A number of motion pictures and film strips are available for rental or for purchase. They require advance scheduling and preplanning to integrate them into the course at the appropriate time.

The educator must always preview the selected media and make certain that the content is consistent with the desired learning activities. Immediately prior to the class, the appropriate equipment must be checked to make sure it is functioning properly. An extra bulb should always be available for all projectors.

Independent Study

In independent study, the student selects a topic or problem of personal interest and seeks out information on the topic or solves the problem independently of the educator.

Clinical Conferences

Clinical conferences with case presentations guide the student to identify experiences and, through analysis, to associate them with previous knowledge gained from didactic material. Criteria for case presentations should include the following patient data:

1. Review pathophysiology of surgical procedure
2. Discuss psychosocial aspects influencing patient's response to surgical experience
   a. Social history
      1) Culture and ethnicity
      2) Family organization
      3) Language
      4) Religion
      5) Socioeconomic status
   b. Mental status
   c. Teaching and learning needs
   d. Pertinent laboratory data
   e. Emotional reaction of patient and significant others
   f. How patient and significant others cope with stress
   g. Nonverbal communication

3. Identify components of nursing diagnosis and patient care plan for intraoperative period
4. Discuss implementation of patient care plan
5. Discuss postoperative outcome, including interpreting impact of surgical intervention

Additional Resources

Additional resources are the course syllabus, bibliographies, and textbooks. The bibliography must be revised annually to reflect current concepts regarding the perioperative role. A tour of the library facilities and a discussion with the librarian during the orientation period will be a valuable asset to the student.

Feedback regarding the students' progress is an important component of the teaching–learning process. Feedback can come from a variety of sources. Clinical conferences, checklists, tests, and evaluations supply the students with information as to their position in relation to the objectives. Frequent feedback also helps the students and the educators measure the quality of the experience and collaboratively create an environment of mutual respect and concern.

The educators must remain informed of new approaches to teaching and include in their repertoire a wide variety of methods with which they are comfortable and that will best achieve the desired outcome.

USE OF PRECEPTORS

Preceptors are an important component of a postgraduate program. The preceptor provides one-on-one teaching in the clinical area and is responsible for reinforcement of theory content during the student's clinical experience. The goal of preceptorship is to improve the clinical experience. A buddy system has the same goal, but is not as effective as a preceptorship.

The difference in the concepts relates to definition of the words *preceptor* and *buddy*.

Preceptor. Teacher, mentor, consultant

Buddy. A fellow soldier or partner

A buddy system merely provides someone with whom to work, someone to show the student how to do tasks. There is no specific accountability or responsibility inherent in being a buddy.

A preceptor is one who makes certain that the student translates theory content into departmental policies and procedures. The preceptor serves as a role model and stimulates the student to identify with an appropriate reference group in developing his or her professional practice. The attitudes, philosophies, and skills of the preceptor are eventually reflected in the student. Therefore, explicit criteria for preceptors should be established and discretion exercised in the choice of these individuals.

Criteria for Preceptorship Appointments

1. Minimum of 1 year experience at current institution
2. Demonstrated clinical competency substantiated consistently with above-average or superior performance evaluations
3. Demonstrated leadership skills (i.e., problem solving skills)
4. Demonstrated communication skills, as evidenced in positive interpersonal relationships through the use of tactful, direct, and sensitive interactions
5. Demonstrated interest in personal professional growth
6. Demonstrated comprehension of the theoretical concepts of adult learning through application to appropriate practice situations
7. Willingness to participate in the program, meet identified responsibilities, and to provide feedback to the student

Prior to the selection of preceptors, the specific responsibilities of the role must be defined and conveyed to qualified candidates. These responsibilities include:

1. Cognizance and affirmation of the purpose and objectives of the course
2. Competence to impart course content in theory and practice
3. Capability to develop the clinical experience collaboratively with the student
4. Accessibility to the student once per week, outside the work setting, to discuss clinical progress and establish future goals
5. Attendance at regularly scheduled preceptor meetings
6. Attendance at weekly student clinical conferences
7. Submit written evaluations on designated students at the end of a clinical rotation
8. Attendance at end-of-quarter conference to evaluate clinical experience and submit recommendations for course content revisions

A workshop covering all aspects of preceptorship should precede assumption of responsibilities by selected individuals. Material for a workshop should include:

1. The role and responsibilities of the preceptor
2. Presentation of the individual and collective needs of the students and formulation of plans to meet them
3. Advantages and disadvantages of educating adults and children
4. Hypothetical problem situations: how to handle them; how to cope with feelings; and how to evaluate the outcome

After the preceptors have been designated, it is important that their work schedule coincide with that of the student's clinical experience. If there are unavoidable scheduling problems, the preceptor must make specific arrangements for a substitute preceptor from among the selected individuals, apprising him or her as to the clinical skills that the student is capable of performing.

Together, the preceptor and the student should develop objectives for the clinical experience by surgical service, and the student should maintain a clinical experience record[5] (Tables 17–2, 17–3, and 17–4). The objectives and the clinical experience record are effective tools for evaluating the student's performance in the clinical setting.

TABLE 17-2. GYNECOLOGY: OBJECTIVES OF THE STUDENT'S EXPERIENCE

A. Objectives: At the completion of the rotation, the student will be able to:

1. Describe the anatomy of the normal female reproductive tract
2. Describe the common gynecologic disorders, including but not limited to the following:
   Cervical carcinoma
   Endometrial carcinoma
   Infertility
   Leiomyomata
   Ovarian carcinoma
   Tubal carcinoma
   Vaginal carcinoma
   Vulvar carcinoma
3. Discuss the classification scheme for malignant tumors in the female pelvis
4. Express the nursing considerations and functions specific to the intraoperative care of gynecologic patients
5. Develop nursing care plans that reflect consideration of an individual patient's specific needs
6. Perform at least one preoperative assessment of a patient scheduled for surgery the following day and participate in the care of that patient
7. Locate the special supplies and equipment needed for gynecologic surgery, according to the printed gynecology equipment list
8. Perform effectively the preoperative assessments and check-in of an outpatient
9. Demonstrate the ability to circulate effectively and independently on any gynecologic surgery
10. Demonstrate the ability to scrub effectively and independently on any gynecologic surgery
11. Demonstrate the use and processing of the special supplies and equipment needed for gynecologic surgery, according to established procedure
12. Evaluate care given in the operating room by making postoperative phone calls to outpatients
13. Describe the use, dosage, and location of drugs used in gynecologic surgery
14. Explain the purpose behind, use of, and medicolegal implications of, the sterilization consent form
15. Describe the various methods of electrosurgery used in gynecologic surgery
16. Establish, maintain, and promote effective relationships with patients, families, and members of the health care team
17. Locate and use, as necessary, appropriate resource materials/personnel in order to provide safe, effective patient care

B. Methodology:

1. It is expected that each student will use these objectives and communicate his or her learning needs to the preceptor during the clinical experience.
2. At the completion of the clinical experience, the student will participate in a performance evaluation based on these objectives and will be asked for feedback about the clinical experience.

TABLE 17-3. GYNECOLOGICAL ROTATION

Operative Procedure	Scrub	Circulate	Observe
Abdominal cases Hysterectomy			
Radical hysterectomy			
Tuboplasty			
Tuboplasty with microscope			
Adnexal surgery			
Ectopic pregnancy			
Vaginal Cases Hysterectomy			
Anterior–posterior repair			
D & C			
Suction abortion (TAB)			
Cervical conization			
Radium insertion			
Combination Laparoscopy–laparotomy			
Pelvic exeneration			
Construction of vagina			
Radical vulvectomy			
Laparoscopy[a]			

[a]Laparoscopy: Indicate Type: fallope ring, tubal cauterization, or PE tube.

Preceptorship is a rewarding experience for both the students and preceptors. Such a collegial relationship enhances the students' clinical experience while providing increased job satisfaction for the preceptor by recognition of staff expertise. Through the experience, a preceptor has an opportunity for professional growth as she/he develops his or her teaching, planning, and supervisory skills.

EVALUATIONS OF THE COURSE

A terminal evaluation of the course by all concerned is important to critique the content of the course and to determine the effectiveness of the teaching methods and activities.

The nurse educator will design a tool (Tables 17–5, 17–6, 17–7) that will effectively assess these two areas and will reflect his or her philosophy of education and views about

TABLE 17-4. SPECIAL EQUIPMENT AND SUPPLY LIST GYNECOLOGY SURGERY[a]

Item	Purpose	Location	Method of Sterilization	Method of Checking	How to Assemble
Laparoscope insufflator					
Laparoscope cart					
Pap smear slides					
Abortion machine					
D & C Set					
Fetuscope					
Leg holder Heavy Leg stirrups					
Ankle straps					
Electrosurgical Generator mono- & biopolar					

[a]To be initiated by preceptor when student accomplishes the task.

TABLE 17-5. STUDENT ASSESSMENT OF INSTRUCTOR AND TEACHING METHODOLOGIES

Each of the categories below deals with the instructor's efficacy in contributing to the student's learning processes. Please indicate your rating of your instructor by circling the appropriate key letter:

- (A) Strongly agree
- (B) Agree
- (C) Neutral
- (D) Disagree
- (E) Strongly disagree

1. The instructor has a thorough knowledge of the subject matter.
   Examples or comments: A B C D E

2. Presentations and explanations were clear and enlightening.
   Examples or comments: A B C D E

3. The instructor communicated clearly by speech, blackboard and other methods.
   Examples or comments: A B C D E

4. The instructor encouraged thought and insight.
   Examples or comments: A B C D E

(continued)

TABLE 17–5. CONTINUED

5. The instructor's lectures were well organized.
   Examples or comments: A B C D E

6. The instructor showed personal interest in the subject.
   Examples or comments: A B C D E

7. The instructor was responsive to questions, discussion, and disagreement
   on issues.
   Examples or comments: A B C D E

8. The instructor showed concern for the student's understanding
   of course material.
   Examples or comments: A B C D E

9. The pace of instruction was reasonable.
   Examples or comments: A B C D E

10. The instructor was able to inspire students and generate enthusiasm.
    Examples or comments: A B C D E

11. The instructor was able to judge the level of class comprehension
    and adjusted teaching methodologies accordingly.
    Examples or comments: A B C D E

12. The instructor was fair and impartial in dealing with the students.
    Examples or comments: A B C D E

13. The instructor's speech skills were adequate for teaching.
    Examples or comments: A B C D E

14. The instructor kept the students informed of their progress and reenforced
    good performance.
    Examples or comments: A B C D E

If you have additional comments concerning the instructor, teaching methods, or course content,
please submit them below:

Thank you.

**TABLE 17-6. STUDENT ASSESSMENT
OPERATING ROOM—POSTGRADUATE COURSE—CONTENT**

1. What suggestions do you have for improving the lecture part of this course? How would you change the order of the presentations?
2. What suggestions do you have for improving the clinical aspects of the course?
3. What suggestions do you have for choosing and using preceptors?
4. Were the 3:00 PM–11:00 PM and weekend experiences valuable? Why or why not?
5. Was the recovery room rotation helpful?
6. What suggestions do you have for improving the methods used during this course for evaluating your performance?

**TABLE 17-7. STUDENT ASSESSMENT
OPERATING ROOM—POSTGRADUATE COURSE—CONTENT**

	(1) Strongly Agree	(2) Agree	(3) Undecided	(4) Disagree	(5) Strongly Disagree
1. Course has clearly stated objectives.					
2. Stated goals/objectives are consistently pursued.					
3. Lecture information is highly relevant to course objectives.					
4. Course material is pertinent to my professional training as an OR nurse.					
5. The course contributed significantly to my professional growth.					
6. I can apply clinical skills and theory learned in this course.					
7. There was sufficient time in class for questions and answers.					
8. Bibliographies for this course are current and extensive.					
9. The content of the clinical experience is a worthwhile part of this course.					
10. In general I learned a great deal from this course.					

Other Comments:

the student. If the educator has set a climate of mutual respect and open exchange of ideas and suggestions, the students will willingly provide feedback.

The educator then uses the feedback from the student to implement changes in the course objectives or in the clinical experience. Evaluation of the course should be a continuous, ongoing process that reflects changes in perioperative nursing practice and in principles of adult education.

REFERENCES

1 Knowles MS. *The Adult Learner: A Neglected Species.* Houston: Gulf Publishing; 1978: 110
2 Kneedler J. *Speciality Nursing Courses: OR.* Denver: Association of Operating Room Nurses; 1976
3 Davis DL, Kneedler J, Manuel B. *The Surgical Experience: A Model for Professional Nursing Practice in the Operating Room.* Denver: Association of Operating Room Nurses; 1976
4 de Tornyay R. *Strategies for Teaching Nursing.* New York: John Wiley; 1976:89
5 Bever S. *Orientation to the Perioperative Role in Gynecology Surgery.* San Francisco: University of California Hospitals and Clinics: 1980

Index

Page numbers followed by an *f* refer to figures. Those with a *t* refer to tables.

Page numbers followed by an *f* refer to figures. Those with a *t* refer to tables.

Page numbers followed by an *f* refer to figures. Those with a *t* refer to tables.

Page numbers followed by an *f* refer to figures. Those with a *t* refer to tables.

Page numbers followed by an *f* refer to figures. Those with a *t* refer to tables.

Page numbers followed by an *f* refer to figures. Those with a *t* refer to tables.